ELECTRON PARAMAGNETIC RESONANCE: TECHNIQUES AND APPLICATIONS

Electron Paramagnetic Resonance:

Techniques and Applications

RAYMOND S. ALGER

U.S. Naval Radiological Defense Laboratory,
San Francisco, California

Illustrated by
ICHIRO HAYASHI

INTERSCIENCE PUBLISHERS

a division of John Wiley and Sons, New York · London · Sydney

Preface

The rapidly developing use of electron paramagnetic resonance (EPR) spectroscopy as an analytical tool brings to the foreground a need for reference information covering experimental methods and techniques. A number of books and review articles adequately treat EPR theory and results; however, detailed descriptions of apparatus and procedures are frequently sacrificed as victims of stringent space limitations. This volume is for the experimentalists and is designed to expedite the entry of physicists, chemists, biologists, and engineers into the rites and practices of the EPR fraternity.

In scope the emphasis is on experimental problems and numerous examples are used to show the status of solutions. Some of the illustrations were selected to indicate the historical interests and development of EPR in various fields of application. While a brief outline of theory is included to establish the nomenclature and to provide a background for the various experimental procedures, such references as P-4, A-6, I-2, L-1, etc., should be consulted for instruction and assistance in interpreting results.

The format of this volume bears the imprint of John Strong's admonition that the ideal way to learn experimental procedures is by direct contact with them in the laboratory. When such learning commences with a book, the liberal use of figures may help bridge the gap between laboratory demonstrations and experience on the one hand and exposition on the other.* Mr. Hayashi's technical skill, untiring efforts, and enthusiastic cooperation in preparing the numerous illustrations made this format possible and his contributions are greatly appreciated.

The plan, to augment the experimental information obtained from the literature by first hand observations of procedures in outstanding EPR laboratories, developed in conversations with M. S. Carstens and E. A. Edelsack of ONR. Their encouragement throughout this endeavor has been very helpful. Through combined ONR and NRDL support, laboratories of 43 institutions were visited in the U.S.A. and Europe to collect experimental techniques, particularly those unpublished details in the sealing wax and string category that frequently spell the difference between success and failure. These sources of information are acknowledged throughout the text by the numbered references. Literature references are

*Paraphrased from the preface to *Procedures in Experimental Physics* by John Strong, Prentice-Hall, New York, 1943.

v

indicated by a composite letter number notation. Since a book of this type is essentially a collection of ideas from many sources, I am deeply indebted to the many originators for permission to use their information. The words courtesy, after, and reference which appear at the end of the figure captions serve two functions: (1) they indicate various degrees of indebtedness for the use of copywrited material and (2) they warn the reader of the liberties exercised in redrawing the figures. "Courtesy" means that the figure is essentially a copy of a copywrited illustration. The referenced authors and publishers have graciously granted permission to use these figures and this courtesy is gratefully acknowledged. "After" means the figure follows the general outline of the original work but alterations ranging from modest to extensive have been introduced to emphasize features of particular concern to this volume. These authors and publishers also have granted permission to use their copywrited material. When the reference number appears alone or accompanied by the word "reference" it means a source of additional information or data in the public domain where no permission was requested. When a reference number appears following the title of a table, it means the information in the table came from a single source and permission has been granted for its use.

The encouragement and cooperation encountered during the laboratory visits was an important factor during the gestation period for this book and this assistance is acknowledged with sincere appreciation. I am also indebted to T. H. Anderson, for numerous helpful suggestions and comments.

RAYMOND S. ALGER

January, 1968

List of Symbols

A	Magnetic hyperfine interaction constant A_x, A_y, A_z, $A_\parallel$, $A_\perp$ (cm^{-1})
AFC	Automatic frequency control
B	Noise bandwidth
c	Velocity of light (2.998 × 10^{10} cm sec^{-1})
C	Information capacity
d	Interionic distance (cm)
D and E	Fine structure coefficients (cm^{-1})
EPR	Electron paramagnetic resonance
F	Quantum number for total angular momentum including nuclear spin
F	Noise factor
FM	Frequency modulation
f	Frequency
f_0	Cavity resonant frequency
f_m	Modulation frequency
e	Electron charge (4.803 × 10^{-10} statcoul)
E	Electric field
g, g_e	Spectroscopic splitting factor = $\dfrac{\text{magnetic moment (in Bohr magnatons)}}{\text{angular momentum (in units } h/2\pi)}$
$g_\parallel$	g factor for H_z applied in the direction of axial symmetry of the crystal (c axis)
$g_\perp$	g factor for H_z applied perpendicular to the c axis
$g_{x,y,z}$	g factor for H_z applied along the coordinate axis x, y, z, respectively
g_I, g_n	Nuclear g factor = $\dfrac{\text{nuclear magnetic moment (in nuclear magnatons)}}{\text{angular momentum (in units } h/2\pi)}$
G	Yield of radicals, i.e., number generated by 100 eV absorbed energy
G	Amplifier gain
h	Planck's constant (6.625 × 10^{-27} erg-sec)
$\hbar$	$h/2\pi$
H	Magnetic field intensity at any instant (G)
H_1	The maximum amplitude of the microwave magnetic field, usually perpendicular to H (G)
H_0	Static magnetic field intensity at the center of the spin packet, i.e., at resonance (G)
H_m	The maximum amplitude of the modulating magnetic field, usually parallel to H (G)
$\Delta H_{1/2}$	Linewidth at half of the maximum intensity (G)

ΔH_s	Linewidth between points of maximum slope (G)
hfs	Hyperfine structure
i	Electric current
I	Spin of nucleus in units of $h/2$
I	Information transferred
J	Total quantum number of the electron shell
k	Boltzmann constant (1.380×10^{-16} erg deg^{-1})
L	Electronic orbital angular momentum quantum number of an entire atom or molecule
m	Rest mass of electron (9.108×10^{-28} g)
m_s	Quantum number governing the component of the spin angular momentum of a single electron along the axis of an applied field
M_I	Quantum number governing the projection of nuclear spin angular momentum on the axis of an applied field
M	Proton mass
M	First moment of area under absorption curve
M_s	Quantum number governing the projection of electron spin on the axis of an applied magnetic field
M_L	Quantum number governing the projection of the electronic orbital angular momentum on the axis of an applied magnetic field
n	Atomic principal quantum number
N^+	Number of spins in higher energy spin state
N^-	Number of spins in lower energy spin state
N	Noise power
N	Total number of spins
NF	Noise figure
P	Power of the radio frequency field
P_0	Incident power or oscillator power
P_s	Signal power
Q	Quality factor (resonator figure of merit)
Q_0	Quality factor, unloaded
Q_L	Quality factor, loaded
Q_x	Quality factor, external
R	Roentgen
rad	Absorbed dose of 100 ergs/g
rf	Radiofrequency
s	Electron spin quantum number
S	Total electron spin quantum number for the atom
S_x, S_y, S_z	Components
S	Saturation parameter
S/N	Signal-to-noise ratio
t	Time
T	Absolute temperature (°K)
T_n	Noise temperature
T_1	Longitudinal paramagnetic relaxation time or spin lattice relaxation time

T_2	Transverse or spin–spin relaxation time
V	Electrical potential
VSWR	Voltage standing wave ratio
W	Linewidth
W_a	Transition probability for absorption
W_e	Transition probability for emission
W_n	Noise power from single port device
β, β_e	Bohr magnaton $= e\hbar/2mc$ (0.9273×1^{-20} erg G^{-1})
β	Cavity coupling coefficient $= Q_0/Q_x$
β_I, β_n	Nuclear magnaton $= e\hbar/2mc$
Γ	Reflection coefficient
Γ_{res}	Reflection coefficient at resonance
Γ_0	Reflection coefficient far off resonance
γ	Gyromagnetic ratio $= e/2mc$
δ	Skin depth
δ	Loss angle when used in tan δ
ϵ	Dielectric constant
ϵ'	Real part of ϵ
ϵ''	Imaginary part of ϵ
ϵ_0	Dielectric constant of free space
θ	Debye temperature
θ	Angle between H and the crystalline field axis
λ	Wavelength
λ_a	Wavelength in free space
λ_c	Cutoff wavelength
λ_g	Wavelength in waveguide
μ	Magnetic permeability
μ_0	Permeability of free space
ν	Frequency of rf magnetic field
ν_0	Resonant frequency
ν'	Wavenumber (cm^{-1})
ν_e	Resonant frequency for electrons
ν_n, ν_p	Resonant frequency for nucleus and protons, respectively
χ	Complex paramagnetic susceptibility
χ'	Real part of χ
χ''	Imaginary part of χ
χ_0	Susceptibility at resonance
ρ	Density of a substance
ρ	Electrical resistivity
η	Filling factor
τ	Time for disturbed spin system to return to within $(1/e)$th of its equilibrium or steady-state value
ω	Angular velocity or angular frequency $= 2\pi\nu$
ω_0	Angular velocity at resonance $= 2\pi\nu$
ω_m	Modulation angular frequency
$\Delta\omega$	Bandwidth

Contents

CHAPTER I

Introduction

Historically scientific techniques tend to follow a fairly regular path of development and in this respect electron paramagnetic resonance (EPR) is no exception. The evolution begins, of course, with "discovery" which for EPR was in 1945, then progresses rapidly through confirmation and testing on well-established systems where prior knowledge indicates that the phenomena should be observable. In spectroscopy these are the days when almost any spectrum is noteworthy, and such spectra begin to appear in the "note" and "letter" sections of the journals, frequently with considerable emphasis on measuring techniques. This is the period when, of necessity, all the apparatus is home built and the experimentalist is usually well acquainted with his equipment and its limitations. Next the horizons are broadened to encompass observations on many new materials. Spectra are published in increasing numbers, and interpretation of the spectra becomes an important factor in understanding these new materials. Gradually the spectroscopy progresses from a phenomenon worthy of study in its own right to a tool of importance in many areas of research. Spectra become so numerous that compilations, catalogues, and indexes are required to keep track of the flood of information and to permit efficient use of the new tool. Commercial instruments begin to appear during these latter stages and the new spectroscopy becomes available to all with "the price." In the final mature stage the tools continue to be refined, measurements are made with greater precision, interpretations are made with greater certainty, and the instrument manufacturers provide an ever increasing array of accessories to lighten the experimental effort.

Compared with other forms of spectroscopy in the electromagnetic domain, i.e., visible, UV, and infrared, EPR is chronologically young; however, it has developed rapidly and now stands in the final mature stage, able to compete both in equipment and interpretation with its elder brethren. Evidence of this maturity can be found in the indexed EPR spectra (H-11), the theoretical spectra compiled in atlases (L-2,L-3), numerous books and chapters describing various aspects of this new spectroscopy

1

(e.g., A-9,G-15,I-3,J-1,L-13,O-3,P-1,P-12,S-21,W-1) and the commercial spectrometers and accessories on the market. Despite this comfortable state of affairs, some experimental problems await better solutions and various satisfactory procedures remain scattered throughout the extensive EPR literature or buried unreported in the mores and practices of various laboratories. These problems and procedures fall into three general categories, namely, men, machines, and materials. We include men because the complexities of EPR can expedite the making of experimental mistakes perhaps more so than other forms of absorption spectroscopy. Hyde (H-28), Squires (S-21), and others hasten to emphasize that the spectroscopist should become intimately familiar with instrumentation and experimental techniques. While this is sound advice in any experiment it is particularly important in EPR spectroscopy where sample preparation, instrument settings, and environmental factors can materially alter the data obtained. In the early days, familiarity with the instrumental capabilities and limitations come naturally because everyone made his own spectrometer. Now that this form of apprenticeship is no longer necessary the neophyte needs some guidance with respect to the limitations, trials, and tribulations of this form of spectroscopy. Machine problems are limited to a relatively small number of experimental situations where existing spectrometers are not adequate. Insufficient sensitivity is the most common complaint and occasionally more stability and resolution are required. Finally, the materials or samples offer a ready supply of problems ranging from inhospitable dielectric properties to insufficient spins. Usually the specimen consists of a host material containing the spins of interest and often experimental success depends on finding the proper combination.

The purpose of this volume is to dispel some of the beginner's problems by presenting the techniques, incantations, rites, and practices that have been effective in several areas of experimental EPR. Always the goal is to provide guidance in fitting the instrumentation and witchcraft to a particular experiment. We have tried to identify the experimental problems indigenous to various types of sample materials; to consider the relative importance of the various EPR and environmental parameters; to indicate appropriate apparatus and measuring techniques; and to demonstrate achievable results with spectra obtained by successful spectroscopists. Usually the procedures followed in various laboratories tend to converge in the case of measurements on a particular type of material so that recommendations follow in a straightforward manner. However, such unanimity is not always present and when divergences of opinion and practice exist, it is usually in an area where the experimental results do not clearly establish the superior approach, either because the rituals are equally effective or because the available data does not admit to a quantitative comparison. Under such circumstances we present both opinions along with supporting evidence pro and con.

1.1 SCOPE

In keeping with the theme, the scope is characterized by matters experimental with only a smattering of theory and results included. The boundaries are further defined by four subject categories:

1. A brief survey of EPR nomenclature, theory, and customs which is intended to establish the language of EPR and to clarify the notation and units involved in presenting data. Hopefully this section will add some meaning and a touch of logic to practices that might otherwise appear to be unadulterated sorcery.

2. A discussion of instrumentation, i.e., spectrometers and associated gear. Here the emphasis is on matching the spectrometer to the experiment so that adequate sensitivity and resolution are achieved with as much convenience as possible. Considerable attention is given to noise problems and techniques for rescuing weak signals from a noise background. While not intended as a guide to home spectrometer construction, numerous details are included for cavities and accessories commonly built in the laboratory.

3. A description of general techniques for measurement and control of the principal spectrometer and environmental parameters, e.g., frequency, field strength, spin concentrations, relaxation times, temperature, etc.

4. Examples of experimental problems, measurements, and results for specific spin systems in gas, liquid, and solid sample materials. The main emphasis is on solids, particularly the radicals of interest to chemists and biologists. Numerous spectra are included; however, they were selected to illustrate the results obtainable with the various measuring techniques and are not intended as a survey of available spectra. References H-11, B-17, and B-26 provide a good introduction to the available spectra.

Hopefully these four areas will serve as a guide book from the time the EPR trail reaches the experiment planning stage, i.e., selecting or setting up the spectrometer and auxiliary equipment, through the various and sundry measurements until the data emerge in recognized form. From then on through the realm of interpretation turn to the periodical literature for the most recent results or to references such as A-9, B-26, I-2, I-3, L-13, and P-12.

1.2 EPR AND ITS USES

A particular atomic or molecular species can often be examined in various regions of the electromagnetic spectrum; consequently, in designing an experiment it is of some importance to know the relative advantages of the various spectroscopies. For example, the simplest atom in the periodic system, hydrogen, absorbs in the vacuum ultraviolet (Lyman series), the visible (Balmer series), the infrared (Pashen and Brackett series), and at microwave frequencies. On a photon energy basis the span from the vacuum ultraviolet about 10^3 eV to microwave frequencies at 10^{-6} eV, covers nine decades which are usually divided into the various spectroscopic regions as shown in Fig. 1-1. In some experiments, such as energy level determinations, the spectral regions are fixed by the energies of interest, but in other cases where the goal is detection of the species, as in chemical reactions or a knowledge of molecular or crystalline environments, a choice is often available. Important considerations in detection are sensitivity, selectivity, and simplicity and these characteristics do not converge on a single part of the spectrum. Generally high-energy photon spectroscopy offers the highest sensitivity. Events involving a single photon can be detected in the vacuum ultraviolet while under ideal conditions of narrow absorption lines about 10^{12} absorbers are the minimum for detection at microwave frequencies. Color centers that absorb in the visible and microwave regions offer another sensitivity comparison. With the relatively broad absorption bands encountered for F centers in the alkali halides, about 10^{16} centers can be observed optically about as readily as 10^{18} centers by EPR. EPR is limited to the detection of unpaired electrons, but in this selectivity it is unexcelled. At shorter wavelengths absorptions are encountered for numerous other species, particularly in liquids and solids which become opaque in the vacuum ultraviolet. Infrared spectra become complicated in organic materials because of the numerous molecular absorption bands. Experimental simplicity usually favors optical spectroscopy because the equipment can be relatively simple and the spectroscopist can see what is going on.

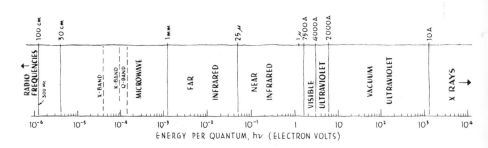

Fig. 1-1. Spectroscopic regions of the electromagnetic spectrum showing the location and energy of the principal EPR absorption bands.

When the environment is of concern, spectroscopy with low-energy photons is most sensitive to small perturbations in the vicinity of the absorber; therefore, infrared and EPR spectroscopy predominate. When magnetic nuclei are present as in the case of hydrogen atoms in organic molecules, EPR becomes extremely sensitive to the unpaired electron's environment. Infrared spectroscopy gives a more complete picture of the sample by including the normal bond absorption in addition to unpaired electrons and thus may save the spectroscopist from an overly simplified interpretation based on the detection of only one species. However, many solids are difficult to analyze in the infrared and the fine environmental details are not resolved.

On the basis of this admittedly brief comparison, EPR appears to be the spectroscopy of choice where its selectivity for unpaired electrons and sensitivity for the absorber environment are the controlling concerns. Although the sensitivity with EPR does not match the higher-frequency spectroscopies, it is high compared to most other methods of chemical analysis. Finally, the advantages of a combined attack using spectroscopy at several frequencies should not be overlooked.

In common with other forms of electromagnetic spectroscopy the experimental information in the EPR spectrum is contained in the location, amplitude, and shape of the absorption bands. Consequently, there are three fundamental measurements, i.e., the determination of these three parameters. The locations marked X band, K band, and Q band in Fig. 1-1 are nominal values for the photon energies in these microwave bands. For experimental convenience the frequency is usually held constant while the magnetic field responsible for the Zeeman effect is adjusted to produce resonance. If the procedure were reversed and the magnetic field remained constant, essentially all of the reported spins could be measured with a decade of frequencies and the organic radicals would be covered by a frequency range of two. Photon energies from roughly 10 to 100 μeV are involved.

The amplitude of the absorption band or more precisely the area under the curve, provides an indication of the number of spins present. As long as the experimental conditions permit a linear relation between numbers of spins and the amplitude, it is a simple matter to obtain relative spin concentrations. Quantitative measurements of spin concentrations are also possible but by the time all the essential precautions have been observed, these measurements become as difficult as any other in the field of EPR. Commercial spectrometers normally have an advertised sensitivity threshold of 10^{11} or 10^{12} spins for a material exhibiting a single line 1 G wide. Unfortunately, the materials most spectroscopists study depart from these conditions, because of either wider lines or multiple lines, or both.

Consequently, it is usually convenient to have 10^{15}–10^{18} spins trapped in the sample.

The third fundamental characteristic, namely, line shape, embraces both the mathematical configuration of the absorption lines and the number of fine structure and hyperfine structure (hfs) components. Herein often lies a wealth of information about the unpaired electron's environment, the nuclei with which it interacts, and the extent of its delocalization. Line shapes frequently have a Lorentzian or gaussian shape and the number of lines can range from one for the simplest environment to hundreds in some organic radicals.

In addition to these EPR parameters there are a number of experimental variables that permit some control over the experiment and through this control may assist in interpreting the results. The various magnetic fields are of central concern: i.e., H, the polarizing field; H_1, the rf field responsible for the spin transitions; and H_m, the modulating field. In addition to their amplitude, their orientation to each other, and to the sample, control the allowed transitions. Other important variables are the temperature, spin concentration, and the sample material. These quantities often determine whether a spectrum can be resolved, particularly into its hfs. All of these parameters will be discussed in detail in subsequent chapters and their control will be illustrated in numerous examples. Some typical ranges covered by these variables are H, 0–15,000 G; H_m, 100 cps to 300 kc; H_1, 10^{-6} to 10^{-1} G; T, 0.5–1000°K; pressure, vacuum to 10^5 atm; total spins, 10^{12}–10^{20}; and materials, metals, semiconductors, dielectrics, gases, liquids, and solids, including biological substances. The material is one of the most versatile parameters, thereby explaining the wide range of scientific disciplines that have embraced EPR.

Initially EPR was almost exclusively the domain of the physicist who studied the behavior of spins in well-ordered systems, i.e., usually single crystals of metals, semiconductors, or dielectrics and sometimes gases. The spins ranged from free electrons in metals and semiconductors to a large variety of the trapped electrons or defect centers that are responsible for many important electronic processes in solids, e.g., color, luminescence, photoconductivity, and the photographic latent image. Where the spin systems were already well known, the measurements contributed to the knowledge of EPR, but in other cases EPR soon made major contributions to models for various centers. This information appeared as interaction coefficients, relaxation times, and energy level diagrams. Also, EPR techniques were applied extensively to paramagnetic ions of the transition elements, rare earths, and transuranic group in suitable host crystals in order to establish energy levels and relaxation times, particularly in connection with laser and maser developments. Crystals were studied as grown and under such external forces as electrical fields and mechanical strains. Examples from the physicists domain appear in Sections 7.1–7.4.

Chronologically the chemists were next in applying EPR on a wide scale, particularly in the study of organic radicals. These radicals appear in many important reactions involved in electrochemistry, photochemistry, radiochemistry, polymer chemistry, and pyrolysis. Other paramagnetic species of principal concern to the chemists are stable radicals, ions, solvated electrons, and triplet-state molecules. EPR allowed the chemist to follow the radicals in reactions without interfering with the reaction, to measure yields in photolysis and radiolysis experiments, to determine the extent of electron delocalization in radicals and ions, and frequently to identify the paramagnetic species. Examples of EPR in chemistry appear largely in Chapters VI and VII, Sections 7.5 and 7.6.

Biology is another discipline with a rapidly developing interest in EPR. Again radical processes attract most of the attention, e.g., in photolysis and radiolysis. Enzyme–substrate reactions are another popular though difficult area for EPR research. With living cells the nondestructive feature of EPR is particularly attractive. For example, photochemical studies have been performed on living plant cells and bacteria. Other examples of EPR in biology appear in Section 7.7.

Applications of EPR are being extended beyond the bounds of research into such areas as process control and clinical analysis. For example, vanadium ion concentrations of a few parts per million in crude oil can poison the catalyst used for catalytic cracking; therefore, an EPR system monitoring the oil on its way to the cracking columns can detect excessive concentrations of vanadium and instigate protection for the catalysts. Other applications ranging from radiation dosimetry to diagnosis of a certain strain of jaundice are receiving attention.

CHAPTER II

EPR Nomenclature, Theory, and Customs

2.1 LANGUAGE AND SCOPE

In opening the 1961 international conference on "Spectroscopie des Radiofréquences" at Brussels, Professor C. J. Gorter commented on the language and practice of EPR as follows:

To non-physicists it is often very confusing that physicists are in the habit of employing two rather different languages when they refer to the interaction between radiation and matter. Namely the language of classical physics of Maxwell and Lorentz (ML) and the quantum language of Planck, Einstein, and Bohr (PEB).

In classical language radiation is an electromagnetic field, the electric or magnetic vector of which acts on the charged particles of which matter is composed. In the quantum language radiation consists of packets called light quanta or photons with energy $h\nu$ and matter has to be in well-defined energy states. When an atom or molecule passes from one discrete state into a lower state, the energy ΔE is carried away by an emitted light quantum $h\nu$ while absorption of such a quantum leads to excitation of the atom or molecule into a state of higher energy. A third process may also occur: the atom or molecule may be stimulated to emit radiation under the influence of a passing light quantum of the same frequency. This is Einstein's stimulated emission.

During the last forty years, the physicist has become used to this dilemma and he employs alternatively the language of Maxwell and Lorentz or that of Planck, Einstein, and Bohr, depending on the kind of problems he is considering. Sometimes—in particular, also in the fields we shall discuss during the present colloquium—he uses an intermediate language, borrowing notions and arguments from the two sides in a bold and often successful but somewhat confusing manner. He can only do so because he knows his rear is well protected. Until 1925 he could merely produce the statement that in the limiting case of high quantum numbers and sometimes also in the case of a system of many particles, the quantum picture leads to the same results as the classical picture does. But thirty-five years ago quantum mechanics had been created by de Broglie, Heisenberg, Schrödinger, and Dirac, which indicates how the interaction between radiation and matter can be calculated in principle—and with the aid of modern computing equipment often also in practice—with all the precision desired, and so far in excellent agreement with observation.

In elementary courses and scientific conversations one, however, persists in the old habits often without specifying which of the languages is being used at any given moment. I shall do the same (G-16).

In describing the interactions between radiation and matter, the quantum language is convenient for indicating EPR requirements; however, the experimental environment involving cavity geometry, coupling holes, and sample placement is easier to visualize by classical electromagnetic fields so the dichotomy is perpetuated.

In keeping with handbook tradition, this section reviews the theory of EPR and microwaves in a tantalizing brevity sufficient to recall the nomenclature and common relationships but insufficient for instruction or detailed interpretation of results. Emphasis is focused on factors which provide guidance for performing the experiment. Discussion follows the phenomenological approach and frequent reference is made to works where pertinent detailed information is available.

2.2 REQUIREMENTS FOR EPR

We now consider the fundamental ingredients for generating electron paramagnetic resonance, namely, the unpaired electrons which constitute the spin, the magnetic field to order the spin system, the radiation field to interact with the electrons, and the selection rules governing these interactions.

2.2.1 The Spin System

Spin systems are frequently represented by energy level diagrams such as the example in Fig. 2-1 which holds for the simplest case of free

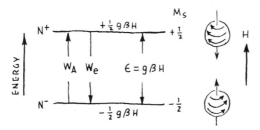

Fig. 2-1. Energy level diagram for simple spin $\frac{1}{2}$ system of free electrons showing populations (N), transition probabilities (W), and schematic representation of spins (P-1,I-2).

electrons in an external magnetic field H. The hieroglyphics at the right indicate schematically the two possible spin orientations conventionally designated by the magnetic moments $= \pm\frac{1}{2}$; N^+ and N^- are the electron populations in the two levels; $g\beta H$ is the energy difference of the Zeeman splitting; and W_a and W_e are the respective absorption and emission transition probabilities. Left to their own devices these electrons will interact with their environment to flip spins and in so doing will create or inelastically scatter phonons until thermal equilibrium is reached at which time the populations will be inversely proportional to the transition probabilities, i.e. (P-1)

$$N^-/N^+ = W_e/W_a = \exp{(\epsilon/kT)} \tag{2-1}$$

where $\epsilon = g\beta H$.

2.2.2   Radiation Interactions with Spin Systems

Einstein was the first to solve the problem of an electromagnetic radiation field interacting with an atomic system and as indicated in Gorter's introduction, the solution involved three processes. When applied to the simple spin system of Fig. 2-1, these processes involve the following transitions expressed in the mixed ML and PEB notation.

1. Spontaneous emission. A spontaneous transition from $M_s = +\frac{1}{2}$ to $M_s = -\frac{1}{2}$ with emission of the corresponding photon independent of the radiation field.

2. Stimulated absorption. Absorption of a photon ($h\nu$) from the radiation field accompanied by a spin transition from $M_s = -\frac{1}{2}$ to $M_s = +\frac{1}{2}$.

3. Stimulated emission. A transition from $M_s = +\frac{1}{2}$ to $M_s = -\frac{1}{2}$ forced by the radiation field and accompanied by the emission of a photon coherent in phase and frequency with the radiation field.

The Einstein transition coefficients are frequency dependent but in laboratory experiments at microwave frequencies, the probability for spontaneous emission can be neglected compared with stimulated emission; however, at optical frequencies, spontaneous transitions become significant (G-15,H-4).

Both stimulated emission and absorption are coherent with the radiation field, and the number of transitions is proportional to the energy density of the radiation field at the particular frequencies. For all practical purposes, the transition coefficients for stimulated absorption and emission can be equated for typical microwave fields.* With this equality and the coherent character of the stimulated transitions, a detectable absorption or emission requires a difference in the spin population of the two energy levels, i.e., $N^- \neq N^+$.

---

* Reference P-1 discusses the slight departure from equality.

Combining the effects of the spin lattice and the radiation field transitions, it is apparent that the phonon interactions in their quest for thermal equilibrium will always tend to keep $N^- > N^+$ while the radiation field tends to equalize the populations. Experimentally, EPR measurements are usually performed with radiation fields too small to appreciably upset the thermal distribution of electrons. Equation 2-1 indicates two possibilities for enhancing the ratio N^-/N^+ and thus the detectable signals (*1*) minimize the temperature T and (*2*) maximize the energy gap ϵ by maximizing the magnetic field H.

2.2.3 Energy Transport

If the radiation field is increased until $N^- = N^+$, there will be no net energy absorption and the spin system is said to be saturated. When the radiation field is removed, the spin system returns to the thermal equilibrium distribution at a rate determined by the ability of the spins to dissipate excess energy. This relaxation process depends on the coupling between the spin system and its environment and is normally described in terms of the following relaxation times.

(a) Spin–Lattice or Longitudinal Relaxation Time (T_1). The two commonly discussed mechanisms for transferring energy from the spin system to the lattice are described as direct and Raman processes. In the direct processes for the two-level system of Fig. 2-1, "relaxation occurs through transfer of energy from a single spin to a single vibrational mode of the crystal lattice which has essentially the same frequency" (G-7). Pake has illustrated the process with a diagram similar to Fig 2-2 (P-1). Low has pictorially described these phonons as on "speaking terms" with the spins (L-13). An examination of the acoustic vibration spectrum for a crystal reveals two weaknesses in the direct process: (*1*) only an extremely small fraction of the acoustic vibrations have the proper frequency for coupling in the microwave range and (*2*) at these low frequencies, the acoustical waves are long compared to lattice dimensions; consequently, the displacement between neighboring atoms is small and the modulation of the local field is slight (P-1). When relaxation is by the direct process, $T_1 \propto 1/H^2T$ (P-1) and is independent of the spin concentration (G-7); therefore, the temperature and magnetic field can serve as variables either for the study or for the control of T_1. Actually, the "direct" process is important only at low temperatures, e.g., below about 4°K.

At high temperatures, the indirect or Raman process predominates. Here a phonon is inelastically scattered in the process of flipping a spin as indicated in Fig. 2-2. Energy is conserved and this process is strongly temperature dependent with $T_1 \propto 1/T^7$ for $T < \theta$, and $T_1 \propto 1/T^2$ for $T > \theta$, where $\theta =$ the debye temperature (L-13).

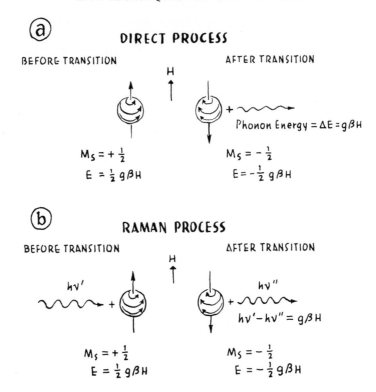

Fig. 2-2. (*a*) Spin–lattice relaxation by the direct process illustrating the creation of a phonon when the spin flips. (*b*) Relaxation by the Raman process where phonon $h\nu'$ is absorbed and phonon $h\nu''$ is emitted as the electron spin flips. (After P-1.)

Experimental results are in fair agreement with theory at high temperatures but not at low temperatures where the direct Process is important. Consequently, there is considerable interest in relaxation measurements at low temperatures. Various concepts have been introduced to aid and abet the above process, e.g., the phonon bottleneck and lattice bath relaxation (L-13 and G-7). Although we may not understand the mechanism controlling the relaxation process, T_1 can be lengthened for experimental convenience or necessity, by working at low temperatures and large energy gaps.

(b) Spin–Spin or Transverse Relaxation Time (T_2). Unpaired electrons can interact with other magnetic dipoles in the vicinity, thereby spreading local disturbances over the entire spin system. Such interactions are not energy dissipating and thus do not contribute directly in returning the spin system to equilibrium; however, the spin–lattice transition may be enhanced if the spin–spin process brings the excess energy to a position for a propitious transition to the lattice. A variety of dipoles are frequently part of an unpaired electron's environment, i.e., unpaired brother electrons, magnetic nuclei native to the lattice, and various impurity dipoles—either electrons or foreign nuclei. Obviously these interactions depend on the dipole concentration as well as their homogeneity. Since the dipole field decreases with the cube of the separation, many of the spin–spin interactions can be eliminated by diluting the environment with diamagnetic atoms. Dipole–dipole interactions are also characterized by a dependence on orientation with respect to the external magnetic field. The importance of both dilution and orientation will be repeatedly encountered in EPR experiments. Other aspects of these spin–spin interactions are considered subsequently in the sections dealing with line shapes, broadening, saturation, and hfs.

2.2.4 Selection Rules

Essentially the only restriction invoked this far in our discussion of radiation field–spin interactions and spin–spin interactions is the conservation of energy. This conservation rule is the basis for the resonance criterion illustrated in Fig. 2-1, i.e.,

$$h\nu = g\beta H \tag{2-2}$$

Now it is time to consider in finer detail the protocol governing the behavior between radiation fields and spins. The polarization of the radiation field with respect to the spin orientation governs the transition probability; consequently, this is an important experimental consideration. We will consider three cases involving spin systems with different degrees of spin–spin interaction.

(a) The Isolated Spin. $\Delta M_s = \pm 1$ (no structure). If Fig. 2-1 is modified to show the energy levels as a function of external magnetic field H, the diagram for a free electron becomes Fig. 2-3. Transitions in either absorption or emission will involve a change in the spin magnetization of $\Delta M_s = \pm 1$ and the spectroscopic selection rules for magnetic dipole transitions of $\Delta M_s = \pm 1$ require a radiation field polarized with the $H_1 \perp H$ in order to optimize the transition. Frequently, this rule is illustrated on a classical basis with a vector diagram of the magnetic fields $H \perp H_1$ and the precessing magnetic moment which experiences a torque due to H_1 and can be flipped when H_1 and s rotate at the same frequency (see Fig. 2-3) (P-2). Another approach is to resort to the conservation of parity which requires that $H_1 \perp H$ for $\Delta M_s = \pm 1$.

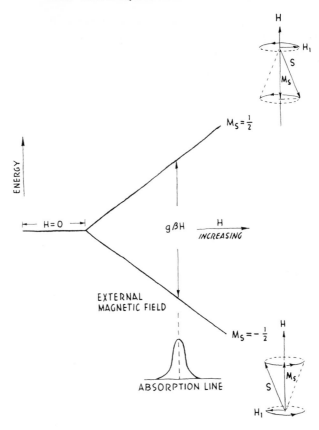

Fig. 2-3. Energy level diagram showing Zeeman splitting for simple free electron spin system in crossed steady (H) and rf (H_1) magnetic fields.

(b) Strong Electron–Electron Dipole Interaction. $\Delta M_s = \pm 1, \Delta M_s = \pm 2$ (fine structures). The triplet-state molecule is a case where strong spin–spin interaction determines the selection rule. In the triplet state, the molecule contains two electrons with their spins aligned parallel so that the total spin $S = \pm 1$ and M_s takes on values of $+1$, 0, and -1. Figure 2-4 is a typical energy level diagram showing the energy as a function of the external field H. With three energy levels, two types of transitions are possible, namely, $\Delta M_s = \pm 1$ and $\Delta M_s = \pm 2$.

For a radiation field of fixed frequency, the conservation of energy causes the $\Delta M_s = \pm 2$ transitions to occur at about half the average H for $\Delta M_s = 1$ transitions (V-1). As before, $H_1 \perp H$ for the $\Delta M_s = \pm 1$ transitions but parity conservation requires $H_1 \parallel H$ for $\Delta M_s = \pm 2$. The

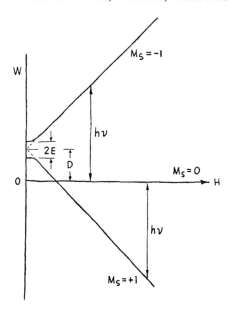

Fig. 2-4. Energy level diagram for the triplet state of naphthalene with H_0 perpendicular to the molecular plane. (Courtesy M-15.)

strength of the spin–spin interaction indicated by the splitting D at $H = 0$ accounts for an appreciable fraction of the energy $h\nu$, e.g., in this case, $D \approx h\nu/3$.

(c) Electron–Magnetic Nucleus Interaction (High-Field Approximation, hfs). $\Delta M_s = \pm 1$, $\Delta M_I = 0$. A very common environment for an unpaired electron contains one or more nuclear magnetic moments. Figure 2-5a illustrates the energy levels as a function of H for interactions with a nuclear spin of $\frac{1}{2}$. The frequency ν required to flip electron spins is far away from the resonance for flipping nuclear spins; consequently, the nuclei normally maintain their alignment during the transition and $\Delta M_I = \pm 0$. With this limitation on the nuclei and aside from triplet states the electrons will make transitions indicated by $\Delta M_s = \pm 1$ and the field should be polarized, with $H_1 \perp H$.

2.3   CONVENTION OF THE SPIN HAMILTONIAN

In the real world of EPR, the unpaired electron seldom finds the simple habitats indicated in Figs. 2-2, 2-3, 2-4, and 2-5. Frequently, the electron interacts with a variety of nuclei and electrons in various degrees so the magnetic field H in Eq. 2-1 becomes the sum of numerous components.

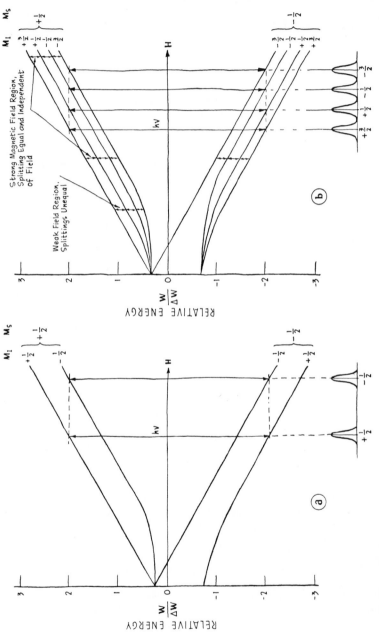

Fig. 2-5. Energy level diagram for (a) $S = \frac{1}{2}, I = \frac{1}{2}$ and (b) $S = \frac{1}{2}, I = \frac{3}{2}$, showing allowed transitions and the resulting hfs (A-10, P-1, B-17).

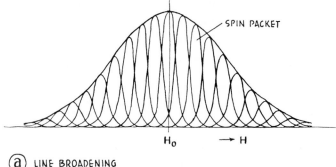

(a) LINE BROADENING

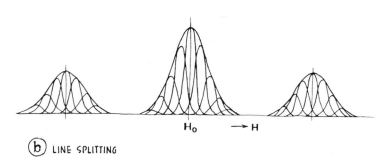

(b) LINE SPLITTING

Fig. 2-6. (a) Combination of signals from spins in slightly different environments to produce a broadened line. (b) Spin packets arranged to illustrate line splitting as encountered in fine structure and hfs.

Furthermore, the observed spectrum contains contributions from many electrons residing in many different local fields. When these fields are nearly the same, the individual electron interactions will develop to form a broad line as indicated in Fig. 2-6. Conversely, substantial differences in the local fields as illustrated in Figs. 2-4 and 2-5 lead to fine structure or hfs in the lines as at b.

In gases and liquids where the rapid motion and tumbling of the molecules tends to average the local field to a common value, we encounter the narrowest lines, but the presence of magnetic nuclei can still lead to rich hfs. Unpaired electrons in solids encounter the most complex interacting fields. Conventionally, the state of affairs has been expressed from the quantum mechanical viewpoint in terms of Hamiltonians. Abragam and

Pryce (A-2) initially and numerous others subsequently described the electronic interactions which contribute to the total energy of the ion by the following Hamiltonian (A-9,A-10):

$$\mathcal{H} = \mathcal{H}^0 + \mathcal{H}_{cr} + \mathcal{H}_{s-o} + \mathcal{H}_{s-s} + \mathcal{H}_Z + \mathcal{H}_{hf} + \mathcal{H}_Q + \mathcal{H}_n + \mathcal{H}_e$$

(2-3)

where

	Energy[a] ν' cm^{-1}	Gauss
$\mathcal{H}^0$ = Free ion or coulomb energy	10^5	
$\mathcal{H}_{cr}$ = Stark crystalline or electrostatic energy	10^4	
$\mathcal{H}_{s-o}$ = Electronic spin–orbit interaction energy	10^2–10^3	
$\mathcal{H}_{s-s}$ = Electronic spin–spin interaction energy	1	10^4
$\mathcal{H}_Z$ = Zeeman energy, interaction of the electron with the external field = $\beta H \cdot (L + 2S)$	1	10^4
$\mathcal{H}_{hf}$ = Dipole–dipole coupling between the electron and the nuclear magnetic moments	10^{-1}–10^{-3}	10^3–10
$\mathcal{H}_Q$ = Quadrupole or higher electrostatic interaction between electron and nucleus	10^{-3}	10
$\mathcal{H}_n$ = Nuclear Zeeman energy, interaction of nucleus with the external field = $g_I \beta_I H \cdot I$	10^{-4}	1
$\mathcal{H}_e$ = Energy of exchange effects between two types of electrons		

[a] In spectroscopy energy is commonly expressed in units of cm^{-1} (wavenumbers) omitting a factor hc, i.e., energy = $h\nu = hc\nu'$. Although gauss are not units of energy they are sometimes used in this fashion through Eq. 2-2, where $H = hc\nu'/g\beta \approx 10^4 \nu$.

Since the energy contribution from the various terms ranges over nine decades, it is not surprising that some interactions fall outside the realm of EPR. In microwave practice magnets, generators, and components for a 1-mm wavelength system are hard to come by; yet at this high frequency the energy only corresponds to 10 cm^{-1}. Obviously, $\mathcal{H}^0$, $\mathcal{H}_{cr}$, and $\mathcal{H}_{s-o}$ involve too much energy for excitation by EPR. $\mathcal{H}_{s-s}$, $\mathcal{H}_Z$, and $\mathcal{H}_{hf}$ involve energies ideally suited to existing microwave practice; consequently, the fine structure, Zeeman splitting and hfs are the main concerns of EPR spectroscopy. At the other extreme, $\mathcal{H}_Q$, $\mathcal{H}_n$, and $\mathcal{H}_e$ are frequently too small to observe in the presence of $\mathcal{H}_Z$. Figure 2-7 is an energy level diagram for the Cu^{2+} ion which is frequently used to illustrate the energy contribution from the various fields. Bearing in mind the wide range of energies from the various terms, it is obvious that the splittings between levels are not to scale. The transitions permitted by the selection rules and the energy available in the microwave field are indicated by the dotted vertical arrows, i.e., a hyperfine structure of four lines.

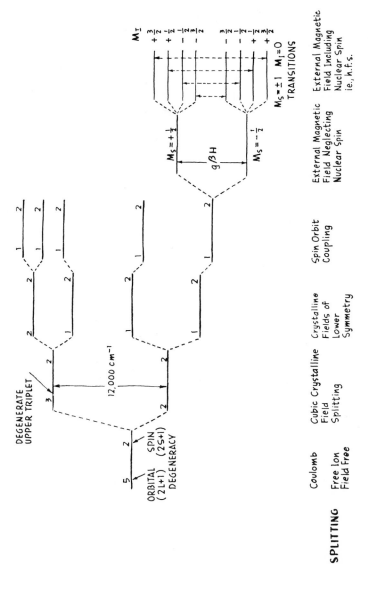

Fig. 2-7. Energy level diagram showing splitting of the ^2D term for Cu^{2+} in crystalline electric and strong magnetic fields. (After A-10.)

Calculations with the total Hamiltonian are very difficult; therefore, a simplified accounting of the more likely interactions is performed with a spin Hamiltonian. Abragam and Pryce developed the spin Hamiltonian and derivations appear in numerous references (B-26,I-2,P-1,etc.). Our reason for dabbling in Hamiltonians is best explained by a quotation from Low (L-13), "The spin Hamiltonian is used to give a shorthand description of the experimental results." Such parameters as the g factor, the zero field splittings, and the hyperfine structure constants are determined experimentally, then fitted to models with the aid of the Hamiltonian. Consequently, reporting the parameters in a standard form simplifies communication and aids the quest for models. The spin Hamiltonian for a principal axis system can be written as (P-1,G-15):

$$\mathscr{H} = D[S_z^2 - \tfrac{1}{3}S(S + 1)] + E(S_x^2 - S_y^2)$$
$$+ \beta(g_x S_x H_x + g_y S_y H_y + g_z S_z H_z) + A_z I_z S_z + A_x I_x S_x$$
$$+ A_y I_y S_y + Q[I_z^2 - \tfrac{1}{3}I(I + 1)] - g_I \beta_I H \cdot I \qquad (2\text{-}4)$$

where S is the effective electronic spin, the β's and g's are the usual magnatons and splitting factors, I is the nuclear spin, and D, E, A, and Q are interaction coefficients to be determined empirically from observed spectra as described in Section 2.5. Reference A-2 should be consulted for details of the effective spin concept. By convention S is assigned a value that makes the observed number of energy levels equal $(2S + 1)$ (P-1). In spin systems where only the lower energy levels are inhabited, the higher levels will not be detected experimentally; consequently, the S determined from the $(2S + 1)$ observed levels corresponds to a fictitious state. As a consequence g may vary considerably from the Landé g factor (L-13). Equation 2-4 can be simplified considerably when the crystalline electric field has axial symmetry (tetragonal, trigonal, or hexagonal) (P-1). If z is the axis of symmetry, then

$$g_z = g_{\parallel}, \quad g_x = g_y = g_{\perp}$$
$$A_z = A_{\parallel}, \quad A_x = A_y = A_{\perp}$$
$$\langle S_x^2 \rangle = \langle S_y^2 \rangle$$

and the spin Hamiltonian becomes

$$\mathscr{H} = D[S_z^2 - \tfrac{1}{3}S(S + 1)] + \beta[g_{\parallel}S_z H_z + g_{\perp}(S_x H_x + S_y H_y)]$$
$$+ A_{\parallel} I_z S_z + A_{\perp}(I_x S_x + I_y S_y) \qquad (2\text{-}5)$$

"This equation can be regarded as one of the most important in EPR of the crystalline state, being the essential link between the measurements of the experimentalist and the general considerations of the theoretician" (I-3).

In many cases Eq. 2-5 reduces to simpler terms as in the following examples:

Case 1. The free electron. $D = 0$, $A_{\parallel} = A_{\perp} = 0$, $g = $ a scalar; therefore, $\mathcal{H} = h\nu = g\beta H_0$.

Case 2. Electron and one type of nucleus. Dilute liquids or gases are examples of this system. At high dilutions, the spin–spin and exchange interaction are negligible, i.e., D is negligible. Rapid tumbling of the molecules averages all anisotropic interactions so the g factor is a scalar (H-7).

Therefore

$$\mathcal{H} = h\nu = g\beta H_0 + \sum A_i M_{Ii}$$

where

$$M_I = -I, -I + 1, \ldots, +I$$

resulting in $(2I + 1)$ hf lines with a spacing between adjacent lines of A/h cps or $A/g\beta$ Oe (P-1).

2.4 PASSAGE EFFECTS

2.4.1 Nomenclature

Common assumptions in EPR measurements are that the radiation fields do not seriously disturb the thermal distribution of electrons N^+ and N^-, and that the spin system is in thermal equilibrium (Section 2.2.2). When these conditions fail, we enter the world of passage effects and encounter a nomenclature designed to specify succinctly the experimental conditions. The important instrumental variables are: (*1*) rf magnetic field strength (H_1); (*2*) magnetic field sweep rate; (*3*) magnetic field modulation frequency; and (*4*) the time between sweeps. Most of the passage effect terms indicate either the magnitude of the time dependent variables with respect to relaxation times T_1 and T_2 or the degree of disturbance in the spin distribution as listed in Table 2-1.

2.4.2 Symmetry Conditions

Reference W-10 should be consulted for a detailed account of EPR behavior under various combinations of the conditions defined in Table 2-1. Here we briefly list a few of the passage effects and describe some of their experimental characteristics so that hopefully they can be recognized and separated from physical effects. In considering passage effects it is convenient to divide the magnetic field H into three components: (*1*) H_0, the field at the center of the spin packet, i.e., resonance; (*2*) $(dH_0/dt)t$,

Table 2-1
Definition of Passage Terms (W-10)

Rapid: $\dfrac{H_1}{dH/dt} \ll \sqrt{T_1 T_2}$ [a]	The time each spin packet is swept through is *short* compared with the mean relaxation time. We have rapid passage conditions, in the Bloch[b] sense.
Fast: $\omega_m T_1 \gg 1$	The time between successive modulation cycles is *short* compared with T_1. Each spin packet does not relax considerably between successive modulation cycles.
Slow: $\dfrac{H_1}{dH/dt} \gg \sqrt{T_1 T_2}$	Not rapid, i.e., "slow passage" in the Bloch sense.
Adiabatic: $\gamma H_1{}^2 \gg \dfrac{dH}{dt}$	The passage through the line is sufficiently slow, so that the magnetization vector S follows the effective magnetic field $H - \omega/\gamma + H_1$ adiabatically (i.e., is parallel or antiparallel to it). Again, see Bloch.[b]
Nonadiabatic: $\gamma H_1{}^2 \ll \dfrac{dH}{dt}$	The passage through the line is so rapid, that the magnetization vector S cannot follow the effective field, but stays almost parallel to the dc magnetic field.
Burnt	Most of the magnetization S has been destroyed ("burnt out") by the microwave field H_1.
Stale	Individual spin packets have reached a stationary state. The magnetization is an almost periodic function of time, with period $\omega_m/2\pi$.
Fresh	Most of the contribution to the signal comes from packets which have not yet been swept through many times.
Scope trace	The signal at the output of the IF amplifier (or crystal detector, if no superheterodyne arrangement is used). This may be observed by an oscilloscope, or sometimes, a recorder.
Recorder trace	The signal at the output of the phase sensitivity detector.

---

[a] T_2 here, and in the following, is essentially T_{2e} of Redfield. [Redfield, A. G., *Phys. Rev.*, **98**, 1787 (1955).] For perfect saturation it is approximately T_1. For imperfect saturation it is shorter. The situation $T_2 < H_1/(dH/dt) < \sqrt{T_1 T_2}$ corresponds to neither slow nor rapid passage. For $\gamma H_1 T_2 > 1$, we have $T_{2e} \approx T_1$, while for $\gamma H_1 T_2 < 1$, the signal is very weak (under saturation conditions). Therefore, this situation is ignored here.

[b] Bloch, F., *Phys. Rev.*, **70**, 460 (1946).

the magnetic field sweep; and (3) $H_m \cos \omega t$, the modulating magnet field. Therefore

$$H = H_0 + \left(\frac{dH_0}{dt}\right) t + H_m \cos \omega t \tag{2-6}$$

Components (2) and (3) determine how much time the rf field has to alter the electron distribution $N^- \to N^+$ and the time between sweeps plus component (3) affect the time available for thermal equilibrium to be restored. Consequently, when the spin distribution is disturbed, the observed spectra become sensitive both to the direction of sweep and time between sweeps. Reference W-10 lists the following symmetry conditions or parity observed when the direction of sweep is reversed in systems obeying the Bloch equations.*

Case A. The usual situation where the spin populations are not appreciably disturbed, when $(dH_0/dt) \to -(dH_0/dt)$.

(1) For scope display

$$S_x \to -S_x, \qquad S_y \to S_y, \qquad S_z \to S_z$$

Therefore, χ' changes sign while χ'' does not.

(2) For recorder trace display, the transformation $\delta \to -\delta$ causes the phase of the modulation signal to invert with respect to the reference signal, so when

$$\left(\frac{dH_0}{dt}\right) \to -\left(\frac{dH_0}{dt}\right)$$

$$S_x \to S_x, \qquad S_y \to -S_y, \qquad S_z \to -S_z$$

Therefore, χ' is unchanged while χ'' is reversed.

Case B. The rf field is strong enough to invert the spin populations and the system does not relax between successive sweeps; then all of the above symmetry relations will be reversed as indicated in Fig. 2-8 where the

---

* Bloch equations:

$$\frac{dS_x}{dt} + \frac{S_x}{T_2} - \gamma H_1 \delta S_y = 0$$

$$\frac{dS_y}{dt} + \frac{S_y}{T_2} + \gamma H_1 \delta S_x - \gamma H_1 S_z = 0$$

$$\frac{dS_z}{dt} + \frac{S_z}{T_1} + \gamma H_1 \delta S_y = \frac{S_0}{T_1}$$

where

$$\gamma = \frac{\omega}{H_0}, \qquad \chi' = \frac{S_x}{2H_1}, \quad \text{and} \quad \chi'' = \frac{S_y}{2H_1}$$

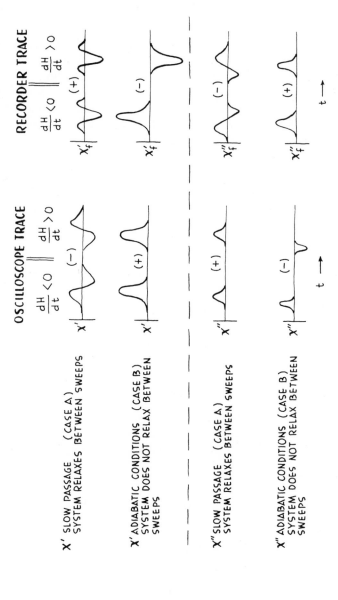

Fig. 2-8. Effect of passage conditions on symmetry of oscilloscope and derivative recorder traces of χ' and χ'': $(+)$ = mirror image; $(-)$ = reversed or inverted image. (After W-10.)

($-$) sign indicates the signal reverses or inverts and the ($+$) means a mirror image so that a symmetrical signal appears unchanged.

2.4.3 Classes of Passage Effects

In between the extreme cases of A and B there are many combinations of the experimental variables capable of distorting the symmetry and spectrum in various degrees. Reference W-10 discusses 11 cases summarized in Fig. 2-9.

Case 1. Slow passage corresponds to a spin system continually in equilibrium and leads to the solution to the Bloch equations given in Section 2.5.4. The remaining 10 cases all involve sweep rates capable of producing rapid passage effects. These rapid cases are further subdivided according to the modulation frequency into "not fast" and "fast" groups. Cases 2, 3, and 4 all involved rapid passage and a long time between field modulation cycles but the passage varies from adiabatic in Case 2 through the intermediate condition of Case 3 to a nonadiabatic passage in Case 4. The "rapid, fast" cases after division into adiabatic and nonadiabatic are further grouped according to the destruction of the individual spin packets, thus involving the rf field intensity with the sweep factors. Therefore, Cases 5, 6, 7, and 8 involve rapid adiabatic passage with a short time between consecutive field modulation cycles but with various degrees of burning. Finally, Cases 9, 10, and 11 are all rapid nonadiabatic passage with a short time between consecutive field modulation cycles and three degrees of burning.

Most of the measurements described in this volume are preferably made operating under Case 1 conditions, i.e., the determination of g values, the hf structure, spin concentrations, and line shapes, but some of the techniques for determining T_1 and T_2 are in the rapid passage category.

2.5 QUANTITIES TO BE DETERMINED EXPERIMENTALLY

2.5.1 Spectroscopic Splitting Factor or g Factor

The spectroscopic splitting factor is defined by the resonance condition $h\nu = g\beta H$; therefore, in terms of the simple energy level diagram of Fig. 2-1, g expresses the proportionality between the magnetic field and the energy difference between Zeeman levels. Two general procedures for determining g are:

1. The direct method where ν and H are measured independently at the resonance absorption peak and g is calculated from $g = h\nu/\beta H$.

2. The comparison method where an unknown specimen is measured along with a system of known g value. Figure 2-10 illustrates this method with spectra obtained at a common frequency in a dual sample cavity.

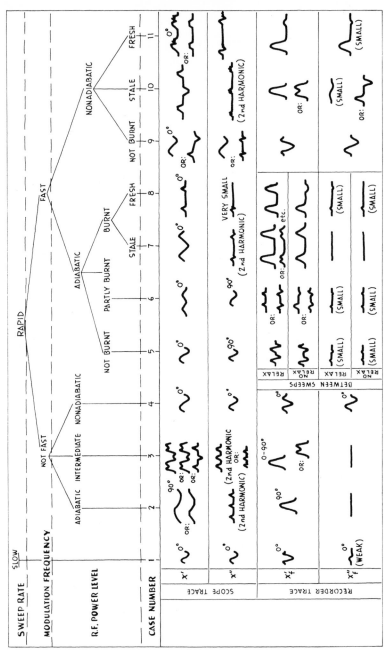

Fig. 2-9. Summary of relationships of the various passage cases. (After W-10.)

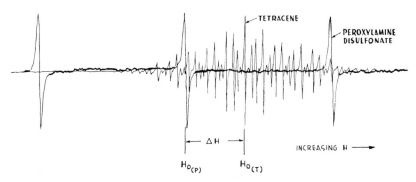

Fig. 2-10. Determination of g values in a dual cavity with a yardstick of known g value and hf splitting. Starting with $g_{\text{tetracene}} = 2.00250 \pm 3 \times 10^{-5}$, measure $h\nu$ to wavemeter accuracy, calculate $H_{0(T)}$ from $h\nu = g_T\beta H_{0(T)}$, determine ΔH from the tetracene hf splitting, and calculate $g_P = g_{\text{peroxylamine disulfonate}}$, $h\nu = g_P\beta H_{0(P)} = g_P\beta(H_{0(T)} - \Delta H)$; therefore

$$g_P = g_T[H_{0(T)}/(H_{0(T)} - \Delta H)] \approx g_T(1 - \Delta H/H_{0(T)})$$

(After V-7.)

Here tetracene is the standard, having a $g_T = 2.00250$, and peroxylamine disulfonate is the unknown.

ΔH is determined with precision from the tetracene hf splitting and $H_{0(T)}$ is obtained from the known g_T combined with a measurement of the resonance frequency (wavemeter accuracy is adequate). Substituting ΔH and $H_{0(P)}$ into the modified resonance equation gives a $g_P = 2.00550$. Both g factors in the example are close to the free electron value of 2.0023, indicating that the spin–orbital and spin–spin interactions are essentially negligible in these systems. While the g values are isotropic and relatively easy to determine for such ion radicals in solution, the information carried in the value of g is useful only in refined measurements capable of revealing small departures from the free electron value.

In crystalline solids the other terms in the Hamiltonian frequently become important and g is no longer isotropic or independent of the field strength. An easy way to visualize the impact of these interactions on the splitting factor is to write the resonance condition as $h\nu = g\beta (H_e + H_i)$ (E-7). Experimentally, g is still determined from the measured values of the resonance frequency ν and the external field H_e. Therefore, the influence of the internal field H_i shows up in the g value. Now g can vary both with the strength and orientation of H_e with respect to H_i. When $H_e < H_i$, the internal field will control the spin orientation and dominate the splitting factor. Conversely, when H_e becomes large enough to swamp H_i, g will approach a constant value. This variation in g with the strength of the external field indicates the desirability of measuring g at more than one field strength.

When the direction of H_e is varied with respect to the crystalline axis, g will change to reflect the changes in the total field; consequently, it is customary to measure the direction components of the splitting factor g_x, g_y, and g_z. When crystalline symmetry permits, $g_\parallel$ and $g_\perp$ will suffice where $\parallel$ and $\perp$ refer to the direction of H_e with respect to the symmetry axis of the crystalline electric field. Because of this orientation dependence, g-value measurements provide a sensitive probe for studying the local field symmetry and such measurements play an important part in the EPR spectroscopy of crystals. Reported magnitudes of the splitting factor vary from about 1 to 8 with the majority in the vicinity of 2.

In the materials where strong crystalline field forces or covalent bonds decouple the spins from the orbital motion, g is close to the free electron value (I-2). Most of the materials of principle concern in this volume fall in this category, e.g., free radicals and trapped electrons.

2.5.2   Fine Structure Coefficients D and E

The electric and magnetic fields internal to a spin system can lift the degeneracy of superimposed energy levels and generate a fine structure which appears when the splitting is small enough so that the levels are populated and the resonance transitions are within the energy range of EPR. Interactions such as spin–orbit coupling, electron spin–spin coupling, and the Stark effect of an asymmetrical crystalline electric field are usually responsible for the fine structure, e.g., the fine structure in Fig. 2-4 was produced by spin–spin interactions in the triplet state of naphthalene molecules. Coefficients D and E as illustrated in Fig. 2-4 are the zero field splitting, i.e., the separations between energy levels when the external magnetic field is zero. According to Eq. 2-5 only the D term is required when the crystalline field has complete axial symmetry; however, the additional E term of Eq. 2-4 is required to describe fields of lower symmetry (B-26).

D and E can be determined directly with a zero field spectrometer or by an extrapolation from high magnetic field measurements. An appropriate zero field spectrometer is described in Section 7.6; however, the necessity of a continuously variable microwave frequency complicates the spectroscopy and diverts most practitioners to the high field techniques. If the spins are precessing about the crystalline field axis, the application of an external magnetic field along the same axis will not change the precession and the energy levels will diverge linearly, as shown in Fig. 2-4 (M-15). If there is an angle θ between the axis of these two fields, competition will ensue and the axis of precession will switch from the crystal

Table 2-2

Evaluation of D from Fine Structure Splitting of a Strong Field Spectrum
(calculated from the first-order term of Eq. 2-7)

Transition	M	$M - 1$	θ	$f_1(\theta)$	$g\beta H$	Remarks
$\Delta M = \pm 1$	1	0	0	2	$g\beta H_0 - D$	$D = g\beta\Delta H/2$
	0	1	0	2	$g\beta H_0 + D$	
	$\frac{3}{2}$	$\frac{1}{2}$	0	2	$g\beta H_0 - 2D$	
	$\frac{1}{2}$	$-\frac{1}{2}$	0	2	$g\beta H_0$	$D = g\beta\Delta H/4$
	$-\frac{1}{2}$	$-\frac{3}{2}$	0	2	$g\beta H_0 + 2D$	
	1	0	$\pi/2$	-1	$g\beta H_0 + D/2$	$D = g\beta\Delta H$
	0	-1	$\pi/2$	-1	$g\beta H_0 - D/2$	
	$\frac{3}{2}$	$\frac{1}{2}$	$\pi/2$	-1	$g\beta H_0 + D$	
	$\frac{1}{2}$	$-\frac{1}{2}$	$\pi/2$	-1	$g\beta H_0$	$D = g\beta\Delta H/2$
	$-\frac{1}{2}$	$-\frac{3}{2}$	$\pi/2$	-1	$g\beta H_0 - D$	
	Any M		$54°$	0	$g\beta H_0$	Splitting vanishes
		$(M - 2)$				
$\Delta M = \pm 2$	1	-1	0	2	$g\beta H_0/2$ [a]	Half field value
	$\frac{3}{2}$	$-\frac{1}{2}$	0	2	$g\beta H_0/2 - D$	$D = g\beta\Delta H/2$
	$\frac{1}{2}$	$-\frac{3}{2}$	0	2	$g\beta H_0/2 + D$	
	1	-1	$\pi/2$	-1	$g\beta H_0/2$	Half field value
	$\frac{3}{2}$	$-\frac{1}{2}$	$\pi/2$	-1	$g\beta H_0 + D/2$	$D = g\beta\Delta H$
	$\frac{1}{2}$	$-\frac{3}{2}$	$\pi/2$	-1	$g\beta H_0 - D/2$	
	Any M		$54°$	0	$g\beta H_0$	Splitting vanishes

[a] For $\Delta M = \pm 2$ transitions $g\beta H = g\beta H_0/2 - D(M - 1)f_1(\theta) - \cdots$.

axis to the direction of the magnetic field as the magnetic field increases. Since both D and E depend on the angle θ, these coefficients can be used to study the internal field symmetry and conversely a judicious selection of θ can simplify the determination of D and E. For example, D is best measured with $\theta = 0$ because E vanishes for this orientation.

Starting with the spin Hamiltonian, Bleaney derived a relation that included the effects of the angle θ on the location of the fine structure absorption line (B-15):

$$g\beta H = g\beta H_0 - D(M - \tfrac{1}{2})f_1(\theta) - (D^2/H_1)f_2(\theta) - \cdots \qquad (2\text{-}7)$$

where $h\nu = g\beta H_0$ is the resonance in the absence of fine structure, the $\Delta M = \pm 1$ transition is from $M \to M - 1$ and

$$f_1(\theta) = 3(g_{\parallel}^2/g^2)\cos^2 \theta - 1$$

Table 2-2 illustrates the relation between D and ΔH, the splitting between outermost lines, obtained with only the first-order term of Eq. 2-7 for several combinations of effective spin and angle θ. Figures 2-11, 2-12, and 2-13 show energy level diagrams corresponding to some of the combinations of S and θ. The proportionalities between D and ΔH listed in Table 2-2 can be derived directly from the geometry of the energy level diagrams as indicated in Figs. 2-11 to 2-13. In order to obtain D it is necessary to measure both g and ΔH. Experimentally there are two procedures.

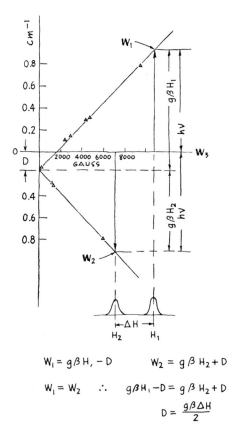

$$W_1 = g\beta H, -D \qquad W_2 = g\beta H_2 + D$$

$$W_1 = W_2 \qquad \therefore \qquad g\beta H_1 - D = g\beta H_2 + D$$

$$D = \frac{g\beta \Delta H}{2}$$

Fig. 2-11. Fine structure in energy levels for Ni^{2+} ion in nickel fluosilicate for H parallel to hexagonal axis: temperature = 90°K. (After P-7.)

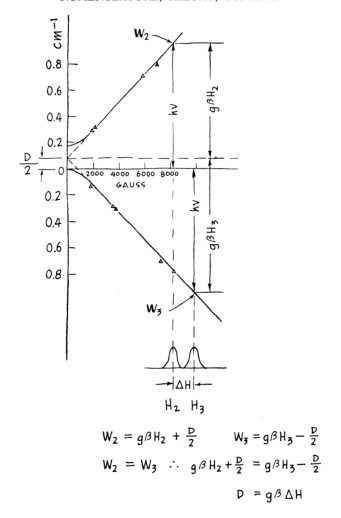

$$W_2 = g\beta H_2 + \frac{D}{2} \qquad W_3 = g\beta H_3 - \frac{D}{2}$$

$$W_2 = W_3 \quad \therefore \quad g\beta H_2 + \frac{D}{2} = g\beta H_3 - \frac{D}{2}$$

$$D = g\beta \, \Delta H$$

Fig. 2-12. Energy levels for Ni^{2+} ion in nickel fluosilicate for H perpendicular to the hexagonal axis: temperature $= 90°K$. (After P-7.)

In the safest method the rf frequency ν and the external field H_0 are measured at resonance for a series of frequencies so that the energy levels W_1, W_2, and W_3 (Fig. 2-11) can be plotted from the observed data. D is obtained by extrapolating W_1 and W_3 to a zero external field where the transition energy $W_1 \leftrightarrow W_3$ or $W_2 \leftrightarrow W_3$ equals D. In this example $D = 0.17$ cm^{-1} for the Ni^{2+} ion in nickel fluosilicate.

The second method requires measurements at only one frequency but

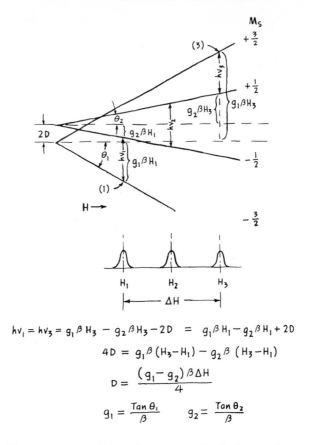

$$hv_1 = hv_3 = g_1\beta H_3 - g_2\beta H_3 - 2D = g_1\beta H_1 - g_2\beta H_1 + 2D$$

$$4D = g_1\beta(H_3 - H_1) - g_2\beta(H_3 - H_1)$$

$$D = \frac{(g_1 - g_2)\beta\Delta H}{4}$$

$$g_1 = \frac{Tan\,\theta_1}{\beta} \qquad g_2 = \frac{Tan\,\theta_2}{\beta}$$

Fig. 2-13. Fine structure coefficient from energy level diagram for system with $S = \frac{3}{2}$ and the magnetic field parallel to the crystalline field axis. (After B-17.)

assumes the energy levels are linear and symmetrical as in Fig. 2-11. From the geometry of the diagram, D is half the separation between the absorption peaks at H_1 and H_2 measured in energy units, i.e., $D = \Delta Hg\beta/2$. Here g must be determined from the slope of W_1 or W_2. Since the slopes are equal in magnitude and the energy levels converge at the zero external field, ordinant lines W_1 and W_2 are readily completed by cut-and-try construction. As long as D is modest compared with $g\beta H_2$, slight errors in construction will have a small effect on the determination of g and the calculation of D from the ΔH. A corresponding diagram for H_0 parallel to the symmetry axis, Fig. 2-12 shows a nonlinearity in W_2 and W_3 at low magnetic field intensities. Now the extrapolated lines intersect the zero field coordinant at $D/2$ and D can be determined from the splitting between the doublet lines from $D = \Delta H g \beta$. ΔH in Fig. 2-12 is only half as large as that in Fig. 2-11 so that both orientations give the same value of D.

When $S = \frac{3}{2}$, the EPR spectrum will consist of a triplet with equal spacings between the absorption peaks, as indicated in Fig. 2-13. Again, D can be determined by either the multiple measurement or the ΔH methods. When D is calculated from the separation between the two outermost peaks, $D = (g_1 - g_2)(\beta \Delta H / 4)$ where the nomenclature follows that of Fig. 2-13. In constructing the diagram to obtain g_1 and g_2 it is convenient to commence with the $M_s \pm \frac{1}{2}$ levels corresponding to the middle absorption peak because the symmetry of the splitting eliminates cutting and trying. Next lines $+\frac{3}{2}$ and $-\frac{3}{2}$ with equal slope (magnitude) are constructed at H_2 and H_1 through the points 3 and 1 so that they intersect on the zero field ordinant.

These general procedures can be applied to systems involving more than two fine structure levels; however, the problem of unraveling the spectrum becomes increasingly complicated, particularly when hfs is also present. In sorting out lines belonging to the various electronic transitions, the variation in intensity from one transition to another can be very helpful. In a given spectrum the intensity of the lines for the various transitions will be proportional to $[S(S + 1) - M(M - 1)]$ (I-1). For example, in the case of Cr^{3+} of Fig. 2-13, where $S = \frac{3}{2}$ and $M = \frac{3}{2}, \frac{1}{2}$, $-\frac{1}{2}$, and $-\frac{3}{2}$, the intensities should be in the ratios of $3:4:3$, and for a more complicated spectrum like Mn^{2+}, which has 5 electronic transitions and $S = \frac{5}{2}$, the ratios are $5:8:9:8:5$.

The magnitude and sign of D depends on the spin species, the host crystal, and the temperature. References A-9, B-26, and P-1 contain numerous examples of D in their tables of Hamiltonian coefficients. A few values are as large as 3 or 4 cm^{-1} but most values are less than 1; small values are about 0.002. EPR measurements alone do not give the sign of D, which can be either plus or minus. Reference L-13 discusses several related experiments which can determine the sign of D including a study of the populations of the various absorption lines at low temperatures where significant differences exist between more populated M_s^- and less populated M_s^+ levels.

While many spin systems exhibit no anisotropic coefficient E, there are other systems where E is significant, although it is generally an order of magnitude smaller than D. When the additional splitting expressed by the E term exists, a pair of converging energy levels do not meet at the zero field ordinant but become nonlinear and exhibit a splitting equal to $2E$, as indicated in Fig. 2-4. In such a system, two absorption lines would occur at zero magnetic field separated by a frequency corresponding to $2E$. When H_0 is parallel to the axis of symmetry (z), the splitting between lines reduces to the previous relation $\Delta H = 2D/g\beta$ but when H_0 is parallel to x or y, $\Delta H = [(|D| \pm |3E|)/g\beta]$ (M-15).

2.5.3 Hyperfine Structure Coefficients A_x, A_y, A_z, etc.

Equations 2-4 and 2-5 contain terms in A to account for the interactions between the electronic and nuclear spins, i.e., the hyperfine interactions. The number of coefficients required depends on the number of nuclei involved, the strength of the various interactions, and the spatial homogeneity of the resultant field. With a constant frequency spectrometer the hf splitting is normally measured in gauss or oersteds; however, A is preferably reported in wavenumbers, i.e., A cm^{-1} = $[(g\beta\Delta H, G)/hc]$.

In the simplest case of an electron satisfying the strong field approximation in an isotropic field of a single nucleus where $A = A_x = A_y = A_z$, the selection rules associated with Fig. 2-5 apply and $(2I + 1)$ hf lines are possible which correspond to $(2I + 1)$ orientations of the nuclear magnetic moments in the external magnetic field. Figure 2-14 illustrates this case with hf spectra for a series of nuclei with moments ranging from $\frac{1}{2}$ to $\frac{7}{2}$. The resonance condition $h\nu = g\beta H_0 + AM_I$ with $M_I = -I, -I + 1, \ldots, + I$ leads to a spacing between adjacent lines equal to A. The nuclear moments have been measured for most isotopes so that we know how many lines to expect. Liquids, gases, and atoms isolated in a glassy matrix or in crystals with exact cubic symmetry are examples of spin systems exhibiting single values of A. Within the limits of the high-field approximation the hyperfine interaction is independent of the external magnetic field strength and the splitting remains constant for all fields.

Spins in a single crystal frequently experience an anisotropic field requiring two or more coefficients to specify the hfs dependence on crystal orientation in the external field. If the crystal exhibits axial symmetry, two coefficients are sufficient, namely, $A_{\|}$ and $A_{\perp}$. By convention, the crystalline axis is assigned the z direction so that $A_z = A_{\|}$, which is measured with the external magnetic field parallel to the z axis. Similarly, $A_x = A_y = A_{\perp}$, which is measured with H external perpendicular to the z axis. When such symmetry is absent, measurements along all three orientations x, y, and z are required. Figure 2-15 shows the variation in hf splitting for the silicon *Pl* center as a function of the crystal orientation with respect to the external fields.

In many instances the unpaired electron interacts with several magnetic nuclei and the hf structure becomes increasingly complex, in some cases blossoming into hundreds of resolvable lines. Such spectra are extremely important sources of information about the extent of interactions or nonlocalization of electrons. Organic radicals provide

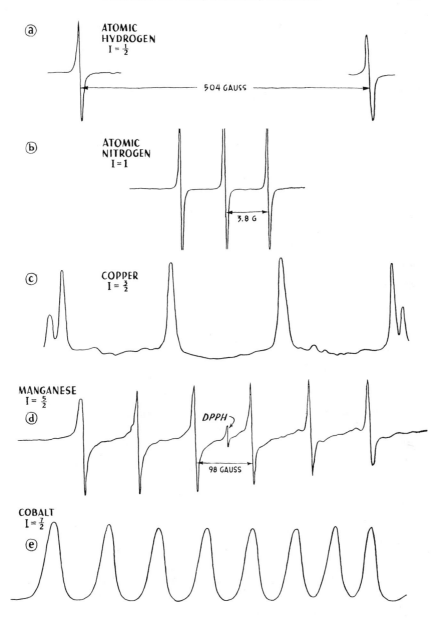

Fig. 2-14. EPR hyperfine structure for interactions with nuclei of various magnetic moments. The number of lines = $2I + 1$. Curves *a*, *b*, and *d* are derivative presentations. Curves *c* and *e* are absorption curves. (*b*, Courtesy U-2; *c*, I-1; *d*, K-5; *e*, B-17.)

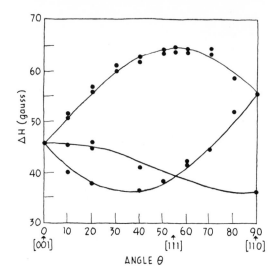

Fig. 2-15. Variation of the hyperfine interaction with the direction of the magnetic field for the Si-*Pl* center at 77°K. ΔH is the separation between the hf line and the corresponding fine structure line. (Courtesy N-1.)

many examples of this type of hf structure because of the prevalence of hydrogen atoms. Here we will consider three types of electron sharing appropriate to organic radicals.

(a) Electron Shared Between Magnetic and Nonmagnetic Nuclei. C—H and O—H bonds are common examples of an electron shared between a magnetic hydrogen nucleus and an atom with no magnetic moment. In this situation the splitting indicates the relative degree of association or amount of time spent in the vicinity of each nucleus. For example, the hf splitting for an electron 100% associated with a proton is 504 G from Fig. 2-14; however, when the electron is associated with a C—H bond, the splitting drops to 20–30 G, indicating that the electron spends most of its time on the carbon. Other examples of splitting for similar shared electron systems are included in Section 7.5.

(b) Electron Equally Shared Between Magnetic Nuclei. If all alignments of the nuclear moments are equally probable with respect to the magnetic field, then each nucleus will contribute $2I + 1$ levels equally spaced and superimposed on levels arising from n other nuclei for a total of $(2NI + 1)$ lines (I-2). For n equally interacting protons the number of hf lines is $(N + 1)$ as illustrated in Fig. 2-16, and amplitudes of the absorption peaks follow the coefficients in a binomial expansion of $(1 + x)^n$, e.g., for $n = 4$ we have $1x^4 + 4x^3 + 6x^2 + 4x + 1$, which gives the same intensities obtained by counting the number of overlapping states in Fig. 2-16, i.e., $1:4:6:4:1$.

(c) Electron Unequally Coupled to Magnetic Nuclei. Continuing with the example of protons in an organic molecule, the maximum number of absorption lines occurs when all couplings are different. Then 2^n lines of equal intensity occur as in Fig. 2-17. This situation is not common because the protons attached to a single carbon generally interact equally with an unpaired electron.

(d) Mixture of Equal and Unequal Couplings. Such mixed couplings are frequently encountered with organic molecules and crystalline solids. Consequently, the spectra can become very complex and difficult to unfold. Figure 2-18 illustrates this point with spectra for two aromatic hydrocarbon anions. In the benzene spectrum the six equivalent protons produce a seven-line hyperfine pattern with intensity ratios of

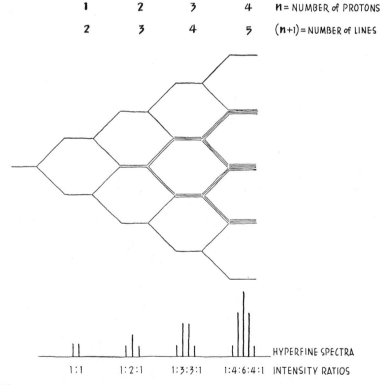

Fig. 2-16. Energy levels and hfs generated by protons interacting equally with an unpaired electron.

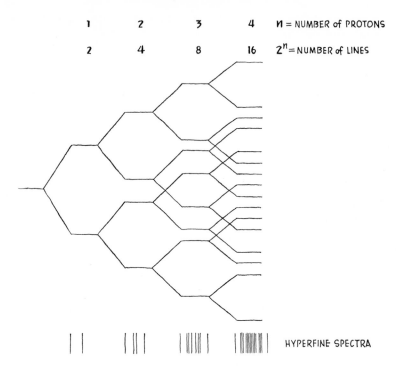

Fig. 2-17. Energy levels and hfs generated by protons interacting unequally with an unpaired electron.

$1:6:15:20:15:6:1$ and a splitting between lines of 3.715 G. In the adjacent naphthalene anion the four equivalent protons produce five lines with amplitudes of $1:4:6:4:1$ and a splitting of 4.84 G. The remaining four protons constitute another equivalent group but with a weaker coupling to the unpaired electron. Consequently, each line of the quintet is split into five lines with a separation between lines of 1.83 G. Obviously, in these aromatic systems unpaired electrons can interact with protons over a sizable distance. Such is not usually the case in saturated aliphatic molecules where the α, β rule is frequently applicable. This rule states the observation that the spectra for saturated aliphatic chain-type molecules indicate that the interaction between electron and nuclei is limited to protons attached to the α and β carbons, where α refers to the nominal sight of the unpaired electron and β refers to the adjacent carbons.

(e) **Constructed Spectra.** Very complex spectra, e.g., over 400 hf lines, have been observed for liquid samples where the lines are well resolved (H-3). However, in solids, the broad lines frequently overlap to the point

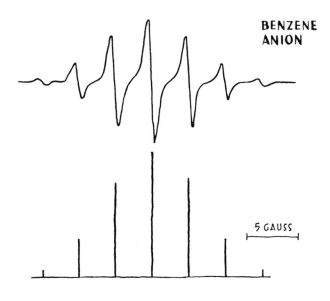

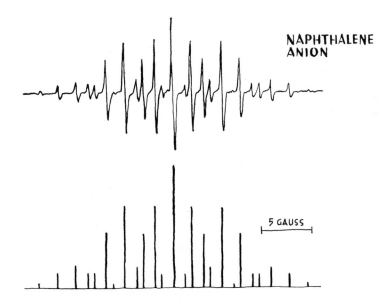

Fig. 2-18. EPR spectra of aromatic hydrocarbon anions: benzene, $A_r = 3.715$ G, $\Delta H = 700$ mG (constructed); naphthalene, $Ar_1 = 4.84$ G, $Ar_2 = 1.83$ G, $\Delta H = 150$ mG. (After H-7.)

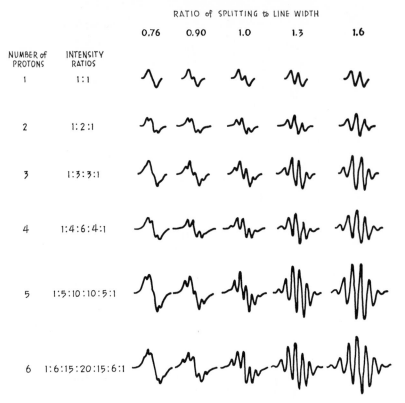

RATIO of SPLITTING to LINE WIDTH

Fig. 2-19. Effect of component separation and linewidth on the hfs produced by equally interacting protons. Gaussian components were used in these constructions. (After A-10.)

of obscuring the structure. Figure 2-19 illustrates how the ratio of linewidth to splitting influences the overall shape of spectra for various numbers of equally interacting protons. These curves were constructed by adding gaussian-shaped absorption curves according to the indicated binomial distribution of amplitudes and ratio of linewidth to splitting. With complex spectra where overlapping of hf lines or the superposition of spectra from several species obscures interpretation, the construction of trial spectra for plausible radicals, assuming reasonable values of the linewidths and splitting, can aid considerably in identification (F-10). References L-2 and L-3 are atlases of theoretically calculated EPR spectra. Each volume contains over 200 spectra arranged in the series listed in Table 2-3. Each series consists of 13–15 curves covering a range of linewidth-to-hf splitting ratios from 0.29 to 5.78 for Lorentzian- and 0.38–

Table 2-3

Number of Lines and Intensity Ratios
used in the Theoretically Calculated
EPR Spectra of References L-2
and L-3

Reference L-2	Reference L-3
1:1	1:5:10:10:5:1
1:1:1	1:6:15:20:15:6:1
1:2:1	1:7:21:35:35:35:21:7:1
1:1:1:1	1:8:28:56:70:56:28:8:1
1:3:3:1	1:2:2:1
1:1:1:1:1	1:2:3:2:1
1:4:6:4:1	1:3:4:3:1
1:1:1:1:1:1	1:4:6:5:5:6:4:1
	1:5:10:11:10:11:10:5:1

7.08 for gaussian-shaped lines. Each series is calculated for both Lorentzian and a gaussian basic line shape.

(f) Conditions for Observing Hfs. Experimentally, several conditions must be satisfied for the observation of hyperfine structure (P-3).

1. Samples must be magnetically dilute. When the average spacing between unpaired electrons is adequate, the exchange interaction or the dipole–dipole interaction between electrons will be negligible compared with the hyperfine interaction with the nucleus, e.g., concentrations less than 10^{-3} mole/liter are suitable for investigating the hfs of radicals in liquid solutions (H-4).

2. The spin–lattice and spin–spin relaxation times T_1 and T_2 should be long enough to avoid line broadening which obscures the individual lines, i.e., $T_1 > 1/\Delta\omega$, where $\Delta\omega$ = the splitting interval in frequency units (W-11).

3. The amplitudes of the microwave or radio-frequency field must be small compared to the splitting interval when expressed in the same units.

4. The splitting interval should be large compared to the side bands generated by field modulation or the field inhomogeneities over the sample area. Observed splitting intervals cover a range from about 500 to 0.05 G; however, most values are greater than 1 G where the requirements on the spectrometer are not generally difficult to meet. In the high-resolution spectroscopy discussed in Section 5.5 the demands for spectrometer stability and uniformity are extremely stringent because spectra containing over 400 lines and line widths as narrow as 17 mG are encountered.

2.5.4 Line Shape and Width (A-10,I-2,O-3)

Line shapes are determined by the types of interactions between the spin system and its environment while the widths depend on the strength of the interaction and the relaxation time. In a simple homogeneous system where relaxation is controlled by spin–lattice interactions and the energy absorbed from the radiation field is distributed so that the spin system maintains thermal equilibrium throughout the resonance process, theory predicts that the line shape should be Lorentzian (O-3,P-14). Under these slow-passage conditions the rate "A" of energy absorption can be obtained in the form* (P-1)

$$A = \chi_0 \omega_0{}^2 H_1{}^2 T_2 / [1 + T_2{}^2 (\omega_0 - \omega)^2]$$

which fits the Lorentzian shape.

In an inhomogeneous spin system the individual electrons find themselves in differing local fields so that resonance does not occur for all the spins simultaneously. If the spin–spin interaction process is slow compared with the relaxation to the lattice, the spin system will not reach thermal equilibrium and the absorption curve will have a gaussian shape.

In addition to these well-defined shapes many spectra appear to be mixtures of Lorentzian and gaussian curves. Consequently, simple rituals for distinguishing Lorentzian or gaussian shapes can simplify unfolding of the spectra. Two such procedures are (*1*) the derivative curve slope method and (*2*) the normalized plot. In the slope method illustrated in Fig. 2-20 the ratio of slopes $b:a$ will be 4:1 for a Lorentzian and 2.2:1 for a Gaussian curve if the sign of the slopes is ignored (B-18). In the normalized plot procedure of Fig. 2-21 the base line is divided into units of "a" where a is the value of χ where the curve reaches a maximum and the ordinant is normalized to unity. The indicated ordinant values will intersect the two curves at the values of a listed in Table 2-4. If the identity

---

* Our discussion has emphasized the microscopic picture of EPR involving the interactions between electrons and their environments. Experimentally, matter is examined in the bulk and observations are made in terms of the macroscopic magnetic moment normally expressed as the complex susceptibility $\chi = \chi' - i\chi''$. The rate of energy absorption is proportional to the out-of-phase component χ'' so that $A = 2\omega\chi''H_1{}^2$. Under slow passage conditions the Bloch susceptibilities become (P-1)

$$\chi' = \tfrac{1}{2}\chi_0\omega_0 T_2 \, [T_2(\omega_0 - \omega)/1 + T_2{}^2(\omega_0 - \omega)^2 + \gamma^2 H_1{}^2 T_1 T_2]$$
$$\chi'' = \tfrac{1}{2}\chi_0\omega_0 T_2 \, [1/1 + T_2{}^2(\omega_0 - \omega)^2 + \gamma^2 H_1{}^2 T_1 T_2]$$

In the absence of rf saturation effects $\gamma^2 H_1{}^2 T_1 T_2 \ll 1$, so

$$\chi'' = \tfrac{1}{2}\chi_0\omega_0 T_2 \, [1/1 + T_2{}^2(\omega_0 - \omega)^2]$$

when the line is narrow $\omega \approx \omega_0$; therefore, $A = 2\omega_0\chi''H_1{}^2$, or

$$A = \chi_0\omega_0{}^2 H_1{}^2 T_2/[1 + T_2{}^2(\omega_0 - \omega)^2]$$

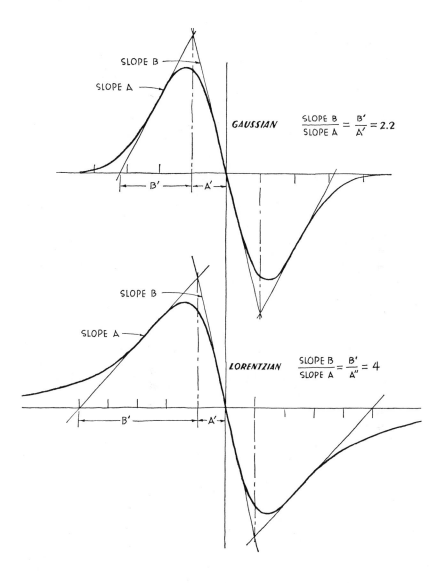

Fig. 2-20. Identification of Lorentzian and gaussian derivative curves by the slope method. (After L-5.)

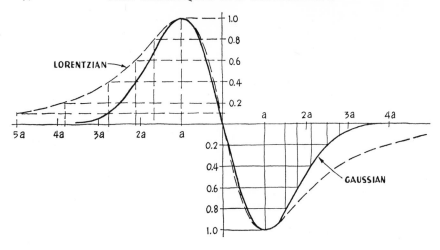

Fig. 2-21. Normalization technique for identifying Lorentzian and gaussian derivative curves. (After H-28.)

is not apparent, a plot of the position (experimental) values of a versus
the Lorentzian or gaussian values will give a straight line when the shapes
match.

    (a) Linewidths. We will see that many interactions influence the line-
width; however, as in all cases of ultimate resolution, the Heisenberg
uncertainty principle sets the ultimate minimum width $\delta E \delta t \geq \hbar = h/2\pi$,
where $\delta E =$ the uncertainty in the energy level E and $\delta t =$ the uncertainty

Table 2-4
Values of Ordinates and Abscissas for
Lorentzian and Gaussian Derivative Curves
(H-28)

Ordinate in % of peak height	Abscissas in units of a where $a =$ half the peak-to-peak distance	
	Lorentzian	Gaussian
100	a	a
80	$1.65a$	$1.5a$
60	$2.10a$	$1.8a$
40	$2.75a$	$2.1a$
20	$3.80a$	$2.5a$
10	$5.0a$	$2.8a$

in the time spent by the election in energy level E. Substituting $h\Delta\nu$ for δE, the uncertainty in the resonance frequency corresponds to a half-bandwidth $\Delta\nu \geq 1/2\pi\delta t = 1/2\pi T$ where T now corresponds to the relaxation time as related to the bandwidth in the usual expressions for Lorentzian curves as shown in Table 2-5. Low coupling forces lead to long relaxation times and narrow lines; conversely, short relaxation times and wide lines result from strong interactions. Either T_1 or T_2 can be the controlling relaxation time but usually the temperature can be lowered to lengthen T_1 until the linewidth is set by T_2. Several examples will indicate the magnitude of limits set by the uncertainty principle. Using the equivalent form $\Delta H_{1/2} = \hbar/g\beta T = (0.568 \times 10^{-7})/T$, from Table 2-5 it becomes apparent that a value of T smaller than about 10^{-11} sec, i.e., a $\Delta H_{1/2}$ of about 5000 G will exceed the range of most magnets and microwave equipment. At

Table 2-5

Characteristics of Gaussian and Lorentzian Curves in Terms of T_2, Assuming T_2 Governs the Linewidth

	Lorentzian line	Gaussian line	Ref.
Normalized equation	$g(\omega - \omega_0)$ $= \dfrac{T_2/\pi}{1+(\omega-\omega_0)^2 T_2^2}$	$g(\omega - \omega_0)$ $= \dfrac{T_2}{\pi} \exp -[(\omega-\omega_0)^2(T_2^2/\pi)]$	I-2
	$g(H-H_0)$ $= \dfrac{2\Delta H_{1/2}}{\pi[(H-H_0)^2 + \Delta H_{1/2}^2]}$	$g(H - H_0)$ $= \dfrac{2}{\pi\Delta H_{1/2}} \exp -\left[\dfrac{(H-H_0)^2}{\pi\Delta H_{1/2}^2}\right]$	A-10
Width at half the maximum intensity	$\Delta\omega_{1/2} = 1/T_2$ $\Delta H_{1/2} = \hbar/g\beta T_2$	$\Delta\omega_{1/2} = \sqrt{\pi \ln 2}/T_2$ $\Delta H_{1/2} = (\hbar\sqrt{\pi \ln 2})/g\beta T_2$	I-2 A-10
Width at point of maximum slope	$\Delta\omega_s = 1/\sqrt{3}\, T_2$ $\Delta H_s = \hbar/\sqrt{3}\, g\beta T_2$	$\Delta\omega_s = (1/T_2)\sqrt{\pi/2}$ $\Delta H_s = (\hbar/g\beta T_2)\sqrt{\pi/2}$	I-2 A-10
Ratio $\dfrac{\text{width } \frac{1}{2}}{\text{width } s}$	$= 1.732$	$= 1.177$	A-10

where
$\omega - \omega_0 = \Delta\omega$
$H - H_0 = \Delta H$

the other extreme the narrowest observed lines have a $\Delta H_{1/2}$ of about 10 mG, corresponding to a relaxation time of about 5 μsec.

In contrast to the sharp lines indicating the definite energy levels of Fig. 2-1 the levels in actual spin systems are broadened in various ways thereby adding to the observed linewidth.

Portis has catalogued the various sources of line broadening as follows (P-14):

Homogeneous:
   1. Dipole–dipole interactions between like spins.
   2. Spin–lattice relaxation.
   3. Interaction of spins with the radiation field.
   4. Motion of unpaired spins in the microwave field.
   5. Diffusion of the spin system excitation through the paramagnetic sample.
   6. Motionally narrowed fluctuations in the local field.

Inhomogeneous:
   1. Hyperfine interactions.
   2. Anisotropy of the splitting of the spin levels.
   3. Dipolar interactions between spins with different Larmor frequencies.
   4. Inhomogeneities in the applied dc magnetic field.

Identification of the broadening category is usually related to the behavior of the spin system as the radiation field intensity is increased to rf saturation, i.e., until the spin concentration in the upper and lower energy levels approaches equilibrium. Three identification routines are considered in the following paragraphs.

(b) Line Shape Response to Saturation. Below saturation homogeneously broadened systems exhibit a Lorentzian absorption curve (A-10). As the rf field intensity is increased, saturation commences at ω_0 where the greatest power is absorbed; therefore, the center of the curve is reduced before the wings are affected. This preferential shrinkage produces an apparent increase in the line width measured at half the saturated maximum (I-2).

Inhomogeneously broadened lines have a gaussian shape which does not change on saturation. All parts of the curve fall simultaneously (A-10, I-2).

(c) Amplitude Response to Saturation. Bloembergen (B-18), Portis (P-14), and others have derived expressions for the saturation behavior of both types of broadened systems. Castner (C-6) expresses the signal measured by the spectrometer in the homogeneous case as $V_R = X/(1 + X^2)$

where $X = \gamma H_1(T_1 T_2)^{1/2}$. Below saturation where $X \ll 1$, the signal V_R is proportional to the field H_1 but when saturation sets in and $X > 1$ the signal becomes proportional to $1/H_1$. Figure 2-22 shows this behavior in a log-log plot of the spectrometer signal V_R versus the reduced radiation field $H_1/H_{1/2}$, where $H_{1/2}$ is the value of the microwave field which makes the saturation parameter at the line center equal $\frac{1}{2}$, i.e.,

$$S(\omega_0, H_1) = 1/(1 + \gamma^2 H_1^2 T_1 T_2)$$

In the inhomogeneous case, the absorption signal becomes

$$V_R \propto X/(1 + X^2)^{1/2}$$

where again the signal below saturation is proportional to H_1; however, in the saturation region where $X > 1$, the signal flattens out and becomes independent of the field as indicated in Fig. 2-22. The explanation for curves between the extreme homogeneous case and complete inhomogeneous case involves the concept of "spin packets" and the index "a,"

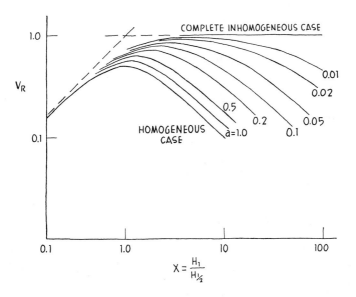

Fig. 2-22. Saturation curves showing the spectrometer absorption signal V_R plotted as a function of the reduced microwave field $H_1/H_{1/2}$, where $H_{1/2} = 1/\gamma(T_1 T_2)^{1/2}$. The various values of "a" lead to a family of curves ranging from homogeneous to inhomogeneous broadening: $a = \Delta H_L/\Delta H_G$, where $\Delta H_L =$ the spin packet width and $\Delta H_G =$ the inhomogeneous envelope width. (Courtesy C-6.)

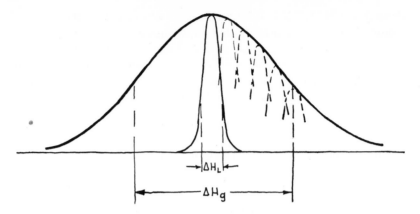

Fig. 2-23. Definitions of spin packet width ΔH_L and inhomogeneous envelope width ΔH_G: $a = \Delta H_L/\Delta H_G$.

which measures the degree of inhomogeneous broadening; "a" is defined by the ratio of the Lorentzian spin packet width to the inhomogeneous gaussian width, i.e.,

$$a = \Delta\omega_L/\Delta\omega_g = \Delta H_L/\Delta H_g$$

This concept is illustrated in Fig. 2-23 where the packet is composed of all spins experiencing the same static field so that they respond as a resonance group with a Lorentzian absorption characteristic and a width $1/T_2$. Since the spin packets are not measurable quantities, $\Delta\omega_L$ and "a" are determined from a study of saturation curves as in Fig. 2-22 (see C-6).

(d) Hole Burning (B-18). Since energy exchange between spin packets is an ineffective process in an inhomogeneously broadened system, it is possible to saturate a few spin packets without disturbing the rest of the absorption curve. Figure 2-24 demonstrates the process of eating a hole in the absorption curve. Curve a is an oscilloscopic presentation of an inhomogeneously broadened line observed with a rf field intensity well below saturation. If the field modulation is reduced to zero and H corresponds to A, the spin packets corresponding to the field at A can be saturated. Since individual spin packets follow the homogeneously broadened saturation curve, their amplitude will decrease with saturation until a hole is burned in the spectrum at A. When modulation is resumed, the hole will appear as in curve b. Such hole burning identifies the inhomogeneously broadened system because in a homogeneously broadened line the whole curve saturates and no hole appears when the test is applied.

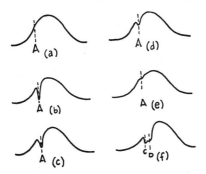

Fig. 2-24. Hole burning in inhomogeneously broadened line: (a) initial line; (b) when H_0 is left at A and the modulation field H_m is reduced to zero, localized saturation develops and appears as a hole when the absorption is subsequently recorded; (c), (d), and (e) show the hole filling in as thermal equilibrium is restored. If the H_m is not reduced to zero during the saturation period, a saddle develops as at (f) because a longer time is spent at the turning points of a sinusoidal wave. Reference B-18 pertains to nuclear resonance but the hole burning technique applies also to EPR. (Courtesy B-18.)

Curves c, d, and e show the absorption line recovering as the relaxation processes restore the spin distributions to thermal equilibrium.

2.5.5   Determination of the Relaxation Times T_1 and T_2

Techniques for determining T_1 and T_2 fall into two categories, direct and indirect. In the direct methods, the spin system is disturbed from equilibrium by an abrupt power input; then the system is observed during the return to equilibrium. Indirect methods involve measurements of parameters that are functions of the relaxation times, e.g., linewidths and saturation line broadening. The choice of method involves both fairly rigid limitations and experimental preferences, where the limitations are set by time resolution of the various methods and the preferences involve choosing between complexity in interpretation or apparatus Direct methods are easier to interpret, particularly for complex line shapes, but the measurements require time and thus fairly long relaxation constants as indicated in Table 2-6. The indirect methods apply to a wide range of relaxation times; however, the ease of interpretation depends on the type of saturation.

The principles of the various techniques are outlined in the following paragraphs but details of the spectrometers and the experimental rituals are reserved for Section 5.4.

(a) Saturation–Recovery. As the name implies, this system involves first saturating the spin system by applying a high-intensity radiation field,

Table 2-6

Region of Relaxation Times T_1 Appropriate for Measurement by Various Techniques

Measuring techniques	Range of relaxation times, sec	Ref.
Direct Methods		
1. Saturation–recovery	$T_1 > 10^{-3}$	
2. Inversion–recovery	$T_1 > 10^{-3}$	C-5
Indirect Methods		
3. CW saturation[a]	$2 \times 10^{-7} < T_1 < 10^{-4}$	C-5
4. Rapid modulation of the saturation factor	$T_1 > 10^{-8}$	H-12
5. Broadening in homogeneous line envelope	$T_1 < 10^{-8}$	C-5

[a] CW = continuous wave.

either as a strong pulse at resonance or continuously as the spectrometer sweeps through the resonance line. At various times after saturation, the recovery of the line is reexamined and here again there are various techniques, e.g. (*1*) the line can be observed throughout the recovery period with a weak monitoring field that does not appreciably disturb the spin distribution, or (*2*) the energy to resaturate the line can be measured by reapplying the strong field as described in Fig. 2-25. In this example of the resaturation method the energy required to resaturate the line is recorded after recovery periods ranging from 5 to 350 sec. At 5 sec, few spins have returned to the lower-energy state so very little energy is required to resaturate the system. In simple spin–lattice relaxation processes, the recovery of the magnetization (*M*) exhibits an exponential time dependence as in the straight line of Fig. 2-26, where T_1 is the time for the signal to drop to $1/e = 0.368$ of its initial value, in this case about 600 sec. This figure also illustrates how the spin concentration effects the relaxation process, i.e., a 27-fold increase in the spin concentration reduced the recovery time by a similar factor; furthermore, the curve is no longer a simple exponential, indicating that relaxation is no longer a simple process.

(b) Inversion–Recovery. In this technique the concentration of spins N^+ and N^- in Fig. 2-1 is suddenly inverted so $N^+ > N^-$; then the system is allowed to relax by normal process to the thermal equilibrium distribution where $N^- > N^+$. During the relaxation process the system is

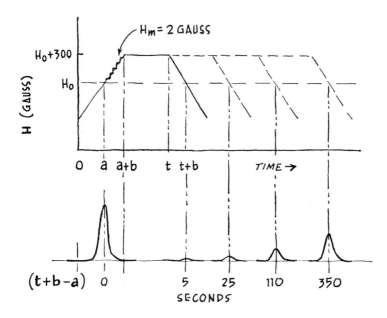

Fig. 2-25. Paramagnetic relaxation of F centers in KCl by the saturation recovery technique. The following measuring sequence was used:

Time	Action
0	The field sweep and time clock are started together.
a	The resonance is swept through and saturated.
$a + b$	The field sweep is stopped at the H value at which relaxation is to be studied.
t	The time clock is stopped simultaneously with the start of the reverse field sweep and the triggering of the oscilloscope.
$t + b$	The resonance is swept through and resaturated and the signal is recorded on the oscilloscope camera.

The a and b values ranged from 1 to 6 sec; t ranged from 5 to 350 sec; $dH/dt = 350$ g/sec; $f_m = 500$ cps; $H_m = 2$ G; $H_1 = 0.01$ G; and the filter time constant $= 0.05$ sec. The spectrometer was a type RS1-X. (After O-2.)

monitored without appreciably disturbing the distribution to yield a recovery curve similar to Fig. 2-27. Immediately after the inversion at time t_0, emission transitions from $N^+ \to N^-$ predominate and energy is received from the sample, as indicated by the sign reversal in Fig. 2-27. At the saturation point, no signal is observed because $N^+ = N^-$, but at longer times the recovery exhibits the behavior already described for the

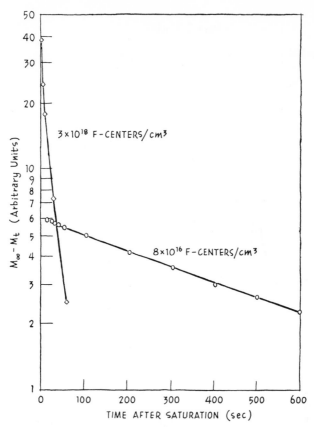

Fig. 2-26. Relaxation of color centers in KCl. At the 8×10^{16} concentration the time dependence is exponential but curvature in the graph for the larger concentration indicates a more complex time dependence. M_∞ = equilibrium magnetization; $T = 1.4°K$. (After O-2.)

saturation–recovery method. Again, T_1 is readily obtained from the magnetization if a plot of log $(M_\infty - M_t)$ versus time yields a straight line. If the recovery is known to be exponential, T_1 can be obtained from the time interval between polarization inversion and the saturation point, i.e., $T_1 = \Delta t / \ln 2$ (V-6). The inversion–recovery method may provide more information than the saturation–recovery technique because phonon interactions may be different in the emission- and absorption-dominated phases of relaxation. For example, a change in slope as the curve passes through the saturation point may indicate the presence of phonon imprisonment or some other change in the relaxation mechanism (C-3).

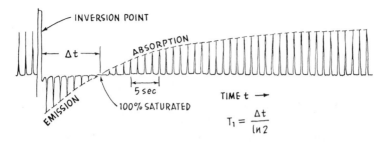

Fig. 2-27. NMR signals from benzene. The polarization was inverted by an adiabatic rapid passage with a strong rf field and monitored throughout the recovery with a weak field that did not appreciably disturb the spin distribution. EPR signals should exhibit a similar behavior during inversion and recovery. (After V-6.)

Two procedures for inverting the populations of N^+ and N^- are (1) adiabatic fast passage and (2) a 180° pulse (C-3), which are described in detail in Sections 5.4.2 and 5.4.3, respectively. Both methods involve a careful balance of the radiation field intensity and passage time or pulse length in order to invert the spin populations before relaxation interactions characterized by T_1 have time to operate or subsequent stimulated emission and absorption transitions can equalize the populations. Here we illustrate this point with the conditions for inverting the spin populations by the adiabatic fast passage technique because it is most commonly encountered in the literature (C-4,L-13). Reference C-5 lists the requirements as follows:

1. Adiabatic transition, $\omega_m H_m \ll \gamma H_1^2$. The passage must be slow compared with the driving frequency H_1 so that the magnetic moment can follow the change in frequency or field (L-13).

2. Fast passage, $\omega_m H_m \gg H_1/T_1$. The passage must be rapid compared with T_1 or T_2 so that relaxation does not occur during the inversion process.

3. Saturation, $\gamma H_1(T_1 T_2)^{1/2} > 1$. The radiation field must be strong enough to complete the inversion before relaxation sets in.

4. Spin diffusion, $\omega_m H_m \gg \Delta H/\tau_D$, where the nomenclature follows Table 2-1.

H_m = modulation amplitude $\qquad$ $H = H_0 + H_m \cos \omega_m t$
$\omega_m/2\pi$ = modulation frequency $\qquad$ $H_m \gg \Delta H$
ΔH = total linewidth
τ_D = the spin diffusion time
H_1 = microwave magnetic field.

In fulfilling these requirements Pake (P-1) points out that "one takes T_1 and T_2 as nature gives them," then selects H_1 large enough to meet the saturation condition (3). Next the sweep rate is selected to satisfy the fast passage requirement (2). If these values of $\omega_m H_m$ and H_1 fail to meet the adiabatic passage constraint (1), a larger value of H_1 becomes necessary. Experimental arrangements for both the fast passage and pulse techniques are described in Section 5.4.

Reference C-5 discusses two other methods used in the fast passage region: (a) M versus ω_m method suitable for short times where $10^{-3} < T_1 < 0.3$ sec and (b) the displacement method for use where $5 \times 10^{-2} < T_1 < 1$ sec. Here M is the magnetization signal magnitude which starts to decrease when the modulation frequency $\omega_m/2\pi$ approaches $1/2\pi T_1$.

(c) Continuous-Wave Saturation. Since the relation between the time constants T_1, T_2, the line shape, and saturation behavior depends on the nature of the line broadening, the ritual for determining T_1 and T_2 for the homogeneous case will be different than for inhomogeneous broadening. Solutions to the Bloch equations and the expressions in Table 2-5 give T_1 and T_2 for the homogeneous case with a minimum of manipulation as follows (H-28)*:

1. Determine that the line shape is Lorentzian.
2. Measure T_2, e.g., from Table 2-5

$$T_2 = (\hbar/\sqrt{3}\, g\beta\Delta H_s) = (1/1.52 \times 10^7 g\Delta H_s)$$

3. Find the value of H_1 which gives the largest obtainable signal. Figure 2-28 shows two ways of handling the measurement of H_1. For curve a, precision attenuators controlling generator output and detector input are adjusted to counteract each other; consequently, the signal remains constant until saturation sets in (B-18).

Curve b is the homogeneous case from Fig. 2-22 where H_1 corresponds to the maximum shown.

4. T_1† is calculated from $T_1 = 1/2T_2\gamma^2 H_1^2$.

---

* The ΔH in Ref. H-28 equals $2\Delta H_s$.
† From Ref. H-28:
Starting with the solution to the Bloch equation for χ''

$$\chi'' = \tfrac{1}{2}\chi_0\omega_0[T_2/1 + \gamma^2 H_1^2 T_1 T_2 + T_2^2(\omega - \omega_0)^2]$$

if the signal is proportional to $\chi'' H_1$, the derivative

$$d\chi'' H_1/d(\omega - \omega_0) = \chi_0\omega_0 H_1 T_2^3(\omega - \omega_0)/[1 + T_2^2(\omega - \omega_0)^2 + \gamma^2 H_1^2 T_1 T_2]^2$$

The maxima of this function occur at

$$(\omega - \omega_0) = \pm\sqrt{(1 + H_1^2 T_1 T_2\gamma^2)/3T_2^2}$$

Maximizing with respect to H_1 at the peaks given above find

$$T_1 = 1/2T_2\gamma^2 H_1^2$$

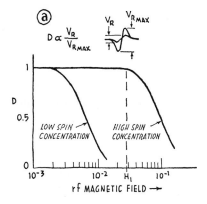

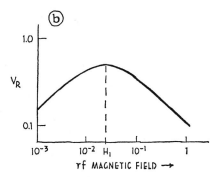

Fig. 2-28. Saturation curves for a homogeneous case and two procedures for determining the value of H_1 to use in evaluating the relaxation time T_1. (*a* After B-18; *b* after C-6.)

When the spin system is inhomogeneously saturated, T_2 is not immediately available from the observed linewidth and either some assumption regarding the spin packet width (e.g., P-14) or determination of the degree of inhomogeneous saturation is required. Castner (C-6) has extended the Portis theory to a method of determining T_2 and T_1 as follows:

1. Plot an experimental inhomogeneous saturation curve in the form of Fig. 2-29, then locate $H_1(V_{R\frac{1}{2}}$, lower) and $H_1(V_{R\frac{1}{2}}$, upper) as shown where $V_{R\frac{1}{2}}$ is one-half the maximum V_R for a given curve.

2. The ratio $H_1(V_{R\frac{1}{2}}$, upper)$/H_1(V_{R\frac{1}{2}}$, lower) determines the parameter (*a*) from the curve in Fig. 2-30.

3. T_2 is obtained from parameter (*a*) and the width of the gaussian curve, i.e., since

$$a = \Delta\omega_L/\Delta\omega_G$$

$$T_2 = 1/\Delta\omega_L = 1/a\Delta\omega_G$$

4. T_1 follows from the saturation parameter and the value of the microwave field $H_{1/2}$ that makes the parameter equal $\frac{1}{2}$, then

$$H_{1/2} = 1/\gamma(T_1 T_2)^{1/2}$$

$H_{1/2}$ uncorrected is obtained from Fig. 2-29 as the intersection of the linear signal below saturation with the horizontal projection from the maximum V_R. The multiplicative correction factor relating the $H_{1/2}$ uncorrected to the true value is a function of parameter (*a*), determined from the appropriate curve in Fig. 2-22, and ranges from 2 for the completely homogeneous case where $H_{1/2}$ corresponds to $(V_{R\max})$ to 1 for the completely inhomogeneous case, i.e., $a = 0$.

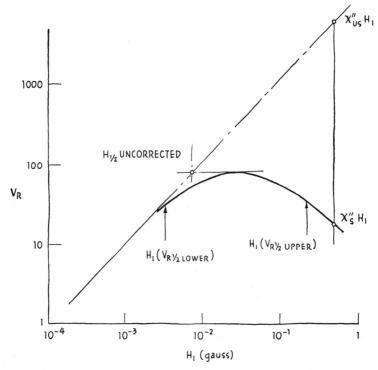

Fig. 2-29. Inhomogeneous saturation curve showing method of determining $H_1(V_{R\frac{1}{2}}$, lower) and $H_1(V_{R\frac{1}{2}}$, upper) which are the values of the rf field where V_R is one-half the maximum V_R. V_R = the spectrometer absorption signal. (Courtesy C-6.)

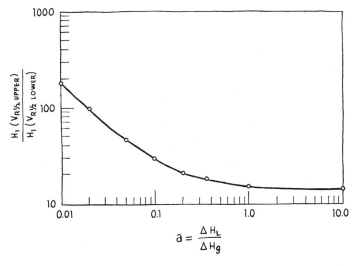

Fig. 2-30. Curve to determine a from the ratio $H_1(V_{R^{1/2}}, \text{upper})/H_1(V_{R^{1/2}}, \text{lower})$. (Courtesy C-6.)

5. Using $H_{1/2}$, corrected $T_1 = 1/\gamma^2 H_{1/2}^2 T_2$.

Because of their experimental simplicity, these CW saturation methods have been widely used (C-3,L-13); however, several precautions deserve mention.

1. In a spin system of two energy levels, the saturation method gives a unique relaxation time but in a many level system the measured T_1 is not unique to any particular pair of levels but gives the rate at which energy is transferred to the lattice via all relaxation processes (L-13).

2. Experimentally, it is important to avoid including χ' in the signal during measurement of the χ'' saturation curve because the dispersion signal does not saturate; consequently, at high power levels a small χ' component could dominate the detected signal.

3. Sample size and geometry should be selected to fit within a uniform H_1; otherwise, saturation will occur in various parts of the sample at different incident power levels (C-6).

(d) Rapid Modulation of the Saturation Factor. Herve (H-12), has described a modulation method to measure relaxation times as short as 10^{-8} sec. This system employs a variable frequency amplitude modulation of the radiation field, e.g., the rf field is strong enough to partially saturate the resonance, the amplitude can be modulated from 0 to 100%, and the modulation frequency covers a range from 500 kc/sec to

30 Mc/sec. With the sample in the cavity, the modulation of the saturation parameter, $(\gamma H_1)^2 T_1 T_2$, involves a variation in the magnetization M_z which is detected by the induction coil outside the cavity as indicated in Fig. 2-31. When the rf field is highly modulated at a sufficiently low frequency, the spin system will have time to relax after each saturating peak in the radiation field. If the modulation frequency is increased, the recovery period will be shortened until ultimately the spin system cannot reach thermal equilibrium between saturating pulses. Then the absorption will decrease in a fashion characteristic of the line broadening mechanism, i.e., homogeneous or inhomogeneous. Figure 2-32 shows experimental curves of signal strength versus modulation frequency for α,α'-diphenyl-β-picrylhydrazyl (DPPH) at room temperature and for a series of rf power levels. Here the curve follows the theoretical expression for a homogeneous broadening case and $T_1 = T_2$, e.g.,

$$S = S_0 \left[\frac{a}{(1+a)} \right]^2 \frac{(\omega_m T_1)^2 [1 + (\omega_m T_1/2)^2]}{[1 + a - (\omega_m T_1)^2]^2 + 4(\omega_m T_1)^2}$$

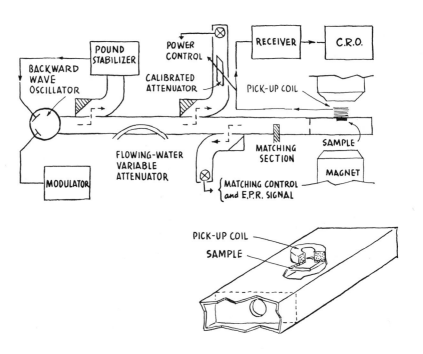

Fig. 2-31. Variable-modulation frequency induction spectrometer for measuring spin–lattice relaxation times by rapid modulation of the saturation factor. (After H-12.)

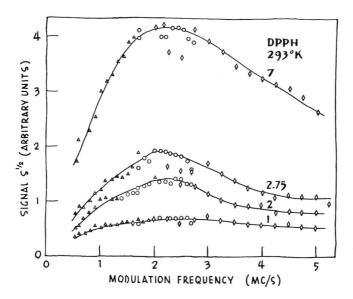

Fig. 2-32. Family of saturation curves for DPPH obtained with the spectrograph power levels indicated on the curves, in watts. The experimentally observed signals agree with the expression

$$S = S_0\left[\frac{a}{1 + a}\right]^2 \frac{(\omega_m T_1)^2[1 + (\omega_m T_1/2)^2]}{[1 + a - (\omega_m T_1)^2]^2 + 4(\omega_m T_1)^2}$$

where a = the saturation parameter $(\gamma H_1)^2 T_1 T_2$ and ω_m = the angular modulation frequency. (Courtesy H-12.)

for the inhomogeneous case, the signal is given as

$$S = S_0 \omega_m^2/[\omega_m^2 + (1/T_1)^2]$$

where the modulation frequency = $\omega_m/2\pi$; a = the saturation factor = $(\gamma H_1)^2 T_1 T_2$, and $S_0 = (2mM_0/T_1)^2$; M_0 = the static magnetic moment; and m = mass of the electron. The original work should be consulted for details and curves for various values of a and the relations of relaxation times to modulation frequency.

(e) Broadening of Inhomogeneous Line Shape (C-5). Under some conditions of temperature or spin concentration, the Lorentzian spin packet width may become comparable to or exceed the gaussian inhomogeneous broadening and the line shape changes to a Lorentzian curve. In this case

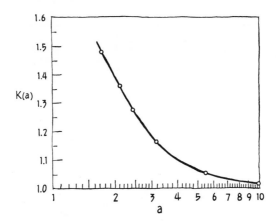

Fig. 2-33. $K(a)$ is the factor representing the ratio of the total peak-to-peak envelope width, ΔH_{PP}, to the Lorentzian spin packet width, ΔH_L, for an inhomogeneously broadened line. (After C-5.)

T_1 can be obtained from the Lorentzian component of the width using the relation

$$T_1 = \frac{2}{\sqrt{3}\ \gamma \Delta H_{PP}}\ K(a)$$

where $a = \Delta H_L / \Delta H_G$ and T_1 is assumed equal to T_2. ΔH_{PP} is the peak-to-peak width of the envelope and ΔH_L and ΔH_G are the Lorentzian spin-packet width and the gaussian inhomogeneous broadening, respectively. Figure 2-33 shows values of $K(a)$ as a function of a. When $a > 4$, then the use of ΔH_{PP} without a correction will result in an error of less than 10% but as a approaches 1, it becomes difficult to obtain accurate values of $K(a)$.

CHAPTER III

Spectrometers: Sensitivity and Resolution

3.1 PHILOSOPHY OF SPECTROMETER SELECTION

Taking a cue from the Mikado whose rule of thumb was "make the punishment fit the crime," we will endeavor in this section to make spectrometers fit the various experimental situations. In the early years of EPR when all spectrometers were home built, one guiding principle appears to have been "maximize the simplicity," at least to the extent consistent with the complexity of the experiment. Now the advent of numerous commercial instruments has changed the picture so that today an EPR laboratory can be set up with a minimum of sweat and effort through the good auspices of a tidy equipment grant or facilities requisition. Sufficient spectrometer styles and accessories are available to fit almost every experimental need; therefore, the affluent scientific community is making a rapid shift to ready-built instruments—understandably a trend destined to continue, particularly in view of high labor costs and the successful commercialization of almost every other field of spectroscopy, e.g., optical, infrared, mass, and beta and gamma ray. Most commercial designs originated as successful instruments in some university laboratory and subsequent years of engineering and development have evolved characteristics such as sensitivity, resolution, and convenience that are difficult for a first-time builder to match and almost impossible to surpass. Lest these remarks become confused with a Madison Avenue sales pitch, let us hasten to state that many "home-built" units still give yeoman's service and there are several situations where "home building" should and will continue, e.g.: (1) when the desirable spectrometer frequency is not commercially available; (2) when ultimate sensitivity requires measures economically impractical in a commercial instrument; (3) when the inherited "homemade" units are adequate; and (4) in the teaching situation where the understanding gained through assembling or refurbishing a microwave bridge bears an importance comparable to the subsequent measurements. Accordingly, our suggestions about spectrometer acquisition reflect the purpose of the EPR spectroscopy. When research is to be

61

maximized with a minimum of labor as in industrial and institutional laboratories, it is best to start with a commercial unit and develop such components or accessories as are necessary. When education is a vital part of the goal, a "home-built" microwave bridge provides an abundance of first-hand experience that injects a great deal of humbling realism into analysis of the data. Of course some discrimination is required in the teaching situation because first-hand experience with microwave fields and electronics which may bring enlightenment to the physicist and engineer may produce more distraction and confusion to the chemist and biologist than the experience is worth. In the universities visited while searching for EPR techniques, it was not surprising to find many physics laboratories equipped with "home-built" units while the chemists and biologists favored commercial systems.

In scope this section makes no pretense of being a construction manual. Various microwave bridges are discussed but emphasis is on selecting the best equipment for the experiment. Since the main points of comparison are sensitivity, resolution, and convenience, attention is focused on the microwave components and factors contributing to the signal-to-noise ratio. For some time the wealth of adequate commercial power supplies, oscillators, amplifiers, phase-sensitive detectors, and other electronic building blocks has eliminated the necessity for the "home builder" to construct these parts; consequently, most of the existing "home-built" spectrometers are an assembly of such units with most of the originality and design attention appearing in the microwave bridge. For the builder, literature references are included for each type of spectrometer to assist in locating construction details. Also, throughout the following chapters spectrometer types and references are listed with examples of data to illustrate the instruments used in various areas of research.

3.2 SPECTROMETER ELEMENTS, BASIC DESIGNS, AND DESIGNATIONS

3.2.1 Basic Elements

Irrespective of their frequency range all absorption spectrophotometers contain four basic elements which describe the main features of the instrument and provide a basis for classification:

1. Source or generator of electromagnetic radiation.
2. Dispersing element.
3. Absorption cell containing the sample.
4. Detector or receiver.

The main characteristic of the source is the frequency, e.g., UV, visible, infrared, and microwave. Common frequencies encountered in EPR are listed in Table 3-1 along with the band designations. Other details such as power level and stability are important but seldom mentioned. The magnetic field functions as the dispersion element with an action that is somewhat unique compared to optical and infrared instruments in that it disperses the response of the sample instead of the frequency spectrum from the source. While the spatial and temporal uniformity are the important field characteristics, they seldom are the limiting factors in EPR measurements; consequently, their values usually are not reported although inferences can be drawn from magnet pole diameters and the width of the gap. Absorption cells fall into two main categories: transmission and reflection cavities. These in turn are classified according to the geometry of the resonating electromagnetic field. Since the microwave plumbing, both in geometry and components, depends primarily on the type of cavity, this element is always mentioned in describing the instrument. Last, the detecting element, namely, a bolometer or crystal and the detecting system (i.e., homodyne or superheterodyne), determine much of the electronics associated with the microwave section. In subsequent sections each of these spectrometer components will be discussed in some detail along with criteria for selecting among the various alternatives. This

Table 3-1

Waveguide Designations and Characteristics[a]

Designations Band JAN[b]	Rectangular waveguide dimension, in. (i.d.)	TE_{10} Operating range			
		Frequency, kMc	Wavelength, cm	Cutoff frequency, kMc	Free space wavelength, cm
S RG-48/u	2.840 × 1.340	2.60–3.95	19.18–8.92	2.078	11.53–7.59
G RG-49/u	1.872 × 0.872	3.95–5.85	12.59–6.08	3.152	7.59–5.12
J RG-50/u	1.372 × 0.622	5.30–8.20	9.68–4.29	4.301	5.66–3.66
H RG-51/u	1.122 × 0.497	7.05–10.0	6.39–3.52	5.259	4.25–3.00
X RG-52/u	0.900 × 0.400	8.20–12.4	6.09–2.85	6.557	3.66–2.42
M —	0.750 × 0.375	10.0–15.0	4.86–2.35	7.868	3.00–2.00
P RG-91/u	0.622 × 0.311	12.4–18.0	3.75–1.96	9.487	2.42–1.67
N —	0.510 × 0.255	15.0–22.0	3.11–1.60	11.571	2.00–1.36
K RG-66/u	0.420 × 0.170	18.0–26.5	2.66–1.33	14.048	1.67–1.13
R RG-96/u	0.280 × 0.140	26.5–40.0	1.87–0.88	21.075	1.13–0.749

[a] Hewlett Packard Catalog No. 24.
[b] Joint Army Navy designations.

brief introduction is for the purpose of establishing a classification system and shorthand notation to be used throughout the remainder of the book. Since no particular designations are universal in the EPR spectrometer industry, the system used here is entirely arbitrary; however, its flexibility should accommodate most of the existing instruments.

3.2.2 Classification

We will label spectrometers according to the type of absorption cell, the system of detection, the plumbing arrangement, and the source frequency in accordance with the notation of Table 3-2. For example, type TH1-X refers to a spectrometer with a transmission cavity, a homodyne detection system, arrangement 1 plumbing, and operation at X-band frequency. Similarly, type RS2-Q refers to a reflection cavity, superheterodyne detection system, arrangement 2 plumbing, and an operating frequency in the Q band. Besides the basic elements most microwave systems contain components suitable for the functions listed in Table 3-3. For example, Fig. 3-1 shows a typical type RS4-X spectrometer with all of microwave components indicated. Since Table 3-2 would soon become unmanageable if the various permutations of all the microwave components were included,

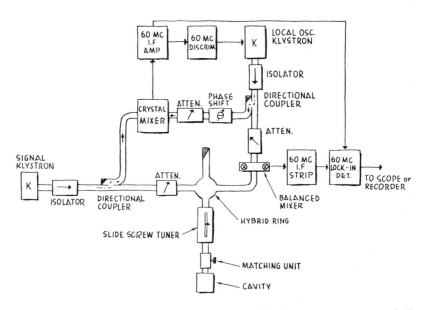

Fig. 3-1. Typical RS4-X spectrometer with essential microwave components indicated. No provisions for frequency measurements are included.

Table 3-2

TRANSMISSION HOMODYNE TYPE 1	TH1 - X K Q	
TRANSMISSION HOMODYNE TYPE 2 with MICROWAVE BUCKING ARM	TH2 - X K Q	
TRANSMISSION SUPERHETERODYNE TYPE 1 with BALANCED MIXER	TS1 - X K Q	
REFLECTION HOMODYNE TYPE 1 KLYSTRON LOCKED to SAMPLE CAVITY	RH1 - X K Q	
REFLECTION HOMODYNE TYPE 2 KLYSTRON LOCKED to EXTERNAL CAVITY	RH2 - X K Q	
REFLECTION HOMODYNE TYPE 3 with BUCKING ARM and BALANCED MIXER	RH3 - X K Q	
REFLECTION SUPERHETERODYNE TYPE 1	RS1 - X K Q	
REFLECTION HOMODYNE TYPE 4 with COUPLER and NO TEE	RH4 - X K Q	
REFLECTION SUPERHETERODYNE TYPE 2	RS2 - X K Q	
REFLECTION SUPERHETERODYNE TYPE 4 with MODULATED ARM and BALANCED MIXER	RS3 - X K Q	

Table 3-3
Some Microwave Components and their Operation

---

1. Attenuators

   a. Function: to control power level in the microwave field.

   b. Range: flap type $\sim$ 0–20 db, rotary-vane type $\sim$ 0–50 db.

   c. Operation: A resistive element in an electric field absorbs energy when it is parallel to the lines of force. Various mechanisms are used to introduce the resistive film into the field, e.g., a glass vane coated with nickel–chromium can be inserted through a slit in the waveguide by flap or guillotine action, or it can be rotated parallel to the field in a circular waveguide for the rotary vane type.

2. Bridge elements

   a. Function: isolates the detector from the rf power supply while keeping the detector sensitive to small changes of power reflected from the cavity.

   b. Range of isolation: depending on the frequency, about 25–45 db between the E and H arms of a hybrid T.

   c. Operation

     (1) Hybrid T: The T consists of four waveguide arms joined so that the E and H arms couple through their respective E or H field to the two side arms, but not to each other. Typically, power from the klystron feeds into the E arm and divides equally between the cavity and a matched load terminating the side arms. The difference in power reflected from the cavity and the termination divides equally between the E arm and the H arm, which contains the detector. When posts, diaphragms, or variable cross sections are introduced to provide the same characteristic impedance in each arm, the device is called a matched hybrid or Magic T.

     (2) Circulator or hybrid ring: The four post variety consists of a waveguide ring with four T junctions in the E plane located around the circumference with spacings of

$$n\lambda/4, \quad n\lambda/4, \quad n\lambda/4, \quad \text{and } (n + 2)\lambda/4$$

where n is an odd integer. Rf power coming down an arm divides at the junction and proceeds in opposite directions around the ring. If the two components arrive in phase at another junction, power goes into the arm; but if they are 180° out of phase, the components cancel. If the spectrometer components are located according to the following ports and spaces (port 1, rf generator, $n\lambda/4$, port 2 matched termination, $n\lambda/4$, port 3 detector, $n\lambda/4$, port 4 cavity, $(n + 2)\lambda/4$, port 1) the incoming power will go down arms 2 and 4 but not 3 while the reflected signal from the cavity goes down 3 and 1. As with the T the input impedances of the four lines are matched.

3. Couplers

   a. Function: to couple power from the main waveguide to an auxiliary guide.

(continued)

Table 3-3 (*continued*)

b. Range:

(1) Multihole coupler: coupling factors from about 3 to 2 db, directivity > 40 db.

(2) Cross-guide coupler: coupling factors of 20 or 30 db.

c. Operation and definitions:

$$\text{Coupling factor} = \frac{\text{forward power in main guide}}{\text{power out of auxiliary guide}} \text{ in db}$$

Directivity

$$= \frac{\text{power out of auxiliary guide with forward power in the main guide}}{\text{power out of auxiliary with reverse power in the main guide}}$$

Power couples from the main guide to the auxiliary through holes sized and spaced to control the direction of power flow, indicated by the directivity, and the division of the power given by the coupling factor. In addition to the multihole and cross-guide couplers, hybrid T's and rings can be used as equal sharing couples.

4. Isolators: Ferrite

a. Function: a nonreciprocal device for transmitting power with low loss in the forward direction while absorbing power going in the reverse direction.

b. Range: loss in forward direction ~ 0.5 db; loss in reverse direction ~ 40–70 db.

c. Operation:

(1) The Faraday rotation type consists of an absorbing vane, a ferrite section in a magnetic field, and a second absorbing vane at 45° to the first. The transmitted wave passing the first vane is rotated 45° by the Faraday effect in the ferrite section so the polarization permits passage past the second vane; however, a similar rotation of the reflected wave brings the wave to the input end with a 90° total rotation and thus an orientation absorbed by the first vane.

(2) In a resonance ferrite isolator at the critical magnetic field and microwave frequency, the electrons in the ferrite can absorb energy from a circularly polarized microwave of appropriate rotation. The transmitted wave has an orientation that is not absorbed; however, the sense of rotation is changed 180° upon reflection so the reflected wave rotates in the proper direction for absorption by the ferrite.

5. Mixers

a. Function: A balanced mixer in a superheterodyne system mixes the signal from the cavity with power from the local oscillator in order to obtain the intermediate or beat frequency.

b. Operation: In a typical hybrid T mixer, the local oscillator couples into the E arm, the signal from the cavity enters the H arm and a pair of matched detector crystals are mounted in the side arms. Power from both sources reaches the crystals but good isolation is maintained between the local oscillator

(*continued*)

Table 3-3 (*continued*)

and the cavity. The output from the two crystals is coupled in push pull through the IF amplifier. Some advantages of balanced mixer detection are (*1*) local klystron noise is eliminated, (*2*) second-order terms proportional to χ'^2 and χ''^2 cancel out, and (*3*) a reproducible procedure is available for tuning to pure absorption (H-7).

6. Phase shifter
   a. Function: to control phase variation.
   b. Range: -360 to $+360$ electrical degrees.
   c. Operation:

   (1) Trombone type: a slide section permits mechanical changes in the length of the waveguide.

   (2) Squeeze section type: Squeezing reduces the cross section and changes the guide wavelength.

   (3) Dielectric vane type: A rotatable dielectric vane in the electric field of a circular waveguide section retards the phase according to the amount of dielectric in parallel with the electric field.

   (4) Ferrite type: The phase length of the ferrite section of the waveguide is varied according to the strength of the applied magnetic field.

7. Terminations
   a. Function: to absorb energy with a minimum of reflection.
   b. Range: peak power 1–100 kW, average power up to 500 W.
   c. Tapered sections of electrically lossy materials absorb the microwave power without setting up large reflections. Air or water cooling controls the temperature.

8. Tuners
   a. Function: to match loads and terminations to the characteristic impedance of the waveguide.
   b. Range: Corrections can be made for voltage standing wave ratio (VSWR) up to about 20.
   c. Operation:

   (1) Slide screw tuner: By adjusting the location and penetration of a probe in a section of slotted line, the amplitude and phase of the induced reflected wave can be adjusted to cancel existing reflections in the system.

   (2) EH tuner: A hybrid-T structure with movable shorts in the E and H arms can be adjusted to establish reflections which cancel undesirable reflections in the remaining arms of the tuner.

---

their presence will be assumed. However, some other pertinent characteristics may be listed without special notation, e.g., the modulation frequency, detecting element, the bridge element, and method of stabilizing the rf generator. Table 3-4 shows how a number of commercially available spectrometers fit into this nomenclature.

Table 3-4
Classification of Several Commercial EPR Spectrometers

Manufacturer	Model	Bridge element	Nearest type
1. Alpha Scientific Laboratories	ALX-10	Circulator	RH1-X
2. Decca Radar Limited	X-1	Coupler[a]	RH1-X
	X-2	Coupler	RS4-X
	X-3	Coupler	RS4-X
3. Hilger and Watts Ltd.	ESR 1	Hybrid T	RH2-X
	ESR 2	Hybrid T	RH2-Q
	ESR 3	Hybrid T	RH2-X+Q
4. Japan Electron Optics Laboratory	JES-P-10	Hybrid T	RH1-X
	JES 3BX	Hybrid T	RH1-X
	JES 3BK	Hybrid T	RH1-K
	JES 3BQ	Hybrid T	RH1-Q
5. Perkin-Elmer Corporation	ESR-1	Circulator	RH1-X
6. Strand Laboratories Inc.	601 A/X	Ferrite circulator	RH3-X
	601 A/K	Ferrite circulator	RH3-K
	602 A/X	Ferrite circulator	RH3-X
	602 A/K	Ferrite circulator	RH3-K
7. Trüb, Taüber and Co.	F 64.5	Ferrite circulator	RS4-K
8. Varian Associates	V-4502, high power	Hybrid T	RH1-X
	V-4502, low power	Hybrid T	RH2-X
	V-4502, super-heterodyne	Hybrid T	RS2-X

[a] Similar to type RH4 coupler arrangement.

3.3 SENSITIVITY

All forms of spectroscopy, including EPR, ultimately encounter theoretical limits in sensitivity and resolution governed by the uncertainty principle; however, before this state is reached, we are stopped in practice by the noise level in currently available components. As usual some sensitivity can be exchanged for resolution and to some extent both can be traded for design simplicity and operating convenience. At most of the laboratories visited in collecting this material, adequate sensitivity and resolution were readily obtained; therefore, when instruments were not obtained by inheritance, operating convenience frequently played an important role in selecting the type. Unfortunately, such good fortune is not universal and

Table 3-5

Experimental Areas Where Existing Spectrometers Are Quite Adequate
and Regions Where Improvements Are Needed

Spin system	Spectrometers, adequate for measurements of	Where improvements are needed
1. Stable paramagnetic atoms, molecules and radicals in		
(*a*) Gaseous state	g, D, hfs, N	
(*b*) Solution	g, D, hfs, N	Stability and sensitivity for very high-resolution EPR
(*c*) Solid-matrix transition elements	g, D, hfs, N, τ	
2. Reactive intermediates or radicals		
(*a*) Gas-phase reactions	g	Sensitivity for G values
(*b*) Liquid-phase reactions		Speed
(*c*) Solid-phase reactions		
Photolysis products	g, hfs, G, D	Sensitivity
Pyrolysis products	g, hfs, N	
Radiolysis products	g, hfs, G	
3. Defects in dielectrics and semiconductors	g, hfs, N, τ	
4. Biological materials		
(*a*) Dry systems	g, hfs, N, G	
(*b*) Aqueous systems		Sensitivity for G where spins limited

some areas of EPR research push existing instruments to their limits without achieving satisfactory sensitivity and resolution. Table 3-5 indicates some fields where existing instruments are quite satisfactory and others where improvements are needed. Sensitivity problems normally arise from low spin concentrations, rf saturation, or a combination of both, i.e., the lack of spin–spin interactions frequently lengthens the relaxation time, thus contributing to rf saturation. Since most of the problem areas involve sensitivity, the following paragraphs will be concerned with procedures for maximizing the signal, minimizing the noise level, and recovering intelligence in a poor signal-to-noise ratio situation. It will become apparent that the design features for improving the signal-to-noise ratio also contribute to high resolution and it is only in the operating procedure that resolution is sacrificed for sensitivity.

3.3.1 Maximizing the Signal

Early in the literature of EPR, expressions were developed showing the relationship of the signal to the various sample and spectrometer parameters (B-17,B-18,F-3,I-2,T-6). For the usual case involving sine wave modulation and no rf saturation the signal power can be expressed as

$$P_s = P_0(4\pi\chi''\eta Q_0)^2/16 \tag{3-1}$$

provided the absorption due to the sample is always small.

Where P_0 = incident power, Q_0 = unloaded quality factor, χ'' = imaginary part of the susceptibility, and η = the filling factor. P_0 is delivered at the spectrometer frequency ν while P_s will have a frequency $\nu \pm f_m$, where ν = microwave signal frequency and f_m = modulation frequency.

Other parameters, involved in establishing the signal level are (*1*) the spectrometer frequency—both χ'' and Q_0 depend on the frequency; (*2*) the sample temperature—χ'' is inversely related to the temperature; and (*3*) the modulation field strength in the case of derivative recording. These parameters along with the conditions of Eq. 3-1 fall into two categories: (*1*) design parameters which include the spectrometer frequency, Q_0, and provisions for mounting samples to optimize the filling factor and (*2*) operational procedures for adjusting the spectrometer to maximize the signal with any particular sample, i.e., rf power level, modulation amplitude, sample temperature, and filling factor. At the spectrometer selection stage we are concerned only with the design parameters ν, Q_0, and the effect of the cavity geometry on η. Frequency selection is discussed at the end of this chapter and all of Section 4.1 is concerned with the selection, design, and construction of cavities. The trend toward higher frequencies and Q_0's in both commercial and homemade spectrometers is indicative of the continuing efforts to maximize the signal. For example, Table 4-5 shows that values of Q_0 for both commercial and homemade cavities are now so close to the theoretical limits that negligible signal enhancement is anticipated from higher Q_0's. Recent efforts have been concerned with absorption cell designs and accessories for conveniently optimizing the filling factor, particularly in difficult samples such as the lossy dielectrics. These developments are considered in subsequent chapters dealing with lossy samples.

Thus far we have mentioned only factors contributing to the signal level; however, the absolute level has little meaning except in reference to the associated noise, i.e., it is the signal-to-noise ratio that counts. If the controlling noise originates in the detector or in some stage in the spectrometer following the sample cell, it becomes practical, at least in principle, to enhance the signal-to-noise ratio by amplification. Several types of amplifiers capable of operating at microwave frequencies have sufficiently low noise figures to be considered for this purpose: tunnel diode amplifiers, reactor diode parametric amplifiers, and masers—listed in the order of increasing complexity and decreasing noise figure (H-13). Figure 3-2 shows typical noise temperatures as a function of frequency for some of these amplifiers. At this writing, several spectrometers are under construction which have maser amplifiers incorporated in their design (19,30).

Also, a commercially available reactor diode parametric amplifier has been successfully used to improve the sensitivity of an existing spectrometer (H-13). Figure 3-3 shows the circuit diagram for the type RH3-X spectrometer and parametric amplifier arranged to measure the effect of rf amplification on the signal-to-noise ratio. A microwave switch permitted the amplifier to be cut in and out of the circuit without disturbing

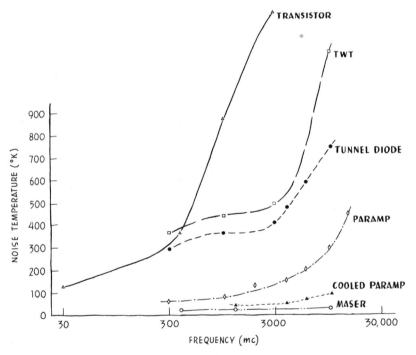

Fig. 3-2. State of the art of low-noise amplifiers showing the noise temperature as a function of the frequency. (Courtesy E-1.)

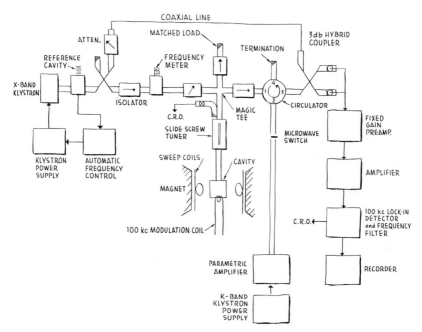

Fig. 3-3. RH3-X spectrometer equipped with parametric amplifier to measure the effect of rf amplification on the signal-to-noise ratio (after H-13).

any of the other components. Measurements were made on a DPPH sample with the post amplifier adjusted to give the same off resonance noise level with the switch closed (Case I) and with it open (Case II). The relative improvement in sensitivity for Case II was between three- and tenfold.*

Typical values with a Texas Instruments Parametric Amplifier, Model X-22A, using a $F_p = 3.2$ were $G_P = 64$, $F_I = 33.2$, $F_{II} = 2.59$, and $F_I/F_{II} = 12.8$ (H-13).

* When all the operating parameters except those relating to the noise figure are considered common, the noise figures provide a measure of the comparative sensitivity of two spectrometers, i.e.,

$$[A_I/A_{II}]_V = [F_{II}/F_I]_P^{1/2}$$

Also $F_I \cong F_D$ applies when the dominating noise source is in the detector–preamplifier, and

$$F_{II} \cong F_P + (F_I - 1)/G_P$$

where A_I and A_{II} are signal amplitudes for Cases I and II, respectively: F_I and F_{II} are the respective noise figures; V and P refer to voltage and power units, respectively; and F_P and G_P are the noise figure and gain of the rf amplifier in power units.

3.3.2 Improving the Signal-to-Noise Ratio

Since sensitivity is a matter of the signal-to-noise ratio, it is just as important to reduce the noise as to enhance the signal. Various EPR practitioners are not in unanimous agreement as to the limiting source of noise; however, the three major candidates listed in descending order of suspicion are:
1. The detector crystal.
2. The microwave generator (klystron).
3. Microphonics.

Apparently, the noise levels are not vastly different in good crystals and klystrons so either component could control the noise level and undoubtedly the controlling source varies from instrument to instrument.* Careful noise measurements are seldom made on homemade instruments, particularly in the majority of situations where sensitivity is not a problem; however, the general suspicion regarding the crystal results from frequent observations that the signal-to-noise ratio frequently changes when another crystal is installed. As long as the noise contributions are about equal for crystal and klystron, only minor gains in the signal-to-noise ratio are available from crystal improvements before the next weakest link comes into play. Consequently, the practice of selecting the lowest noise components on a cut-and-try basis is quite common. Pake has remarked that "Coping with spectrometer noise is an art within which highly successful practitioners can find large areas of controversy or disagreement. Experimental data under well controlled conditions are not common. It is therefore advisable to view pontifications on the subject including those of this article with vigorous independence of mind" (B-21).

(a) **Noise Nomenclature.** Before launching into methods of reducing the noise contributions from the various spectrometer components it appears appropriate to list a few of the definitions pertinent to the noise vocabulary (B-8,S-4,B-13).
1. Mean noise power $W(f)$: mean available power per unit of bandwidth at frequency f.
2. White noise: the noise is white if $W(f)$ is a constant at all frequencies, which means in practice over the frequency range of interest.
3. Noise bandwidth for white noise: B in Fig. 3-4.
4. Thermal noise power:

$$F_{det}kTB \tag{3-2}$$

---

* Also, the dominating noise generator depends on the power level. At low powers, i.e., at fractions of a milliwatt crystal noise is apt to predominate while at high powers the klystron is believed to be the limiting noise source.

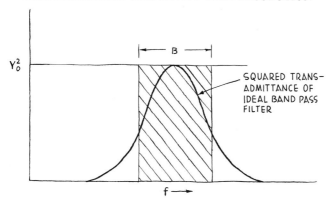

Fig. 3-4. Illustration of noise bandwidth for white noise: B = width of rectangle having an area equal to the area of the squared transadmittance curve.

where k = the Boltzmann factor, T = temperature in degrees Kelvin, B = bandwidth, and F_{det} = detector noise.

5. The noise temperature T_n: the temperature at which thermal noise power is equal to the available noise power W_n output from a single port device. $T_n k = W_n$. Therefore, $T_n = 7.25 \times 10^{22} W_n$, where W_n is in watts per cycle and T_n is in degrees Kelvin.

6. Noise ratio:

$$r_n = T_n/T = W_n/kT, \qquad r_n \text{ in db} = 20 \log (W_n/kT) \qquad (3\text{-}3)$$

7. The excess noise ratio $= r_n - 1$.

8. Signal-to-noise ratio:

$$\text{S/N} = \frac{V_s^{\,2}}{V_n^{\,2}} = \frac{\text{mean squared signal}}{\text{mean squared noise}} \qquad (3\text{-}4)$$

9. Noise factor of a system:

$$F = (S_s/N_s)/(S_0/N_0) = \frac{\text{input signal-to-noise}}{\text{output signal-to-noise}} \qquad (3\text{-}5)$$

An ideal network adds no additional noise and has an $F = 1$, noise figures are frequently expressed in decibels, and the standard temperature is 290°K.

10. Noise figure: NF $= 10 \log F$.

(b) The Detector Crystal. Silicon crystal diodes are currently the mainstay for EPR detectors. Table 3-6 indicates the type of information available to characterize commercial diodes, e.g., losses, noise figure, and test frequency. The noise figure for a particular crystal varies with frequency,

Table 3-6

Characteristics of Some Silicon Mixer Diodes[a]

Desig-nation	Type or electrical equivalent	Band	Test fre-quency f, Mc	Overall noise figure NF_0,db	Con-version loss[c] L_c, db	Output noise ratio, NR_0	IF Imped-ance ohms, Z_{IF}	VSWR
MA-4172	IN21WE	S	3060	7.0	5.5	1.5	350–450	1.3
MA-4174	IN23WE	X	9375	7.5	6.0	1.4	335–465	1.3
MA-4610A	Back diode–low-noise doppler mixer diode	X	8800	12[b]		3	50–200	2.0
MA-4624A		K_e	13,300	12[b]			50–150	2.0
MA-4625A		K_u	16,000	12[b]			50–150	2.0

[a] From Microwave Associates, Inc., *Catalog SF 4002*, Feb. 1965.
[b] 20 kc IF.
[c] $L_c = 1/\text{gain}$.

power level, and temperature. Furthermore, the signal-to-noise level depends on the past crystal treatment, on changes with time, and varies considerably from crystal to crystal. Minimizing the noise therefore involves: (*1*) locating a crystal with a high signal-to-noise ratio; (*2*) choosing operating parameters for minimum noise; and (*3*) careful usage to prevent a gradual reduction in the S/N ratio. A consideration of the various types of noise will indicate where these factors come to bear in the battle against noise. The noise in junction diodes is conveniently considered in terms of the three classical noises of electronic devices, i.e., thermal, shot, and $1/f$ noise. Expressions for the fluctuations in current (i.e., the noise), derived by using several methods to allow for the effects of charge carrier diffusion and recombination, are in agreement and give a noise power

$$W(f) \approx 4kTg_dB - 2eIB \qquad (3\text{-}6)$$

where the first term is identical with the Nyquist thermal noise developed in a passive resistor and the second term matches the shot-noise term for a vacuum diode (B-8,S-4): k = Boltzmann factor, T = absolute temperature, g_d = ac conductance of the junction, e = electronic charge, and I = dc current.

As usual, thermal noise is characteristic of thermal equilibrium and involves the interactions between the free moving charges (holes and electrons) and the vibrating atoms of the crystal while shot noise involves

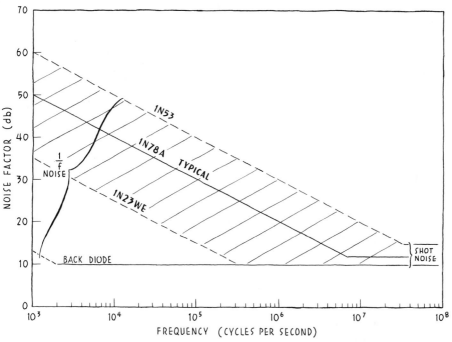

Fig. 3-5. Noise factor of a typical back diode compared with several standard mixer-type crystals. The shaded area indicates the kind of spectral variation obtainable with a hypothetical batch of IN78's. $1/f$ noise becomes effective in the back diode only below about 2 kc in contrast to 200 kc or higher for the other crystals. (Courtesy Microwave Associates, Inc.)

the random arrival of independent charged particles. Both shot and thermal noise sources generate white noise in the frequency range of normal observations so the two types of noise are indistinguishable in outside circuits. However, Eq. 3-6 indicates a basis for determining the predominate noise, i.e., thermal noise is proportional to T while shot noise is proportional to I; therefore, experimentally the temperature and current can be used to determine and to some extent control these noise components. Where $1/f$ noise appears as in the flicker noise of vacuum tubes or as contact noise, it is attributed to slowly varying changes in the conduction of the system, frequently assumed to involve some inhomogeneities in manufacture. In recent years refinements in design and construction have substantially reduced the $1/f$ noise* in crystal detectors (S-4); however, it is usually the

---

* Strictly speaking, the noise is proportional to $1/f^{\Delta}$ where Δ may vary from about 0 to 1.5, but for our purposes, the general use of unity is adequate (B-8).

dominating source at low frequencies. Figure 3-5 shows the general behavior of diode noise as a function of frequency. At low frequencies, e.g., below 1 kc, the $1/f$ component predominates while at higher frequencies shot and thermal noise become the controlling factors. Returning now to the three factors involved in minimizing the noise it becomes apparent that the search for a crystal with a large signal-to-noise ratio involves first minimizing the $1/f$ and the shot noise. Figure 3-5 shows that the first step is to select a modulation frequency that reduces the $1/f$ noise to negligible proportions—thus the general trend to 100 kc or higher modulating frequencies. Further reductions in the noise level rest largely in the crystal manufacturers' hands and they have made considerable progress in recent years, particularly in crystals for S-, X-, and K-band frequencies. Therefore, the second step involves selecting the best of the diodes available with good signal to noise characteristics at the modulation frequency. Doppler diodes have been developed and selected for such low-frequency performance; therefore, they are the most likely candidates currently available. Three types are (1) silicon point contact diodes, (2) back diodes, and (3) Schottky-Berrior diodes.* All of the spectrometers in Table 3-2 except type TH1 permit biasing the crystal to the optimum power level for minimizing the shot noise independently of the signal level. Since this operating procedure is virtually universal, it is mentioned here only to emphasize the desirability of using the best value for the crystal involved. Normally this will be the smallest power consistent with operation in the linear detection region for the crystal. When both the $1/f$ and shot noise have been reduced below the level of thermal noise, it becomes practical to think about the crystal operating temperature. All of the spectrometers encountered while collecting information for this volume operate with the crystal at room temperature and because the large majority of these instruments had an ample S/N ratio, the complications involved in cooling the detector would not be particularly welcome. Nevertheless, critical cases may ultimately require refrigerated detectors.

The question of detector temperature becomes involved in determining the ultimate sensitivity of a spectrometer because the expression usually derived assumed the limit is reached when the signal equals the thermal noise of the detector. If the $1/f$ and shot noise are neglected and the expression for the signal (Eq. 3-1) is equated to the thermal noise power in the detector

---

* Back diodes are preferred by most of the EPR workers who have tried them. The major portion of the theoretically available noise improvement at low frequencies is realized by the use of these diodes (Dr. Uhlir of Microwave Associates, private communication).

$$P_0(4\pi\chi''\eta Q_0)^2/16 = F_{det}kTB \qquad (3\text{-}7)$$

and the minimum signal is

$$4\pi\chi''\eta Q_0 = 4(F_{det}kTB/P_0)^{1/2} \qquad (3\text{-}8)$$

where F_{det} = the noise figure, k = Boltzmann's constant, T = absolute temperature, and B = the bandwidth. An order of magnitude reduction in the room temperature noise power would require operation at about 3°K, a temperature that introduces considerable experimental complexity, because of both the changes in the crystal properties at low temperatures and the added problems of using liquid helium as the refrigerant.

Finally a note of caution is in order regarding protection of the best point-contact diodes. Usually such crystals lose sensitivity if the contact area is enlarged by subjecting the diode to excessive power, even though it remains below the burnout rating. The contact area is very small and thermal equilibrium is reached in a very short time, e.g., less than 10^{-7} sec; therefore, very short pulses of excessive rf power can soften the tungsten point and broaden the contact area (M-10). Since the sensitivity may change slowly over a long period of time, the loss may go unnoticed unless comparisons are occasionally made to a little-used check crystal. Discretion often dictates leaving the less demanding measurements to "lesser" crystals while the "exceptional" crystal remains in safe storage except when its superior signal-to-noise ratio is required. The signal-to-noise improvements already mentioned have substantially reduced the need for such hoarding techniques; however, an occasional comparison between crystals is desirable to check their health from a sensitivity standpoint.

(c) The Microwave Generator. When the detector crystal noise has been minimized, the next point of attack is usually the microwave generator which is usually a klystron. Klystron noise can appear as amplitude modulation or frequency modulation; however, the second type usually predominates (H-27). Two spectrometer conditions accentuate the problem with FM noise, i.e., a closely balanced microwave bridge and a high-Q cavity. When a reflection spectrometer operates with the bridge closely balanced, FM noise becomes a problem because slight changes in klystron frequency alter the power reflected from the frequency-sensitive cavity arm sufficiently to constitute a sizable fraction of the power going to the detector. Similarly, a high-Q cavity is very sensitive to slight frequency changes. Hyde has derived an approximate expression showing the dependence of FM noise on cavity Q and bridge balance for the case of small frequency deviations and a cavity near match (H-27).

$$\Delta V \approx Q^2 \delta^2 V_1{}^2 / 2V_2 \tag{3-9}$$

where V_2 = voltage reflected at resonance; ΔV = the change in V_2 corresponding to a klystron frequency change expressed by the frequency tuning parameter δ which deviates from zero; V_1 = the voltage incident on the resonant cavity; and Q = the cavity quality factor, which is a large term squared. Two examples will help to illustrate where FM noise can be virtually ignored and where it should receive attention. Superheterodyne spectrometers normally operate with the bridge nearly balanced to avoid overloading the IF amplifier and with a high-Q cavity to make the sensitivity high and worth the added complexity of the superheterodyne system; therefore, special attention is normally given to klystron FM noise. At the other extreme several simple type TH1 spectrometers with modest- or low-Q cavities are operating satisfactorily without the customary provisions for stabilizing the klystron frequency (12,42). Because of the broad transmission band, slight frequency changes do not appreciably alter the amplitude of the transmitted rf signal.

Efforts to eliminate FM klystron noise fall into three general categories: (1) stabilizing the klystron power supply; (2) stabilizing the klystron thermal and mechanical environment; and (3) locking the klystron frequency to a frequency reference. Well-regulated commercial power supplies are adequate, particularly with high-frequency modulation or superheterodyne systems. In some of the earlier systems with modulation at frequencies near the fundamental or harmonics of the power lines it was desirable to operate the klystron filaments from batteries to avoid modulation from the power lines (I-2). However, this precaution is no longer necessary.

Stabilization of the klystron temperature is essential for the long-time stability required for high-resolution and high-sensitivity measurements. A variety of arrangements, including oil baths, water jackets, forced air, and natural convection, have been used successfully to cool klystrons. Since the goal is a constant klystron temperature, the constancy of the coolant temperature is more important than the cooling material. At low powers, e.g., below 15 mW, natural air convection is adequate, particularly if heat-dissipation fins are attached to the klystron and the ambient air temperature remains constant for times that are long compared with the length of a continuous spectrometer measurement. When forced air cooling is required for higher-powered tubes, both the air temperature and the possibility of vibrations should be considered. Microphonic noise sources are considered in more detail in the next section so here we will only anticipate sufficiently to warn that both high-velocity air and vibrations from the fan are potential sources of klystron vibration. Therefore, low-velocity fans mechanically isolated from the microwave components are preferred. Since water is normally required to cool the magnet, it is usually convenient to use water cooling for the klystron, either by commercially available clamp on coolers or by home-built baths. With any of these cooling arrangements short-time fluctuations in the temperature can be damped out by attaching the klystron to a source of thermal capacity, e.g., a liquid bath or block of metal.

While stable power supplies and constant temperatures suffice for stable cavity conditions and short runs, all commercial and most home-built spectrometers now lock the klystron frequency to one or more of three references: (a) a high-Q reference cavity; (b) the sample cavity; and (c) a crystal-controlled frequency standard. Each reference offers some advantages and some inconveniences for various experiments; consequently, it is sometimes desirable to change references. Some of the advantages are as follows:

A. Automatic frequency control (AFC) locked to separate reference cavity:

1. The spectrometer can be tuned to observe either the absorption or dispersion signal.

2. Adequate power can be maintained for good automatic frequency control (AFC) irrespective of the power limitations in the sample cavity.

3. Lossy samples do not effect the Q of the frequency control cavity and thus the frequency stability.

B. AFC locked to sample cavity:

1. Operationally this is the simplest locking system. Since only two elements have to be synchronized, the cavity does not have to be tunable.

2. If the cavity resonance frequency shifts for any reason such as temperature changes or bubbles in the cooling liquid, the source frequency follows the change.

C. Klystron locked to crystal oscillator:

1. This system has the same advantages as the separate cavity plus a possible further reduction in noise because both the frequency and phase can be locked. In superheterodyne systems particularly the local oscillator can be locked in a fixed phase relationship and precisely at the IF frequency away from the main klystron.

2. The frequency stability specification for this system in commercial units is slightly higher (a few parts in 10^7) than for cavity lock systems (1 part or better in 10^6). See the Appendix.

3. Splitting factor measurements are simplified because the frequency is normally known for the crystal oscillator.

The Pound circuit is the classical method of locking the klystron to a frequency-controlling cavity and the advantage of such stabilization, particularly over long time periods, is well established (P-16). Experience with crystal oscillator frequency control is relatively sparse and while the system provides good long-time frequency stability, the effect on FM klystron noise is not well established. It is not difficult to phase-lock a klystron but Coles (19) observes that it can be very difficult to achieve a marked improvement in the noise level because the noise in the best klystrons is already very low and it is easy for the feedback to make the noise worse.

Digressing briefly from the noise question, it should be noted that the crystal oscillator phase-locking system can be combined with the cavity-locking procedure to retain the high stability of crystal control while eliminating the difficulties arising from a shift in the cavity resonance frequency. The frequency of the crystal oscillator can be controlled over a few megacycles by a feedback voltage proportional to the departure from the cavity resonance, i.e., now the sample cavity AFC controls the reference frequency standard instead of direct klystron control. In this combined system some of the possible precise frequency control is sacrificed for long-time stability at the cavity resonance frequency; however, in a super-heterodyne system the two klystrons remain locked together in phase.

(d) Microphonics, Mechanical Instabilities, and Spurious Electrical Transients. The obvious solution to these problems is to select a spectrometer with a minimum susceptibility to microphonic disturbances and to mount the instrument on a firm footing in a location free from mechanical and electrical disturbances. In practice few spectrometers are or can be located in such ideal environments so a compromise is usually achieved between the acceptable noise and the effort required for further isolation. Fortunately, most of the microphonics can be avoided by using a spectrometer with high-frequency modulation, i.e., few mechanical vibrations occur in the 100-kc range. Preferred locations are usually on the lowest floor in a building, free from vibrating machinery both inside and out and supplied with an electrical line free from electrical transients. The authors installation is a good example of what to avoid, i.e., the spectrometer is located on the fourth floor close to an escalator that keeps the floor vibrating continually. Furthermore, the electrical power comes from a shipyard where heavy machinery imposes respectable transients on the mains, particularly at shift changes and lunch breaks. Despite these disturbances, quiet times can be found when it is best to run the most crucial spectra.

Some of the more likely sources of mechanical disturbances and possible remedies are as follows:

1. Adjustable components such as cavity matching and tuning devices: At low temperatures where these adjustments are made remotely, it is customary to allow considerable clearance between moving parts in order to insure free operation. Such devices should be spring loaded or otherwise constrained from shifting or vibrating. Some construction details are considered in Chapter 4.

2. Cooling fans, vacuum pump: These should be mounted on supports that are separate from and isolated from the microwave portions of the spectrometer.

3. Bubbling cryogenic fluids: These disturbances are most severe with internal dewars, i.e., when the tip of the dewar and the cryogenic liquid extend into the cavity. Such bubbling generates noise by two effects: (*1*) mechanically the bubbles can move the sample into regions of slightly different rf magnetic field, thereby altering the signal level; (*2*) the presence of bubbles alters the cavity's dielectric properties and thus the Q. The bubbling problem can be handled by a variety of rituals and, as usual, the best procedure for a given experiment depends on the available signal level and thus the amount of convenience that must be sacrificed to reduce the noise. Sample motion is virtually never acceptable; therefore, some type of rigid support is required (see Fig. 7.5-14). Large bubbles or a bumping liquid can move light glass vials and support rods; consequently, additional weight, bracing, or restraint is frequently required. Some commercial dewars come with collets to provide this support. The second precaution involves keeping the bubbles small or eliminating them altogether. With liquid helium the bubbles are usually small and not as much of a problem as liquid nitrogen, at least in the dewar arrangements of Fig. 7.6-4. A few sharp points in the tip of the dewar will accentuate boiling and thus keep the bubble size and bumping at a minimum. Of course where noise is a serious problem, the bubbling should be eliminated during the measurement interval. Figure 3-6 illustrates several techniques for avoiding bubbles in liquid nitrogen by cooling below the boiling point. Arrangement *a* is probably the most convenient since it provides continual cooling with a minimum of equipment and nitrogen consumption. Arrangement *b* is also continuous but helium gas is not always readily available; *c* has been used with short periods of evacuation between spectrometer runs but long runs would require more care to avoid excessive cooling of the nitrogen. Dewars should be suitably covered so that water vapor and CO_2 cannot enter and form snow which swirls around in the liquid.

When the modulation is at audio frequencies, cavities and components in the modulation field require consideration to avoid microphonics,

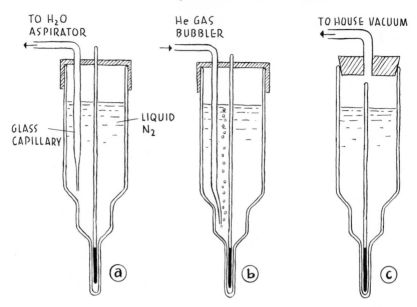

Fig. 3-6. Techniques to avoid the formation of nitrogen bubbles or to keep the bubbles small: (*a*) nitrogen entering through capillary evaporates in vacuum produced by water aspirator and cools main body of liquid (17); (*b*) the rationale for the He bubbles is not immediately obvious but the method is reported to work; (*c*) this is a simple evaporation arrangement.

e.g., rigid cavity walls and supports for coils. Hollocher (5) found some of the stray signal induced by the modulation coils could be nullified by locating aluminum sheets ($\frac{1}{8}$ in. thick for 6 kc modulation) between modulation coils mounted on the magnet poles and the cavity. After locating the optimum position by cut and try, the sheets were taped to the magnet pole.

3.3.3   Rescuing the Signal from the Noise

After the signal has been maximized and the noise minimized, the final step is to extract the signal from the noise and this brings us into the field of information transmission. Communications people, both in their terrestrial activities and in space exploration particularly, apply herculean efforts to recover information in situations where the noise level is many times larger than the signal; consequently, we may profit by an examination of these efforts now and particularly in the future. In an idealized communications system the Shannon–Hartley law expresses the relation between information transfer and the controlling parameters (S-4)

$$I = t\omega \log\left(1 + P_s/N\right) \qquad (3\text{-}10)$$

where I = information, t = time, ω = bandwidth, P_s/N = signal power/ noise power, and the information capacity of the system $C = I/t$.

(a) Tradeoffs. In this idealized case, time, bandwidth, and the signal-to-noise ratio can be traded about to achieve the desired information transfer, noting that P_s/N is least effective because it occurs in a log term. In principle, as long as P_s/N is finite, the time can be lengthened to transmit any level of information. In practice our circuits do not reach this ideal so information is not always recoverable; however, the barters suggested by Eq. 3-10 do apply and are very useful. P_s and N are both related to the bandwidth so that the values are developed in consort. Recalling the frequency characteristics of the noise, i.e., $1/f$ noise and the white spectrum of shot and thermal noise, the center of the pass band is selected to minimize the $1/f$ noise. Next, ω is made wide enough to include most of the signal contributing to P_s but extra width is excluded to keep N as small as possible. Finally, the time is adjusted to give reasonable information transfer. Two factors limit the available time: first, the signal may have a transient existence as in the case of short-lived radicals which may last only fractions of a second; second, the stability of the electronic circuits sets an upper limit on t. The gradual drifts observed in existing spectrometers and occasional large-noise spikes constitute a form of very-low-frequency noise that does not cancel out in practical integrating times. Consequently, the practical exchanges permitted by Eq. 3-10 are rather limited. Current efforts to improve I involve attacks on all three of the limiting parameters; however, the most significant results in EPR spectroscopy concern P_s/N and t.

(b) Phase-Sensitive Detector. A signal buried in noise is easier to find when some characteristics of the signal are known, e.g., in spectrometers with field modulation both the frequency and phase of the signal are known so that it is practical to discriminate against both the noise outside the band pass ω and the noise within the band pass but out of phase with the signal. The phase-sensitive detectors used to perform this discrimination are available as industrial commercial units, have been described in the literature, and are standard practice in commercial spectrometers as well as in most home built units (I-3,S-8). Other names applied to these units are lockin amplifiers, and synchronous detectors. Briefly, the operation is as follows:

1. The incoming signal along with the accompanying noise is amplified to a convenient level in a low-noise preamplifier.

2. A reference signal from the spectrometer 100 kc modulator is used to lock a tuned amplifier to the signal frequency, thereby permitting a very narrow band pass without the possibility that the signal can drift out of the pass band. At this point noise outside the pass band is removed.

3. The next section is a balanced mixer where the (signal + noise) beats against the reference signal. This mixing action results in an output signal $f_0(t) = \frac{1}{2}f(t)\cos\delta$, where $f(t)$ is the input and δ is the phase angle between the input and the reference. Obviously $f_0(t)$ has a maximum value at $\delta = 0$ (negative at $180°$) and goes to zero at $\delta = 90°$. Therefore, when the signal and reference are in phase a large portion of the total noise will be removed by the cosine factor.

4. Now the signal is filtered to smooth out additional noise, amplified in a dc amplifier if necessary and recorded.

Up through step *3*, phase-sensitive detection is concerned with increasing signal-to-noise ratio for each individual cycle; however, step *4* permits an increase of the time to include many cycles, thereby increasing the information transferred. When noise is a problem, the spectrometer is normally swept through the absorption line at a slow rate, e.g., the signal level does not change for several seconds so that the detector can easily have 10^6 uniform cycles of signal, which gives a good average when ferreted out of the noise. Information on the discrimination possible with such systems is not readily available but the synchronous detectors used in radio astronomy are reported capable of detecting signals 40 db below the input noise level.

(c) Coding. The spectrometers described thus far have used single-frequency sine-wave modulation and the information is carried in changes in the amplitude of the carrier, i.e., in communication parlance, amplitude modulation (AM). Also from communication theory it is known that other types of modulation are superior for transmitting information in situations where noise is a problem, e.g., pulse code modulation (PCM). Here we mention only a few elementary characteristics of coded systems but they will demonstrate the ease with which cost and complexity can escalate for slight improvements in transmitted information. To use a code the receiver must know something about the message and considerable prior information is required for a correct translation with an elaborate code. The EPR situation is ideal from this standpoint because the modulation pattern is available at the receiver so that only the absolute amplitude remains unknown. Some considerations in designing a coded system are:

1. Reliability. A code should be selected which has a low probability of being accidentally produced by the noise. Lengthy codes using large blocks of signals achieve this reliability at the expense of time and bandwidth, i.e., an involved modulation pattern is less apt to be duplicated by the noise spectrum; however, it will take time to transmit. We have already mentioned that in EPR 10^6 c are readily available for one point on the absorption curve and this can be extended by an order of magnitude if necessary.

2. *Efficiency.* A complex code introduces bandwidth and the attendant noise. This additional noise is not catastrophic if the signal-to-noise ratio can be maintained roughly constant as the bandwidth grows, which means the coded signal should occupy all frequencies in the pass band as effectively as the noise. One obvious method of satisfying this efficiency requirement is to modulate the carrier with a white noise spectrum. Such modulation would not violate the reliability requirement because it is extremely unlikely that one random noise pattern will duplicate another.

3. *Economy.* Almost any giant code tends to approach the channel capacity expessed by the Shannon-Hartley equation (B-8). Unfortunately the rate of approach is very slow, being logarithmic with code length; therefore, in communications it is usually more economical to use more bandwidth and signal power than excessively complicated codes.

The desperate spectroscopist now toying with thoughts of codes, decoders, and computers deserves some indication of the effectiveness of coding techniques, i.e., how far can a signal be buried in the noise and still be rescued by these techniques? Unfortunately, the EPR situation departs sufficiently from the usual communications situation to make a direct answer difficult. The most efficient general communication practice involves PCM using a binary code or some other system that requires only the determination of the presence or absence of a pulse, i.e., a requirement usually much easier to achieve than determination of signal amplitudes. In the EPR situation essentially two modulations are involved: (*a*) the microwave carrier can be modulated with any code and style of modulation instead of the conventional 100-kc sine wave; but (*b*) the sample absorption superimposes a slowly varying amplitude modulation on the code. The elaborate code in (*a*) can be used to separate the signal from the noise but the information of interest is locked in the amplitude modulation. Techniques developed for the radar problem of bouncing signals off the moon, Venus, or some other target on the fringe of detectability can be applied to step (*a*); however, the additional requirement for accurate amplitude measurements goes beyond radar requirements. The radar people have turned to computers for assistance in separating the signal from the noise. In the EPR situation the modulation pattern consisting of the frequencies, phases, and relative heights of blocks of signal are known; therefore the computer can use all three characteristics to discriminate against the noise.

(d) Computers. One type of computer is gaining rapid acceptance in the battle against certain types of noise in EPR spectroscopy. Variously known by such "Madison Avenueisms" as Enhancetrons and Time Averaging Computers these analyzers can make significant improvements in the signal-to-noise ratios where a series of repetitive signals is available. In essence these units are an adaptation of the pulse-height analyzers long associated with nuclear spectroscopy. The incoming signal is (1) divided into 1024 channels, (2) digitized, and (3) stored in the magnetic memory. By sweeping the spectra repeatedly with the analyzer synchronized to the magnetic field the sum of the amplitudes at 1024 field points can be accumulated in the memory. Improvement in the S/N ratio results because the signals add linearly while random noise averages toward zero; thus, S/N improves in proportion to the square root of the number of signal repetition. There are two important situations in EPR spectroscopy where comparable improvement in the S/N ratio is not possible by conventional filtering over a long time period. The first occurs when the spin species is short lived and does not exist long enough to permit adequate filtering. When such radicals can be generated repeatedly as in photolysis experiments, a large number of replications can replace the filtering time required to average out the noise. The second occurs when the spectrometer is not stable over the time required to filter out the noise. For example, a fairly common dilemma encountered in quantitative measurements of spin concentrations occurs when a rapid scan of the absorption line is too noisy and spectrometer instabilities cause the base line to drift during the course of a slow scan. Again, the computer can add many rapid scan spectra to eliminate the noise and the base line will not have time to drift during each individual scan. Examples of the improvement in S/N for these two situations are shown in Fig. 3-7. Particularly in photolysis experiments the averaging technique often makes the difference between a successful observation and failure. While the hfs in Fig. 3-7 is definitely improved, the results are not as spectacular as those for the radical decay observations.* One type of noise eludes the simple computers, namely, noise that is synchronized with the scanning field such as that which could result from impurities in the cavity, reproducible idiosyncrasies in the magnetic field, or rate of scan. Such contributions to drift will add right along with the signal in these analyzers; however, a more elaborate procedure and a digital computer can remove repetitive noise. For example, Alpha Scientific Company (43) has programmed the output of an EPR spectrometer into a digital computer and subtracted out the synchronize drift before adding the signals. Historically digital computers have been used to average recurrent signals at least since radar echoes from the planet Venus were detected.

---

* For specifications of typical instruments, see the Appendix.

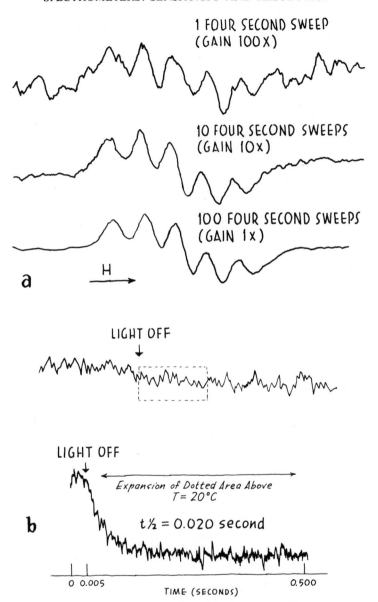

Fig. 3-7. (*a*) Enhancement in signal/noise for the spectrum of DPPH in benzene, single scan, average of 10 scans and average of 100 scans. (*b*) Enhancement in a photolysis experiment: decay spectrum of light-induced cumene hydroperoxide free radical. [(*a*) courtesy 40; (*b*) courtesy V-5.]

Once the spectrometer is hitched to the computer, a number of possibilities arise: (*1*) the decoding mentioned above, (*2*) time-integrated determinations from a series of runs, (*3*) quantitative evaluations of spin concentrations by integrating curves, and (*4*) identification. Identification can be used to rescue signals from noise in various ways: (*1*) when the noise has a regular pattern, it can be identified and thus excluded; (*2*) when the signal shape is known, it can be favored; and (*3*) when only combinations of certain spectra are acceptable, the computer can be programmed to acknowledge only signals that can be synthesized from a library of spectra. In one sense any interfering signal can be considered as noise and within this definition interfering paramagnetic species in a sample act as noise generators. One computer possibility for recovering a signal from this type of noise is illustrated in Fig. 3-8. Photoexcitation experiments frequently produce several paramagnetic species whose spectra overlap like the *d*-phenanthrene triplet state and the peroxide radical. If we are interested in the triplet state, the radical falls into the regular-pattern noise generator category. When the two species are produced or decay at different rates, the computer of average transients can discriminate against one of the rates, thereby achieving a fair separation of the spectra as indicated in the lower trace.

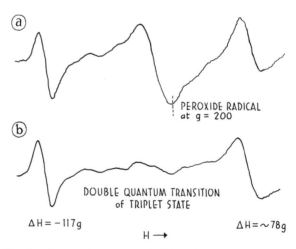

Fig. 3-8. Overlapping spectra separated with an integrator of average transients. (*a*) Spectrum of *d*-phenanthene molecule in the triplet state and a peroxide radical from the solvent obtained with the integrator in the field-sweep mode. (*b*) Spectrum of the triplet state observed with the integrator set to discriminate against the longer-lived radical, i.e., the transient integrator in the transient-field sweep mode. Temperature, 77°K, solvent = 4 parts methylcyclohexane to 1 part cyclopentane (aerated). (Courtesy 40.)

The more conventional noise problem involves random noise and hopefully a signal with some known features. Radicals have characteristic spectra which frequently are well known and are being collected into reference lists.* Such spectra could be incorporated in a computer library, and the computer could be programmed to sort through the library until an unknown spectrum were matched. Presumably the library would permit tentatively identified weak-signal spectra to be improved because the library spectrum could be used to further discriminate against noise. Computers are currently in use or being programmed to unravel spectra in other branches of spectroscopy, e.g., β- and γ-ray spectroscopy and mass spectroscopy. Their use in EPR to unravel spectra and to search through the noise for weak signals is only a matter of time and need. Obviously, when computers are involved, the raw data will be abstracted from the spectrometers in digital form ready to be fed into the computer.

3.4 RESOLUTION

3.4.1 Requirements for a High-Resolution Spectrometer (H-3)

As mentioned at the beginning of this section resolution and sensitivity are linked together so that efforts to improve sensitivity through enhanced signal-to-noise ratios also contribute to better resolution. Normally the limits of spectrometer resolution are encountered only with liquid samples where the spin concentration has been diluted in order to avoid line broadening. Hausser suggests a practical limit for line widths in hydrocarbon radicals on the order of 10 mG and relates that line widths of 17 mG have been observed (H-3). In these observations the incident power on the cavity was about 10^{-5} W and the total absorption was distributed over hundreds of hf lines so the most critical spectrometer property was sensitivity. Other requirements are homogeneity and stability of the magnetic field and the frequency of the microwave oscillator to better than 1 part in 10^6. In the past, recording such complex spectra has required up to 15 hr so that long-time stability is essential. Existing spectrometers can meet the required stability for short times but the long-time requirement is still a problem.

3.4.2 Resolution Enhancement with Filters

This section summarizes briefly the enhancement methods developed and described in Ref. A-7. When line shapes are known, this information can be used to improve the resolution of overlapping lines. For example, most EPR lines are roughly Lorentzian or gaussian; therefore,

* J. H. B. Bielski and J. M. Gebicki, *Atlas of Electron Spin Resonance Spectra*, Academic Press, New York (in preparation).

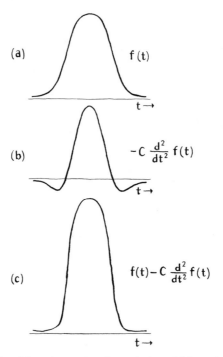

Fig. 3-9. Example of line sharpening through the addition of a second-derivative component. Addition of derivative *b* to line *a* cancels part of the wings and accentuates the height, thereby reducing the effective width of line *c*: $f(t)$ = line shape function; *c* = constant (dependent on width of line). (Courtesy A-7.)

sharpening techniques derived for these shape functions can often materially enhance the resolution. The general procedure involves mixing a series of derivative terms with the original shape function as indicated qualitatively in Fig. 3-9 where only the second-derivative component is added. Allen, Gladney, and Glarum derive the following Taylor expansions for the sharpened spectrum operator $G(t)$ of gaussian and Lorentzian line shape functions $f(\tau)$.

a. Gaussian line:

$$f(\tau) = (1/W)(\ln 2/\pi)^{1/2} \exp(-\tau^2/W^2/\ln 2)$$

$$G(t) \approx F(t) - \left(\frac{W^2}{4\ln 2}\right)\frac{d^2F(t)}{dt^2} + \frac{W^4}{32(\ln 2)^2}\frac{d^4F(t)}{dt^4} + \cdots \qquad (3\text{-}11)$$

b. Lorentzian line:

$$f(\tau) = (W/\pi)1/(W^2 + \tau^2)$$

$$G(\tau) = F(t) - \frac{W^2}{2}\frac{d^2F(t)}{dt^2} + \left(\frac{W^4}{24}\right)\frac{d^4F(t)}{dt^4} + \cdots$$

$$- W\frac{dH(t)}{dt} + \left(\frac{W^3}{6}\right)\frac{d^3H(t)}{dt^3} + \cdots \qquad (3\text{-}12)$$

where W = linewidth, $\tau = t' - t$, and the experimental spectrum is represented by a vector in the time domain with real components $F(t)$ and imaginary components $H(t)$. Only the ratio of derivative coefficients are of interest for construction of a sharpened curve.

Because of its simplicity the gaussian line sharpening expression is easiest to use and the results have been adequate, even when applied to synthetic spectra constructed with Lorentzian line shapes (A-7). Figure 3-10 shows the effect of filtering a gaussian (curve *1*) to the second derivative (curve *2*) and to the fourth derivative (curve *3*).

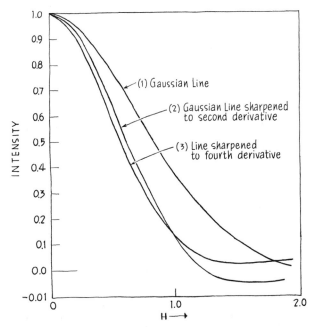

Fig. 3-10. Sharpening a gaussian line (*1*) by addition of a second and fourth derivative: curve (*1*), e^{-H^2}; curve (*2*), $e^{-H^2}(1 - \frac{2}{3}H^2)$; curve (*3*), $e^{-H^2}(1 - \frac{14}{15}H^2 + \frac{4}{15}H^4)$. (Courtesy A-7.)

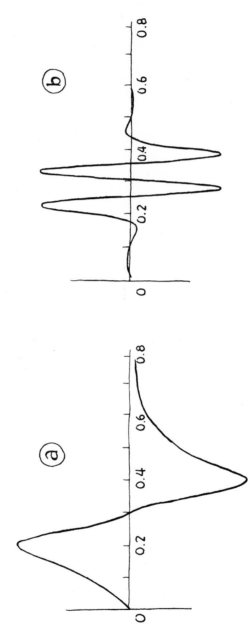

Fig. 3-11. (a) Synthetic spectrum composed of two lines of equal intensity and 0.10 units half-width located at positions 0.25 and 0.35. (b) Resolution achieved by digital filtering of (a) to the fourth derivative.

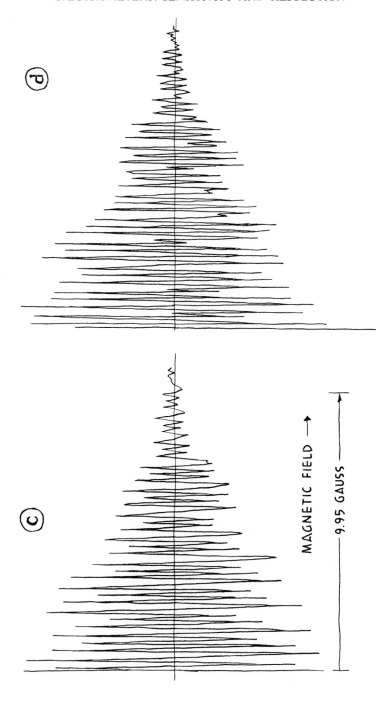

Fig. 3-11. (c) Experimental spectrum of $K^+(benzophenone)^-$. (d) Result of filtering spectrum (c) to second derivative. (Courtesy A-7.)

Two procedures have been used to perform the sharpening: (*1*) digital filtering with a computer to perform the operations in Eq. 3-11 and (*2*) analog filtering with an electrical circuit. Figure 3-11 shows a synthetic spectrum filtered to the fourth derivative and an experimental spectrum filtered to the second derivative with the digital computer. In the first case sharpening the spectrum resolves the doublets completely, thus simplifying splitting measurements. In the benzophenone example a spectrum that initially appears to be a series of triplets becomes a series of quartets after sharpening.

Figure 3-12 shows circuits suitable for mixing in a second-derivative component to sharpen the usual first-derivative presentation (*a*) or an integral input (*b*) where typical values of the circuit components are indicated. R_1 sets the amount of derivative mixing, R_{ring} prevents ringing and permits optimum sharpening with negligible signal distortion, and C_{damp} reduces the high-frequency gain and thus the exaggeration of high-frequency noise. The spectra for DPPH in benzene solution illustrate various degrees of sharpening for both derivative- and absorption-curve presentation, ranging from optimum center spectrum to excessive with destructive overshoots.

Resolution enhancement is achieved at the sacrifice of signal-to-noise ratio. Typically the ratio decreases by a factor of 5–10 with the circuits of Fig. 3-12; consequently, the technique is best suited for strong signal situations. Optimum resolution is achieved when all the spectral lines have the same shape and width; however, unequal lines can be treated. Again, two procedures are available: (*1*) the sharpening can be adjusted for some average width, arithmetic, geometrical, or weighted; or (*2*) one line-shape function can be selected so that the sharpening process will discriminate against all other lines.

3.5 CHOICE OF SPECTROMETER CHARACTERISTICS

Here we are concerned with the three design features used in our code for spectrometer designation, namely, the frequency, class of cavity, and the detection system. The considerations involved in making a choice are discussed in detail in the literature and since the various authors generally agree, we will give only the conclusions and make reference to supporting evidence. Some basis of comparison is involved in any selection so three yardsticks will be used, i.e., the effect on (*1*) sensitivity, (*2*) resolution, and (*3*) convenience.

3.5.1 Spectrometer Frequency (F-3,I-2)

(a) Sensitivity. Feher's paper (F-3) is one widely quoted reference on this subject and Ingram (I-2) also gives a complete discussion. The

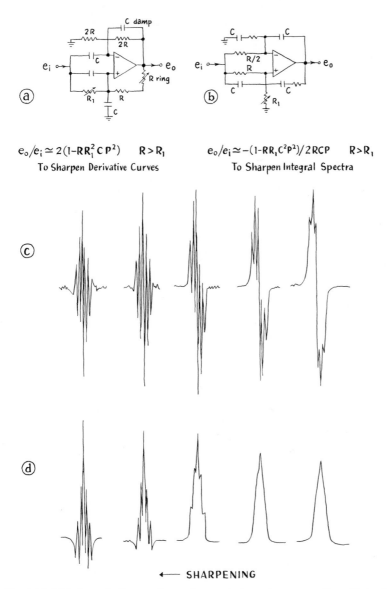

$e_o/e_i \simeq 2(1 - RR_1^2 C P^2)$ $R > R_1$

To Sharpen Derivative Curves

$e_o/e_i \simeq -(1 - RR_1 C^2 P^2)/2RCP$ $R > R_1$

To Sharpen Integral Spectra

⟵ SHARPENING

Fig. 3-12. (a) Schematic diagram for analog resolution enhancement filter. (b) Analog filter for sharpening integral lines. (c and d) Filter output vs second-derivative mixing coefficient for derivative and absorption lines, respectively. The center spectrum represents optimum sharpening. For gaussian lines $RR_1C^2 \approx (\tfrac{2}{3}W)^2$ and for Lorentzian lines $RR_1C^2 \approx (\tfrac{2}{3}W)^2$ to W^2. Typical values for the circuit components are $C = 4\mu F$; $C_{damp} = 0-4\,\mu F$; $R_{ring} = 0-5\,M\Omega$; $R_1 = 0-5\,M\Omega$; $R = 10\,M\Omega$. For operational stability, the small unlabeled resistors should be greater than the output impedance of the input voltage source. The differential operational amplifier is a model GAP R; W = linewidth. (Courtesy A-7.)

common EPR spectrometer frequencies listed in Table 3-1 range from about 300 Mc to 36 kMc and theoretically the sensitivity for a particular instrument design increases with the frequency. However, the available gain depends strongly on the type of sample being measured, the available power from the generators, and the noise level in the various components, particularly the detectors. Some understanding of frequency effects in various operating situations can be obtained by examining the frequency dependence of the various parameters in Eq. 3-1. For a crystal detector operating in its linear range the output is proportional to $(P_s)^{1/2}$; therefore, the signal voltage is proportional to $\chi'' \eta Q_0 (P_0)^{1/2}$.

Hyde (H-29) has considered these four quantities for a series of sample properties, i.e., size, dielectric loss, and saturability, observed in a series of rectangular TE_{102} cavities scaled according to the frequency. He finds $Q_0 \propto \omega^{-1/2}$ and $\chi'' \propto \omega$; however, η and $(P_0)^{1/2}$ are related to ω in a more complex manner, e.g., when there is no rf saturation, $(P_0)^{1/2}$ is independent of ω but for saturable cases $(P_0)^{1/2} \propto \omega^{-3/4}$; $\eta \propto \omega^3$ for limited samples when there is no dielectric loss, but η is independent of ω when the cavity can be filled with the sample. For lossy samples of a thickness sufficient to reduce Q to two-thirds of the empty loaded Q he finds $\eta \propto (\epsilon'')^{-1/3}$. Table 3-7 summarizes the frequency dependence for six typical samples.

Case 1. Minimum Total Number of Spins. This case is of interest, particularly where the available sample is not adequate to provide an efficient filling factor in the larger cavities, e.g., in single-crystal work with very small crystals. When there is no dielectric loss or rf saturation, the signal increases according to the well-known $\frac{7}{2}$ power of the frequency. Obviously, under these conditions there is a substantial advantage in

Table 3-7

Dependence of EPR Signal Height on Microwave Frequency for
Various Types of Samples (H-29)

Case	Limited sample	Di-electric loss	Satu-rable	Q	$(P_0)^{1/2}$	χ''	η	Total signal
1	Yes	No	No	$\omega^{-1/2}$	—	ω	ω^3	$\omega^{7/2}$
2	No	No	No	$\omega^{-1/2}$	—	ω	—	$\omega^{1/2}$
3	Yes	No	Yes	$\omega^{-1/2}$	$\omega^{-3/4}$	ω	ω^3	$\omega^{11/4}$
4	No	No	Yes	$\omega^{-1/2}$	$\omega^{-3/4}$	ω	—	$\omega^{-1/4}$
5	No	Yes	No	$\omega^{-1/2}$	—	ω	$(\epsilon'')^{-1/3}$	$\omega^{1/2}(\epsilon'')^{-1/3}$
6	No	Yes	Yes	$\omega^{-1/2}$	$\omega^{-3/4}$	ω	$(\epsilon'')^{-1/3}$	$\omega^{-1/4}(\epsilon'')^{-1/3}$

going to high frequencies, e.g., the gain is a factor of 40 in going from a 3-cm X band to a 1-cm R band.

Case 2. Constant Filling Factor. When there is no limitation on the available sample size, each cavity can be loaded to the optimum filling factor. The sensitivity is determined by the minimum measurable spin density—namely, in the absence of dielectric loss and saturation only Q_0 and χ'' depend on the frequency; consequently, the signal is proportional to $\omega^{1/2}$. Now, going from a 3-cm to a 1-cm band increases the sensitivity by a factor of 1.7. Many of the organic and biological materials studied in the past were either amorphous or multicrystalline and thus members of this constant filling factor category. Sensitivities quoted for several of the commercial instruments listed in Appendix I indicate a frequency enhancement of about 2 or 3 between the X band and Q or K band.

Cases 3 and 4. Saturable Samples. These cases introduce the effects of rf saturation into the minimum total spin and minimum spin concentration cases, respectively, and in both instances the advantage of high frequencies is reduced. In Case 4 the signal decreases slightly with increasing ω.

Cases 5 and 6. Lossy Samples. These are discussed in modest detail in Section 7.7; however, we will note here that the losses usually involve electric dipoles interacting with the electric component of the rf field in a resonance interaction so that the loss tangent frequently reaches a maximum at a frequency which might well be avoided with the EPR spectrometer. Unfortunately, the most significant dipole, namely "water," has a broad peak which extends over the entire microwave region; therefore, either a great deal of the frequency enhanced sensitivity must be sacrificed to operate below the peak or other measures must be invoked to cope with the dipoles. This loss appears in the filling factor term by the presence of the dielectric loss (ϵ'').

In summary, Table 3-7 shows a substantial enhancement in sensitivity with increasing frequency for samples of limited size over the range where $\eta \propto \omega^3$. Under the other conditions, high spectrometer frequencies are relatively unimportant and may even reduce the sensitivity.

(b) Resolution. In contrast to sensitivity, the spectrometer resolution depends less directly on the frequency than sensitivity, e.g., where the high-field approximation is valid, hf splitting and linewidth are independent of frequency. Consequently, the frequency becomes a matter of concern only in the few cases where the associated magnetic fields cannot be maintained with sufficient stability for high-resolution work.* At times

* For example, a magnet homogeneity of one part in 10^5 G limits the resolution at the Q band frequency to 120 mG, at the X band to 35 mG, and at 300 Mc to about 1 mG.

it is convenient to have two frequencies available as when dealing with a wide variety of samples or when differentiation between hf splitting and variations in the g value (I-2,A-13), i.e., hf splitting is independent of frequency where changes in g are frequency dependent.

(c) Convenience. X-band spectrometers have long enjoyed an advantage in convenience over higher-frequency instruments both in ease and economy of construction and in the preparation of many types of samples. However, these advantages have been weakened by the appearance of commercial Q- and K-band spectrometers and an expanding selection of high-frequency components. Dimensional tolerances both in cavity construction and sample preparation and location become increasingly stringent at the higher frequencies. Also, the available space limits the use of dewars or other paraphernalia inside the cavity to X-band or lower frequencies. One factor that may compel the use of high frequencies is the minimum energy $h\nu$ required to induce transitions between energy levels. In a few cases the X-band frequencies are not energetic enough and shorter wavelengths are required.

3.5.2 Choice of Absorption Cell

There are three general sample cell arrangements: transmission (T), absorption (A), and reflection (R). Each of these cells can be further subdivided into (1) resonant cavities, (2) waveguide cells, and (3) slow-wave circuits, e.g., the helix, comb, or meander line. In principle, similar results can be achieved with all nine of the possible permutations; however, practical convenience has limited general use to three or four combinations.

(a) Sensitivity. Applying the yardstick of sensitivity Ref. W-21 concludes that the theoretical optimum sensitivities of the three cavity systems are identical, and this analysis is well supported by experimental results. Starting with the expression for maximum sensitivity equivalent to Eq. 3-1

$$\delta Q/Q_0 = -4\pi\chi''\eta Q_0 \qquad (3\text{-}13)$$

they find a change in the detector voltage for the transmission, absorption, and reflection cavities to be

$$\delta V_L = -\tfrac{1}{2}E_g\pi\chi''\eta Q_0 \qquad (3\text{-}14)$$

for absorption and

$$\delta V = -j\tfrac{1}{2}E_g\pi\chi'\eta Q_0 \qquad (3\text{-}15)$$

for dispersion.

Similarly, when the analysis is extended to the waveguide and the slow-wave structures, the same expression for absorption evolves. In the paralance of slow-wave structures (S-9) $Q/2$ is analogous to $2\pi SN$ where $S \equiv c/V_g$ is the velocity of light c divided by the group velocity V_g of the circuit and $N \equiv (L/\lambda_0)$ is the number of free-space wavelengths λ_0 in the length L of the slow-wave circuit. Generally these structures in reasonable sizes will have a sensitivity inferior to good cavities because $2\pi SN$ is less than $Q/2$; however, the loss in sensitivity is not enormous and may be worth tolerating to achieve some of the other characteristics of these structures.

(b) Resolution. Resolution is a secondary factor in selecting the cavity system. As is discussed in Chapter IV, a high cavity Q is important when the frequency is stabilized by locking the generator to the sample cavity because the frequency stability is one factor limiting the resolution. While there is no differentiation between transmission and reflection cavities on this score, the slow-wave structures are wide-band devices and would require another arrangement for AFC, e.g., a type RH2 spectrometer or a crystal-locked klystron.

(c) Convenience. Convenience and familiarity have a way of becoming entwined so that separation is not always possible. In the early days of EPR spectroscopy, some schools had a tradition of transmission cavities while others specialized in reflection systems. Upon graduation the students carried the familiar cavity styles to new research assignments. Since the transmission and reflection cavities are capable of essentially equal performances, the choice was not a matter of strong feeling and some laboratories contained both types of systems. Gradually the trend has been toward a predominance of reflection cavities and several of the schools with strong transmission cavity traditions have switched to a standard practice of using reflection cavities. The universal use of reflection cavities in commercial spectrometers undoubtedly contributes to this trend.

Arguments in favor of transmission spectrometers pertain to construction simplicity and economy and to ease of operator training, which are all virtues for beginning students. For example, the type TH1 spectrometers are frequently operated without AFC, thus eliminating one part of the tuning ritual. Furthermore, the detected rf power must go through the cavity, thus avoiding confusion from unscheduled reflections. Finally, the transmission cavity is a fail safe device in that frequency shifts, loss of sample, or any change that causes a shift away from cavity resonance will result in a drop in the rf power reaching the detector so that the bolometer or crystal will escape damage (12). In contrast, a similar shift with a reflection cavity sends more power to the detector.

Unfortunately, the TH1 type is not completely safe because all of the rf power can go to the detector and with samples that require high-power levels, the detector has to be protected either with an attenuator which sacrifices signal along with the excess power or with a bucking circuit such as the one in type TH2 where the tuning procedure is essentially as complicated as that for a reflection cavity. Furthermore, the coupling hole for the bucking arm permits some of the signal to escape, thus reducing sensitivity. TH1 spectrometers can measure only the absorption component but both absorption and dispersion measurements are possible with type TH2.

Reflection cavities are generally preferred in cryogenic studies because they are slightly more convenient for fitting into dewars and the single rf connection provides a smaller heat leak. When the type RH1 is equipped with a circulator instead of the magic T, very little signal escapes back toward the klystron; therefore, the reflection system can be slightly more efficient than a transmission cavity with equal size inlet and exit coupling holes. Of course a very small inlet hole and a large exit hole can be used to achieve higher sensitivity, provided that the sample characteristics (i.e., rf saturation) limit the power level to values that are available through the small hole. While the transmission systems can be made as versatile and about as sensitive as the reflection spectrometer, the transmission systems are no better and their virtue of simplicity gets lost in the steps required to match reflection cavity performance.

Compared to cavities, slow-wave structures are not extensively used at present so that their advantages and conveniences have not been widely explored. According to Ref. S-9 these structures offer the advantages of a wide frequency range, simplified measuring procedures, circularly polarized fields, and extreme accessibility. Resonance spectra can be examined over a wide frequency range in a single apparatus without adjusting the structure, thus facilitating such measurements as zero-field splitting, adiabatic fast passage by frequency sweep, and studies of spin diffusion and cross relaxation involving the application of two or more signals of different frequencies. Of course, a source such as a backward-wave oscillator or traveling-wave maser is required to provide the variable frequency. The broad band features also simplify the circuitry because no special stabilization and AFC is required for the signal source. Frequency shifts do not introduce a mixture of χ'' and χ'. Finally the open helix, comb, or meander line structures permit considerable freedom in sample mounting and allow ready access for the application of external fields or forces. Values of $4\pi SN$ ranging from about 1200 to 2000 are given in illustrative examples in Refs. W-21 and S-9; therefore, when some of the advantages of accessibility compensate for the modest equivalent Q, slow-wave structures should be considered.

3.5.3 Detection—Homodyne Versus Superheterodyne

The choice between homodyne and superheterodyne detection is primarily a matter of balancing sensitivity and resolution against convenience. It is generally acknowledged that a superheterodyne system provides the maximum sensitivity and resolution available; however, under some circumstances the homodyne systems may have equal sensitivity and adequate resolution. It is also generally acknowledged that a homodyne system is easier to construct and operate, enough so that the majority of the worlds supply of spectrometers, both commercial and homemade, are of this type. For most measurements homodyne detection is adequate and its extensive use indicates the importance of convenience and simplicity.

(a) **Sensitivity.** The question of sensitivity centers on the best method of minimizing the $1/f$ crystal detector noise, i.e., the dominating noise at low power levels. At high power levels where klystron noise predominates, the detecting systems no longer control sensitivity. Superheterodyne systems commonly operate with an intermediate frequency of 30–60 Mc extracted from the crystal. At the time of Feher's classic discussion of detecting systems (1957) the common homodyne modulation frequencies were in the audio range from about 20 to 6000 cps. Under these conditions Feher (F-3) showed that the superheterodyne detector offered at least an order of magnitude more sensitivity than the homodyne system at all power levels examined between 10^{-7} and 10^{-1} W. During subsequent years the modulation frequency has been substantially increased until today 100 kc is standard on most commercial spectrometers and home-built instruments operating at 400 kc (12) and 1 Mc (42) are in operation. Furthermore, there has been considerable improvement in crystals manufactured for low-frequency applications thereby limiting further the advantage of the superheterodyne high frequency. In a 1962 discussion Hyde (H-27) carefully compared homodyne and superheterodyne systems operating at the same power level, modulation limits, and integration response time and found that the two systems were equally sensitive at a power level of about 1 mW. At high power levels, the extreme care required to balance the microwave bridge for superheterodyne operation makes high sensitivity more reliable with the homodyne detector, e.g., at 100 mW incident power Hyde, using 100 kc homodyne detection, found that the signal-to-noise ratio was three or four times better than with superheterodyne detection and 400 c modulation. Superheterodyne detection is still the most sensitive in the microwatt power region; therefore, it is an important consideration where rf saturation in the sample limits operation to this power range.

(b) Resolution. High-resolution spectroscopy can require superheterodyne detection if the lines are extremely narrow. Since the sensitivity of the superheterodyne systems does not depend on the modulation frequency, this frequency can always be kept below the value where line broadening occurs. Frequencies between 100 and 1000 cps are frequently used and the corresponding values of $\Delta H = \Delta \nu (h/g\beta)$ are 35 and 350 μG, respectively, compared with 35 and 350 mG for 100-kc and 1-Mc modulation. As mentioned in Section 3.4 the narrowest observed lines are about 17 mG wide, thus below the limits for high-frequency modulation. Of course, low-frequency modulation is also possible with homodyne detection at a sacrifice of sensitivity. Unfortunately, the dilute spin concentrations required for high-resolution measurements usually require maximum sensitivity. Lines narrow enough to require these considerations are found only in liquid samples; consequently, homodyne detection has sufficient resolution for all solid samples.

(c) Convenience. Compared with the usual homodyne spectrometer, the superheterodyne system is complicated by additional circuitry and a more stringent requirement on balance of the microwave bridge. Hyde mentions three reasons for closely balancing the bridge: (*a*) to keep the microwave signal level at the crystal detector small compared with the power from the local oscillator so that the local oscillator AM noise does not modulate the IF carrier; (*b*) to avoid saturation of the IF amplifier; and (*c*) to keep the microwave carrier low so as to avoid IF carrier modulation by $1/f$ noise (H-27). Experience indicates that the microwave signal carrier voltage must be balanced an order of magnitude closer in the superheterodyne than in the 100-kc homodyne detector (H-27). Consequently, detuning factors such as refrigerants bubbling in the cavity or microphonics pose more of a problem for this balance. Of course, microphonics are a problem at the low-modulation frequencies required for high-resolution work but this limitation applies to both types of detection. Also, 100-kc modulation can be used with superheterodyne systems to minimize microphonic problems. As discussed in Section 4.1, 100-kc modulation involves some complexity in transmitting the modulation into the cavity; therefore, cavity construction is simplified and there is more freedom of design with low-frequency modulation. This latitude in cavity design is frequently an important factor favoring superheterodyne spectrometers for use with cavities in liquid helium dewars.

In summary, superheterodyne detection should be used when:

a. Lines narrower than about 60 mG are to be resolved.

b. It is impractical to get high-frequency modulation into the cavity.

c. The highest sensitivity is required in the microwatt power range.

Otherwise, homodyne systems are adequate. Generally, increased sensitivity and flexibility involve more complicated plumbing and tuning procedures. It is frequently convenient to have both a simple and an elaborate spectrometer or an instrument that can be operated in several modes, e.g., RH1, RH2, and RS2, in order to readily adapt the simplicity of measurement to the problem.

CHAPTER IV

Components

4.1 CAVITIES

Few parts of the spectrometer exhibit the ingenuity and individuality encountered in the resonant cavity where the particular experiment frequently sets unique requirements and the experimenter is free to interject his own innovations. Laying aside the pride and prejudice of personal inventions there appears to be no single universal cavity that is superior for all occasions. Consequently, most laboratories gradually acquire a collection of cavities capable of meeting diverse requirements. Here we will consider briefly the function, design, and construction of cavities, covering most EPR requirements.

4.1.1 Function of the Cavity

In the EPR spectrometer, the cavity (*1*) establishes the spectrometer frequency, (*2*) contributes substantially to the sensitivity, and (*3*) may be an important factor in the resolution. Actually, *1* and *3* are related in the sense used here, e.g., most spectrometers are of the fixed frequency variety operating with some type of automatic frequency control (AFC) locking the oscillator frequency to the cavity either directly or by means of an auxilliary cavity. High-resolution spectroscopy requires a frequency stability better than 1 part in a million over times ranging up to a number of hours (H-3); therefore, an extremely sharp cavity resonance is required to permit the AFC to detect small changes in frequency. Conversely, spectrometers of type TH1 and TH2 which operate without AFC require cavities with relatively broad resonance peaks so that slight frequency variations will not drastically alter the signal.

While frequency and resolution have their place, the main reason for using a cavity is to increase the spectrometer sensitivity by controlling the rf magnetic field distribution and intensity. In an ideal infinite wave guide the E and H fields move along together in phase while in a cavity the standing waves form field patterns with electric and magnetic nodes separated so that a sample can be located at the maximum H while introducing a minimum loss due to interactions with the electric field. When the sample does not appreciably effect the losses in the cavity and no rf saturation occurs, Eq. 3-1 shows that the sensitivity is proportional to the quality factor, Q, i.e., the minimum detectable $\chi''_{min} \sim 1/Q_0 \eta P_0^{1/2}$ (A-9, H-7,L-13), where Q_0 is the Q of the cavity in the absence of paramagnetic losses, $\eta =$ the filling factor, and $P_0 =$ the oscillator power. Under the conditions where Eq. 3-1 is valid, Q is more important to sensitivity than the rf power level. In addition to Q, the following characteristics are encountered in describing and identifying cavities (G-6):

1. Resonant wavelength.
2. Selectivity factor, i.e., Q also called quality factor.
3. Mode interference.
4. Methods of tuning and coupling.

(a) **Cavity Nomenclature.** At this point a brief excursion into definitions and cavity nomenclature may alleviate confusion later on. The literature abounds in both British and U.S. mode nomenclature plus a hybrid mixture so that several systems have been known to creep into a single volume, particularly the multiple-author type. Cavities are designated by the pattern of the internal electromagnetic field as either transverse electric $TE_{l,m,n}$ modes, where the electric field E has no z component, or as transverse-magnetic $TM_{l,m,n}$ modes where the magnetic field H_1 has no z component (M-12). The subscripts l, m, n are integers which further define the field patterns by the number of repetitions in the E and H fields along the coordinates indicated in Fig. 4-1. For a rectangular cavity with dimensions a, b, and L aligned with the x, y, and z axis:

$l =$ the number of half-period variations of E and H along x,
$m =$ the number of half-period variations of E and H along y,
$n =$ the number of half-period variations of E and H along z.

Similarly, for the cylindrical cavity with coordinates θ, ρ, and z, and dimensions D and L the integers are defined as:

$l =$ number of full-period variations of E_ρ (for TE modes) or H_ρ (for TM modes) with respect to θ;
$m =$ number of half-period variations in E_θ (for TE modes) or H_θ (for TM modes) with respect to ρ;
$n =$ number of half-period variations in E_ρ (for TE Modes) or H_ρ (for TM modes) with respect to z (M-12).

The cavity mode nomenclature is expressed as given in Table 4-1. We will use the USA (*1*) nomenclature.

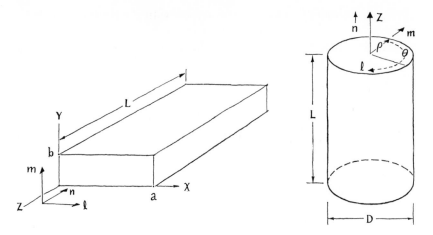

Fig. 4-1. Cavity coordinants and mode nomenclature subscripts for rectangular and cylindrical cavities (M-12).

There is no theoretical limit to the number of modes that can be excited in a cavity; however, in EPR spectroscopy the preference is generally limited to the modes numbered in Table 4-1.

Table 4-1

Table of Equivalents for Cavity Mode Nomenclature

	Great Britain	USA (*1*)	USA (*2*)
	H mode	TE Mode	TE Mode
	E Mode	TM Mode	TM Mode
Rectangular cavities			
	$H_{n,m,l}$	$TE_{l,m,n}$	$TE_{m,n,l}$
	H_{011}	TE_{101}	TE_{011}
	H_{012}	TE_{102}	TE_{012}
	$E_{n,m,l}$	$TM_{n,m,l}$	$TM_{m,n,l}$
Cylindrical cavities			
	$H_{l,m,n}$	$TE_{l,m,n}$	$TE_{l,m,n}$
	H_{011}	TE_{011}	TE_{011}
	H_{111}	TE_{111}	TE_{111}
	$E_{n,m,l}$	$TM_{n,m,l}$	$TM_{m,n,l}$

Other quantities to be used in our discussion of cavities are defined in Table 4-2.

(b) Selectivity Factor Q. The usual definition of the quality factor is (M-12,M-2)

$$Q = 2\pi \frac{\text{energy stored}}{\text{energy dissipated per cycle}} \tag{4-1}$$

and the various Q's listed in Table 4-2 differ only in the sources of dissipation included in the denominator. In an ideal unloaded cavity the stored energy can be expressed as an integral of the power density over the volume of the cavity. The varying magnetic field induces a current flow in a thin shell of skin depth δ and the energy dissipated can be calculated from a surface integral as indicated in Eq. 4-2 (G-6) where

$$Q_0 = 2(\lambda_0/\delta)(\iiint H_1{}^2 \, d\tau / \lambda_0 \iint H_1{}^2 \, |d\sigma|) \tag{4-2}$$

where H_1 = the rf magnetic field, $d\tau$ = an element of volume in the cavity, $d\sigma$ = an element of surface, and δ = skin depth in gaussian units, i.e.,

$$\delta = \sqrt{\rho/2\pi\omega}$$

In view of the rather fascinating field distributions for H_1 in many modes of cavity resonance it is fortunate that considerable design guidance can be obtained from Eq. 4-2 without carrying out the integration. If the goal is to maximize Q_0, the cavity geometry, magnetic field distribution and cavity material should be selected to maximize Eq. 4-2. As a starting point for geometrical considerations, the magnetic field H_1 is frequently approximated by a constant so that Eq. 4-2 becomes (M-2)

$$Q_0 \simeq \frac{\text{volume of the cavity}}{\delta \times \text{surface area of the cavity}} \tag{4-3}$$

On this basis a sphere is an ideal geometry with simple cylinders and cubes following in that order. Complicated designs with protuberances or reentrant surfaces will have lower ratios. Dimensionally Eq. 4-3 calls for large cavities since the volume increases faster than the surface, but in EPR spectroscopy many other factors will set a limit on the size.

Both expressions 4-2 and 4-3 show that Q_0 is inversely proportional to the skin depth which is in turn an inverse function of the electrical conductivity of the cavity walls; therefore, the best conductors yield the largest quality factors. Table 4-3 illustrates the dependence of Q_0 on cavity material, with values computed for several common conductors at room temperature.

Table 4-2

Definitions, and Equations for Cavities:
Parameters Describing the Coupling of the Cavity to the Waveguide[a]

Parameter	Coupling coefficient	Standing wave ratio	Reflection coefficient
Symbol	β	VSWR	Γ
Defining equations and expressions	$\beta = Q_0/Q_x$ $= \dfrac{Q_0}{Q_L} - 1$	VSWR $= E_{max}/E_{min}$	$E_{max} = \lvert E^+ \rvert (1 + \Gamma)$ $E_{min} = \lvert E^- \rvert (1 - \Gamma)$ $\lvert \Gamma \rvert = \dfrac{\text{VSWR} - 1}{\text{VSWR} + 1}$
Range of values	0 to ∞	1 to ∞	0 to 1
For critically coupled cavity, $R = Z_0$	$\beta = Q_0/Q_x =$ $Z_0/R = 1$	VSWR $= Z_0/R$ $= 1$	$\lvert \Gamma \rvert = 0$
For overcoupled cavity, $R < Z_0$	$\beta = Z_0/R$	VSWR $= Z_0/R$ $= \beta$	$\lvert \Gamma \rvert = \dfrac{\beta - 1}{\beta + 1}$
Range of values	1 to ∞	1 to ∞	0 to 1
For undercoupled cavity, $R > Z_0$	$\beta = Z_0/R$	VSWR $= R/Z_0$ $= 1/\beta$	$\lvert \Gamma \rvert = \dfrac{1 - \beta}{1 + \beta}$
Range of values	0 to 1	∞ to 1	1 to 0

[a] Where
Q_0 = quality factor, unloaded
Q_x = quality factor, external
Q_L = quality factor, loaded
E_{max} = maximum value of $\lvert E \rvert$ along waveguide or line
E_{min} = minimum value of $\lvert E \rvert$ along waveguide or line
E^+ = voltage of incident wave at receiving end
E^- = voltage of reflected wave at receiving end
Z_0 = characteristic impedance of waveguide or line
R = equivalent resistance of cavity
VSWR_0 = standing wave ratio at resonance, i.e., ν_0

Skin depth $= \delta = (\rho/\pi\mu\nu)^{1/2}$, meters
1. For nonmagnetic metals:
$$\mu = \mu_0 = 1.26 \times 10^{-6} \text{ henry/meter}$$
2. For copper:
$$\delta_{meter} = 0.0662\nu^{-1/2}, \qquad \delta_{inch} = 2.61\nu^{-1/2}$$

Wavelengths for rectangular waveguides:
1. Free space wavelength, $\lambda_a = c/\nu$
2. Cutoff wavelength, $\lambda_c = 2b$

where λ_c = maximum free space wavelength that can be transmitted in a rectangular pipe of width b.

Table 4-3

Relative Q Computed from
the Resistance of Several
Metals[a] (W-23)

Metal	Q
Silver	1.03
Copper	1.00
Aluminum	0.78
Brass	0.48
Gold	0.84

[a] Relative to copper.

Since the specific resistance of a metal normally consists of two terms, a thermal term proportional to the temperature and a temperature-independent residual term resulting from the presence of impurities and irregularities in the metal lattice, a further increase in Q results when the cavity is constructed from distortion-free very pure metals and when it is operated at low temperatures. Table 4-4 illustrates the gain in Q at low temperatures observed in several plated cavities operating in the TE_{111} mode. The modest increases observed for the gold- and silver-plated cavities probably indicate the presence of impurities or irregularities in these coatings.

Pursuing skin depth and resistivity considerations to the limit leads to the intriguing concept of a superconducting cavity with a phenomenally large Q. For example, lead-coated linear accelerator cavities developed at Stanford (44) have a superconducting Q which is 10^5 times that of copper at room temperature. Other cavities loaded with very low-loss dielectric materials like quartz and Teflon have reached Q's of 10^6. Unfortunately

---

3. Guide wavelength, λ_g

$$\lambda_g = \lambda_a/[1 - (\lambda_a/2b)^2]^{1/2}$$
$$= \lambda_a/[1 - (\lambda_a/\lambda_c)^2]^{1/2}$$

Wavelengths for cavities at resonance (see Fig. 4-1 for nomenclature).

1. Rectangular cavity

$$\lambda_a = 2/[(l/a)^2 + (m/b)^2 + (n/L)^2]^{1/2}$$

2. Circular cylinder

$$\lambda_a = 2/[(2X_{l,m}/\pi D)^2 + (n/L)^2]^{1/2}$$

where $X_{l,m} = m$th root of the Bessel function $J_l'(X) = 0$ for the TE modes and $X_{l,m} = m$th root of the Bessel function $J_l(X) = 0$ for the TM modes; for TE_{011}, $X_{l,m} = 3.832$ and for TE_{111}, $X_{l,m} = 1.841$.

Table 4-4

Q_L Dependence on Temperature and Material for a 12-kMc
Cylindrical TE_{111} Cavity (R-8)

Cavity material	Q_L at 295°K	Q_L at 77°K	Q_L at 20°K
Copper plate on brass	4,300	15,000	19,600
Silver plate on brass	6,200	9,300	11,000
Gold plate on brass	3,700	4,900	5,200
Zinc plate on brass	3,000	6,200	10,700

superconductivity imposes a number of stringent requirements that can
easily nullify the advantages of a high Q. First, the microwave resistance of
superconductors depends on both the frequency and temperature as
illustrated in Fig. 4-2. According to the "two-fluid" model this behavior
is discussed in terms of two sets of electronic states, the resistanceless care-
free superconducting state and the normal state of conduction in non-
superconductors (P-11). When the temperature drops below the transition

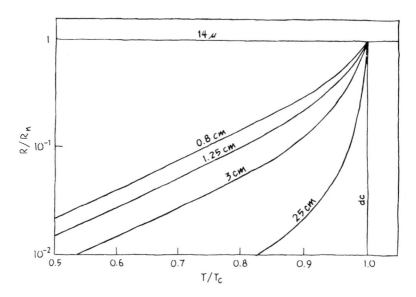

Fig. 4-2. Temperature variation of resistance of superconducting tin at various
frequencies (values given in wavelengths): T_c = transition temperature for onset of
superconductivity; R_n = surface resistance of normal metal at the same frequency
and at a temperature just above T_c. (Courtesy P-11.)

temperature T_c, some electrons enter the superconducting state, carry current without resistance, "short circuit" the normal electrons, and cause the dc resistance to drop to zero, as indicated in Fig. 4-2. When an ac field is applied, it not only interacts with the superconducting electrons to alter their course but also experiences a loss of power through interactions with some of the normal electrons. Consequently, the microwave resistance decreases slowly with temperature. Reduction of the normal electrons to a negligible concentration requires temperatures considerably below T_c. Second, many of the soft superconductors, i.e., Sn, Pb, and Hg, revert to normal conductivity in the modest magnetic fields required for EPR at microwave frequencies. Therefore, the possible materials are limited to hard superconductors like Nb–Zr or Nb_3–Sn whose critical fields are well above H_0. Fabrication is considerably more difficult with these alloys than with the single elements. Third, superconductors are superb magnetic shields; consequently, some new arrangements will be required to get H_0 and H_m into the cavity. Fourth, the fabulous Q's can be obtained only with extremely low-loss dielectrics; consequently, this excursion into superconductivity becomes an academic matter for the many situations where sample losses exceed the cavity wall losses.

Digressing for one further thought, it should be noted that a superconducting cavity should be a very sensitive device for frequency stabilization and control.

Finally, Eq. 4-2 indicates that a judicious selection of the H_1 field pattern will augment Q_0. The induced currents responsible for the losses in the cavity are proportional to the component of the magnetic vector H_1 perpendicular to the walls (K-8); therefore, the ideal field distribution would have small values of this field at the walls and large intensities out in the center of the cavity, e.g., the TE_{10n} cylindrical modes are commonly used where high Q's are required because of this favorable field distribution. Table 4-5 lists theoretical values of Q_0 for several cavity geometries and modes of oscillation along with values measured for well-constructed cavities.

To be useful in spectroscopy the cavity must contain a sample and some arrangement for coupling energy in and out of the cavity. Therefore, the quality factor of importance during measurements is the loaded Q. Since the success of EPR spectroscopy hinges on detecting changes in Q due to energy absorbed by the spin system, this form of loss is encouraged; however, other forms of loss in the sample should be minimized.

The coupling parameter β relates Q_L to Q_0 as indicated in Table 4-2, i.e.,

$$Q_L = Q_0/1 + \beta \qquad (4\text{-}4)$$

Table 4-5

Examples of Theoretical and Experimental Values of Q_0 for Various
Cavities and Modes of Excitation

Cavity geometry	Mode	Frequency, kMc	Material	Q_0 Theoretical	Q_0 Measured	Ref.
Rectangular	TE_{101}			8,900	7,000	S-24
Cylindrical	TE_{011}	10	Ag plate on Invar	27,400	~24,000	M-12
Cylindrical	TE_{011}	2.8	Ag plate on bronze	55,000	~46,000	M-12
Cylindrical	TE_{111}	24	Ag	8,200	~8,000	M-12
Cylindrical	TE_{112}	24	Ag	9,500		M-12
Cylindrical	TE_{113}	24	Ag	10,200		M-12
Cylindrical	TE_{011}	24	Cu		23,850	B-35

for a reflection cavity or

$$Q_L = Q_0/(1 + \beta_1 + \beta_2) \qquad (4\text{-}5)$$

for a transmission cavity.

Maximum power is transferred when the cavity is critically coupled, i.e., when the cavity losses are equal to the coupled impedance and $\beta = 1$ or $\beta_1 = \beta_2 = \frac{1}{2}$. Most spectrometers are operated near this condition; therefore, Q_L will normally be about equal to $Q_0/2$. This cursory statement about the coupling parameter is included here only to complete the picture of factors controlling the cavity Q. More details are included in the design section.

Another expression for the quality factor is based on the resonance characteristics of cavities, namely, the "bandwidth Q"

$$Q_B = f_0/(f_1 - f_2) \qquad (4\text{-}6)$$

where f_1 and f_2 are the frequencies above and below f_0, respectively, where the power to the cavity is one half the value at resonance, i.e., f_0. When Q_B is greater than 10 as is generally the case with cavities, Q_L and Q_B are essentially the same (W-24). The bandwidth Q is pertinent both for experimental measurements of Q and for determining the frequency control obtainable by locking the spectrometer automatic frequency control to a cavity. Figure 4-3 shows the hyperbolic curves for the band-

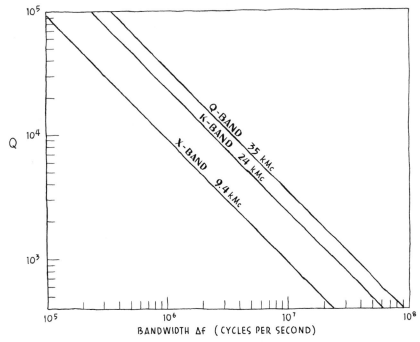

Fig. 4-3. Cavity bandwidth (Δf) as a function of cavity Q.

width $\Delta f = (f_1 - f_2)$ plotted as a function of the cavity Q for three nominal spectrometer frequencies. Depending on the spectrometer frequency, the bandwidth becomes very large for values of Q below 400–800.

4.1.2 Resonant Modes and Fields

In principle every cavity has an infinite number of resonant frequencies and can exhibit a large number of field patterns or modes of oscillation. Therefore, cavity selection or design involves some consideration of the requirements for exciting the desired frequency and discrimination against unwanted modes (W-23). The expressions for resonant frequencies of rectangular and cylindrical cavities in Table 4-2 illustrate the frequency possibilities for any fixed set of dimensions, i.e., the mode integers can form an infinite variety of combinations and as the frequency gets higher, these resonant frequencies fall closer together. The number N of possible modes having a resonant frequency less than f is approximately

$$N = (8\pi/3)(Vf^3/c^3) \tag{4-7}$$

where V is the cavity volume in cubic centimeters and c is the velocity of light in meters per second. If a volume and frequency corresponding to a conventional rectangular TE_{101} cavity is substituted into Eq. 4-7, e.g., 10 cm^3 and 10^{10} c, N would be about a million. Actually the problem is not as prodigious as the general considerations might indicate; usually only a few degenerate or closely adjacent modes require elimination. When venturing away from tested cavity designs, a chart of neighboring modes simplifies the selection of a suitable resonance condition. These charts give the relationship between resonance frequency, the cavity shape, and dimensions for the various modes of oscillation.

(a) **Rectangular Cavity, $TE_{l,m,n}$ Modes.** If cavity dimensions a, $b = K_1a$, and $L = K_2a$ are inserted into the resonant wavelength equation in the footnote to Table 4-2 for a rectangular cavity, a little rearrangement gives the resonance frequency

$$f_0 = K/a \qquad (4\text{-}8)$$

where

$$K = \{(c^2/4)[l^2 + (m/K_1)^2 + (n/K_2)^2]\}^{1/2}$$

For a cavity with a fixed mode and shape, i.e., constant K_1, K_2, l, m, and n, K is a constant and Eq. 4-8 describes a hyperbolic curve. The chart of TE modes becomes a family of nesting hyperbolas, as shown in Fig. 4-4.

(b) **Circular Cylindrical Cavity.** A similar rearrangement of the resonance expression for the cylindrical cavity gives

$$(Df)^2 = (cX_{lm}/\pi)^2 + (nc/2)^2(D/L)^2 \qquad (4\text{-}9)$$

When $(Df)^2$ and $(D/L)^2$ are used as coordinates, Eq. 4-9 results in the family of straight lines plotted in Fig. 4-5. Mode integers l and m control the line intercept at the ordinate through the mth root of the Bessel function X_{lm} and integer n establishes the slope of the line.

References W-23, M-12, and G-6 contain further information on mode charts, including plots of the mode shape factor $(Q\delta/\lambda)$ to assist in selecting dimensions for the optimum Q. For example, in cylindrical cavities the maximum $Q\delta/\lambda$ occurs for a ratio of $D/L = 1$ in the TE_{011} mode and 1.25 in the TE_{111} mode. These D/L ratios can be used in selecting the operating points. Since the shape factor has a broad maximum, the D/L ratio can be varied in this vicinity to avoid conflicting modes as suggested by the rectangle in Fig. 4-5.

The design and use of a resonant cavity requires due consideration of the magnetic and electric field patterns of the various modes, i.e., the H

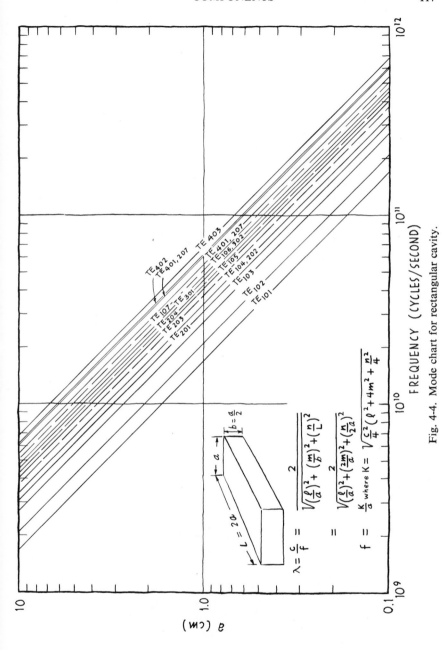

Fig. 4-4. Mode chart for rectangular cavity.

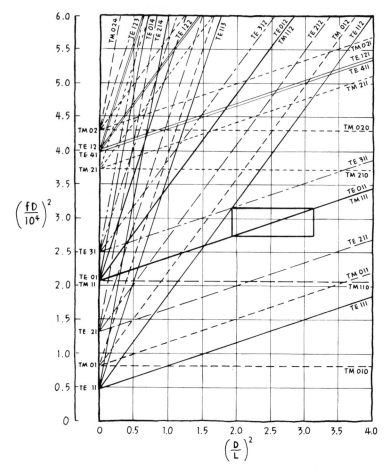

Fig. 4-5. Mode chart for a circular cylindrical cavity of diameter D and length L. Frequency f is in megacycles per second. (Courtesy W-23.)

and E fields in the cavity volume and the current distribution I in the walls. Proper attention to the pattern permits excitation of the desired mode, interference with undesired modes, efficient location of samples, and the location of openings into the cavity. Here we consider in some detail the fields for the cavities listed in Table 4-1 and refer to the literature for information on other modes. Figure 4-6 shows the fields in a rectangular TE_{102} cavity. Usually the external magnetic field is parallel to the Y axis; therefore, both components of the resonant field H_{1x} and H_{1z} contribute to the $\Delta M = \pm 1$ transitions. These field lines form squared circles around the electric lines of force which have only a y component.

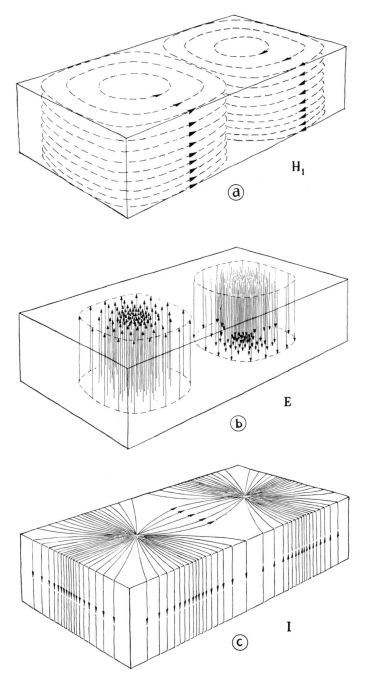

Fig. 4-6. Schematic field distributions in a rectangular TE_{102} cavity: (a) magnetic field, H_1; (b) electric field, E_1; and (c) wall currents, I.

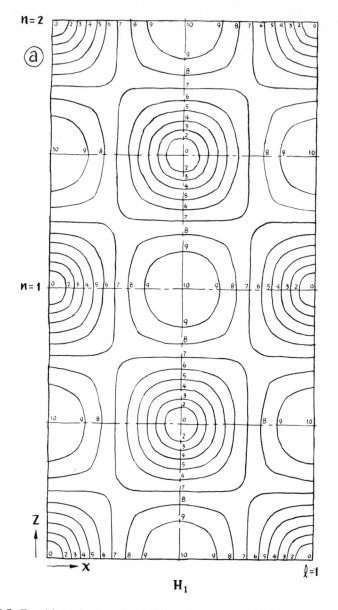

Fig. 4-7. Equal-intensity lines for electric and magnetic fields in rectangular TE_{102} cavity (M-12).

(a) Magnetic field in x–z plane, i.e., $H_1 = (H_x{}^2 + H_y{}^2 + H_z{}^2)^{1/2} = (H_x{}^2 + H_z{}^2)^{1/2}$

$$H_x = (k_1 k_3/k^2) \sin k_1 x \cos k_2 y \cos k_3 z$$
$$= \tfrac{1}{2} \sin (\pi x/a) \cos (\pi z/a)$$
$$H_y = (k_2 k_3/k^2) \cos k_1 x \sin k_2 y \cos k_3 z = 0$$
$$H_z = [-(k_1{}^2 + k_2{}^2)/k^2] \cos k_1 x \cos k_2 y \sin k_3 z$$
$$= -\tfrac{1}{2} \cos (\pi x/a) \sin (\pi z/a)$$

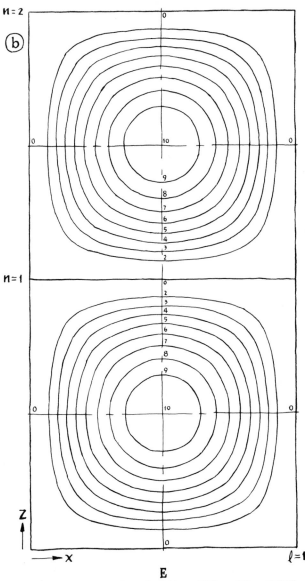

Fig. 4-7. (b) Electric field in x–z plane, i.e., $E_1 = (E_x^2 + E_y^2 + E_z^2)^{1/2} = E_y$ where

$$E_x = -(k_2/k) \cos k_1 x \sin k_2 y \sin k_3 z = 0$$
$$E_y = (k_1/k) \sin k_1 x \cos k_2 y \sin k_3 z$$
$$E_z = (1/\sqrt{2}) \sin (\pi x/a) \sin (\pi z/a)$$
$$E_z = 0$$

For geometry where $L = 2a$ and $b = a/2$

$$k_1 = l\pi/a = \pi/a; \quad k_2 = m\pi/b = 0; \quad k_3 = n\pi/L = \pi/a$$
$$k^2 = k_1^2 + k_2^2 + k_3^2$$

therefore

$$k = \sqrt{2}\,(\pi/a)$$

Figure 4-7 contains normalized field intensity plots for both $|H_1|$ and $|E_1|$ in the xz plane along with the equations describing these fields. The magnetic field reaches a maximum where the electric field is zero and vice versa, except at the corners where both fields go to zero. All of the $|H_1|$ maxima are equally effective positions for coupling the resonance field into the cavity by the usual iris techniques or for mounting the para-

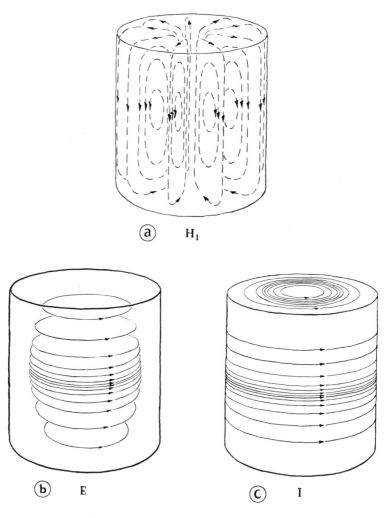

Fig. 4-8. Schematic field distributions in a cylindrical TE_{011} cavity: (a) magnetic field, H_1; (b) electric field, E_1; and (c) wall currents, I.

magnetic sample. Lossy samples, mounting devices, and interior modulating coils should be restricted to regions where $|E_1|$ is zero or nearly so, such as the midplane of the cavity. The $|H_1|$ plot can be used in conjunction with Fig. 4-6a to obtain the current distribution in the cavity walls. Since the induced current flow is perpendicular to the magnetic field lines and the current density is proportional to the field intensity, the densities and directions will appear as in Fig. 4-6c.

Field patterns in other TE_{10n} cavities can be obtained by repeating the patterns in Figs. 4-6 and 4-7 for the required number of half-wavelengths.

Figure 4-8 shows a TE_{011} cylindrical cavity with the electric and magnetic field loops perpendicular to each other. Along the cavity axis $|H_1|$ reaches a maximum and $|E_1|$ goes to zero as shown in Fig. 4-9; therefore, the axis is an ideal location for samples and their supports. Since the magnetic field intensities are relatively low at the cavity walls, losses from induced currents are small and this resonant mode has a large Q. In the end plates I_θ reaches a maximum at slightly under midradius and is zero both in the center and at the walls (K-8). Similarly, I_θ reaches a maximum at the middle of the cylindrical walls.

Figures 4-10 and 4-11 show the field lines and field intensity distribution for the TE_{111} mode in a cylindrical cavity. This mode is analogous to the rectangular TE_{101} mode except for the curvature in both the E and H field lines introduced by the cylindrical walls. Maximum magnetic field intensities develop at positions adjacent to the wall as indicated. These positions or the ends of the cavity are prime locations for the samples. This mode offers the advantage of the smallest cavity size for any dominant mode, a useful characteristic at low temperatures where dewars limit the available space.

Appendix A of Ref. G-6 contains numerous field diagrams for the various TE and TM modes propagating in circular and rectangular wave guides. These can be converted to cavity mode diagrams by registering the E_1 and H_1 nodes 90° out of phase along the z axis. Reference K-8 contains over 30 plates showing current distributions in the cavity walls for various resonant modes in cylindrical cavities.

4.1.3 Cavity Selection

Selection of a cavity for a particular experiment frequently involves a number of compromises and departures from the ideal cavity with the maximum Q; therefore a number of modest Q cavities are in satisfactory service. The designer's problem is to know how much perfection is required and when Q can be traded for simplicity and economy. Here we list a few of these considerations and discuss the relative merits of the cavities in Table 4-1.

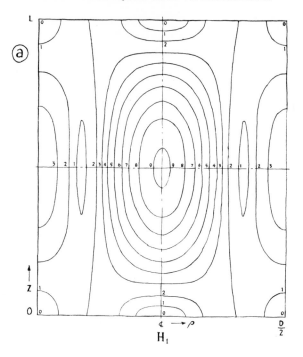

Fig. 4-9. Equal intensity lines for electric and magnetic fields in a cylindrical TE_{011} cavity (M-12).

(a) Magnetic field in r–z plane for $\theta = 0$ and $\rho = r$

$$H_1 = (H_r^2 + H_\theta^2 + H_z^2)^{1/2}$$
$$H_r = (k_3/k)J_l'(k_1r) \cos l\theta \cos k_3z$$
$$= (\text{const})J_0'(7.664r/D) \cos \pi z/L$$
$$H_\theta = -l(k_3/k)[J_l(k_1r)/k_1r] \sin l\theta \cos k_3z = 0$$
$$H_z = (k_1/k)J_l(k_1r) \cos l\theta \sin k_3z$$
$$= (\text{const})J_0(7.664r/D) \sin \pi z/L$$

Usually the magnet determines the space available for a cavity by the gap between the poles and the uniformity of the field. If the magnet is to rotate around the sample, cavity geometries and waveguide runs are further restricted.

Sample considerations involve size, shape, and electrical properties. Equation 3-1 shows that the filling factor and the Q are equally effective in determining sensitivity; therefore, when the sample dictates, it may be desirable to sacrifice Q for an advantageous filling factor.

Environmental factors, such as temperature, illumination, irradiation, pressure, and electrical potentials, sometimes tip the scales to favor a

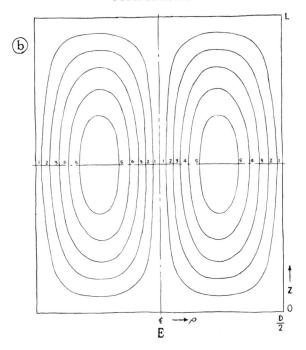

Fig. 4-9. (*b*) Electric field in r–z plane for $\theta = 0$

$$E_1 = (E_r^2 + E_\theta^2 + E_z^2)^{1/2}$$

$$E_r = -l(J_l(k_1 r)/k_1 r)\sin l\theta \sin k_3 z = 0, \qquad k_1 = 2x_{lm}/D$$

$$E_\theta = -J_l'(k_1 r)\cos l\theta \sin k_3 z, \qquad k_1 = (2 \times 3.832/D)$$

$$= -J_0'(7.664 r/D)\sin(\pi z/L), \qquad k_3 = n\pi/L$$

$$E_z = 0, \qquad k^2 = k_1^2 + k_3^2$$

particular geometry and often determine the details of construction, e.g., the number and type of samples frequently determine the selection between internal and external dewars and therefore the most suitable resonant modes. Also the EPR variables under measurement have their effect, particularly when standards or yardsticks must be included in the cavity.

The three common EPR cavity modes exhibit the following advantages and weaknesses.

(a) **Rectangular TE$_{10n}$ Mode.** (*1*) This mode fits in a narrower magnet gap than any other mode. Normally the thickness b is the width of the appropriate waveguide but the resonance frequency does not change if the

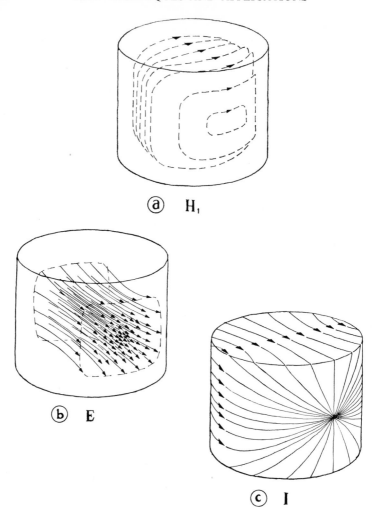

Fig. 4-10. Schematic field distributions in a cylindrical TE_{111} cavity: (a) magnetic field, H_1; (b) electric field, E_1; (c) wall currents, I.

cavity is made thinner to accommodate the magnet gap or thicker to accept large samples or internal dewars.

(2) Rotating the magnetic field with respect to the sample axis is usually achieved by rotating the sample in the cavity. A rotating magnet can be used with the sample orientation of Fig. 4-12a, although rotating the high-frequency modulation field H_m may become a little problem because of lack of symmetry.

(3) Samples with size and geometry sufficient to fill the entire b dimension as indicated in Fig. 4-12b provide the optimum filling factor, i.e., thin-sheet type samples are ideal. When samples are dielectrically lossy like water, the product of the filling factor and loaded Q, i.e., ηQ_L, can be made higher for this cavity than for the cylindrical modes (S-23); therefore, rectangular cavities are attractive for biological and aqueous solution specimens. Comparisons between samples are conveniently made in TE_{104} cavities with the specimens located as indicated in Fig. 4-12c. The second position may be reserved for a yardstick in quantitative measurements of the number of spins in the unknown sample or for a standard in determining g values.

(4) Rectangular cavities are commonly used for measurements over a wide range of temperatures with either internal or external dewars. The small cross section ab will fit modest-sized external dewars.

(5) Access for inserting samples and dewars or for introducing illumination is fairly convenient through appropriate openings in the four narrow walls of the cavity.

(b) Cylindrical TE_{011} Mode. (1) When a narrow magnet gap is involved, this mode may be ruled out because of the large cavity diameter.

(2) The symmetrical geometry is ideal when the magnet is to be rotated. Also, the symmetry of the rf field is an advantage when the sample is to be rotated.

(3) Because of the high Q this cavity is ideal when the sample is limited to a small specimen with low dielectric losses. Small samples are mounted in the high H_1 field along the cavity axis while large samples can be located around the walls as indicated in Fig. 4-12d; however, the modest magnetic field strengths next to the wall reduce the effectiveness of this location.

(4) Temperature control with external dewars may well generate a space problem because of the cavity size; however, this mode is optimum for internal dewars because large holes can be drilled in the ends of the cavity without destroying the Q.

(5) Access to the interior either through the ends or the side walls is excellent because the small wall currents permit numerous access slits. Since there are no radial or axial currents, the ends can be completely separated from the cavity walls; consequently, this mode is very practical for an adjustable-frequency cavity. A minor advantage is the ease of machining and cleaning, especially when the ends are removable.

(c) Cylindrical TE_{111} Mode. (1) This mode gives the smallest possible cylindrical cavity, therefore, it is advantageous for narrow pole gaps and external dewars.

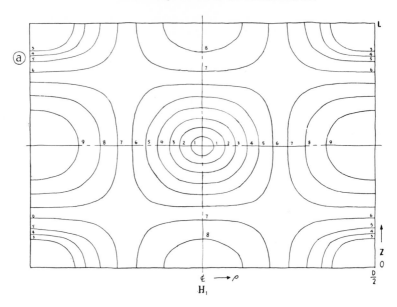

Fig. 4-11. Equal intensity lines for electric and magnetic fields in a cylindrical TE$_{111}$ cavity where $(D/L)^2 = 2$.

(a) Magnetic field in r–z plane when $\theta = 0$ and $\rho = r$

$$H_1 = (H_r{}^2 + H_\theta{}^2 + H_z{}^2)^{1/2}$$
$$H_r = (k_3/k)J_l'(k_1 r) \cos l\theta \cos k_3 z$$
$$= 0.637 J_1'(3.682r/D) \cos \pi z/L$$
$$H_\theta = -l(k_3/k)[J_l(k_1 r)/k_1 r] \sin l\theta \cos k_3 z = 0$$
$$H_z = (k_1/k)J_l(k_1 r) \cos l\theta \sin k_3 z$$
$$= 0.637 J_1(3.682r/D) \sin \pi z/L$$

(2) Rotating magnets and samples encounter the same complications found with the rectangular TE$_{101}$ mode because the fields are analogous.

(3) Where temperature control of the sample is crucial and the sample is being warmed significantly by the microwave power, e.g., in pulse relaxation experiments, the good thermal contact possible with samples mounted against the cavity wall make this mode superior to the TE$_{011}$ for temperature control.

(4) Ease of construction and cleaning are comparable to other cylindrical cavities but accessibility is limited by the relatively few positions where holes can be cut in the walls without disturbing the current flow.

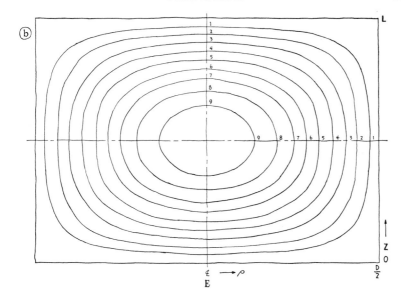

Fig. 4-11. (*b*) Electric field in r–z plane when $\theta = 0$

$$E_r = [-lJ_l(k_1 r)/k_1 r] \sin l\theta \sin k_3 z = 0$$
$$E_\theta = -J_l'(k_1 r) \cos l\theta \sin k_3 z$$
$$\quad = -J_1'(3.682 r/D) \sin(\pi z/L)$$
$$E_z = 0$$

4.1.4 Design Factors

(a) Openings and Joints in Cavities. Since usable cavities are never perfect enclosures, it is necessary to locate holes and joints where they will produce a minimum disturbance in the cavity fields. The rule is "minimize the interruption of the currents flowing in the cavity walls," which means that holes should be located at points of minimum current intensity and cuts should follow the lines of current flow. Figure 4-13 shows suitable locations for cuts in three cavities in accordance with the current-flow diagrams in Figs. 4-6, 4-8, and 4-10. In the rectangular TE_{102} mode, construction joints along the center lines indicated are parallel to the current flow and therefore are not very critical. Joints at other positions require excellent electrical contacts to minimize ohmic losses, e.g., in cavities formed by attaching ends to a piece of waveguide. The rectangles indicate points of minimum current density suitable for sample

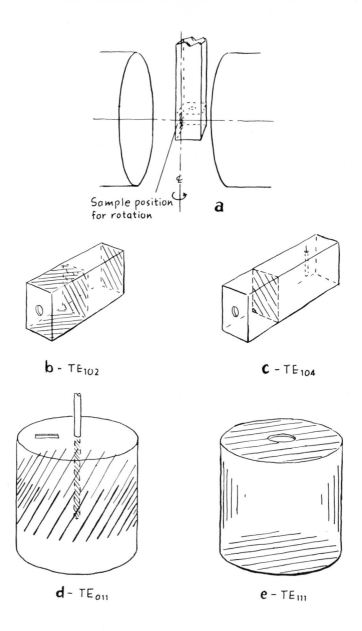

Fig. 4-12. Location of samples for optimum filling factor, i.e., located in regions of maximum magnetic field intensity.

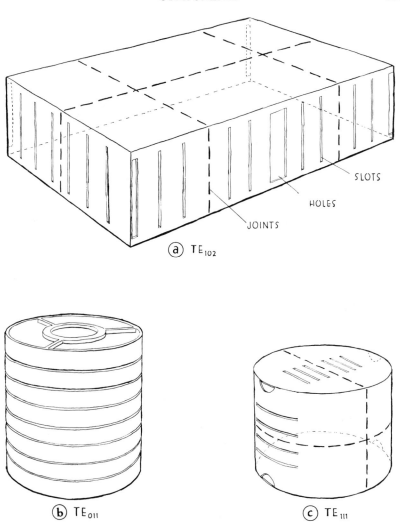

(a) TE_{102}

SLOTS

HOLES

JOINTS

(b) TE_{011}

(c) TE_{111}

Fig. 4-13. Location of slots, cuts, and holes to minimize interference with cavity wall currents.

access holes. Losses due to the electromagnetic field leaking through these holes are normally reduced by a waveguide extension too small in cross section to propagate the cavity resonant frequency. A series of parallel slots in the edges of the cavity frequently provide access for illumination or high-frequency modulation of samples attached to the walls. Slots about $\frac{1}{16}$ in. wide and spaced to remove half the surface are adequate.

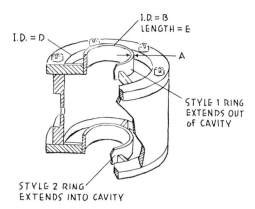

Fig. 4-14. Open-ended cylindrical TE_{011} cavity showing two end modifications that sacrifice very little Q. (After T-1.)

A cylindrical TE_{011} cavity places few restrictions on joints because it can be cut anywhere along the cylinder or ends as long as the cuts are as indicated in Fig. 4-13b. Since no currents cross the junction between the cylindrical wall and the end, no electrical contact is required. Furthermore, most of the end material can be removed without great loss of Q. For example, Ref. T-1 describes a series of cavity modifications in which about 90% of the end-plate area was removed with less than a 30% drop in Q. Figure 4-14 and Table 4-6 summarize some of the results of

Table 4-6

Change in Cavity Q with Opening Dimensions for the TE_{011} Cavity in Fig. 4-14 (T-1)

Style	Dimensions, in.				v_0, Mc	Q_L	Per cent of end open
	A	B	D	E			
1	$\frac{1}{16}$	0.850	1.90	0.5	8951	3000	90.6
1	$\frac{1}{16}$	1.125	1.90	0.5	8953	4080	89.6
1	$\frac{1}{16}$	0.938	1.90	0.5	9021	4920	90.3
1	$\frac{1}{16}$	1.031	1.90	0.5	8971	4688	90.0
1	$\frac{1}{32}$	1.094	1.90	0.5	8961	3815	93.6
2	$\frac{1}{16}$	1.031	1.67	0.5	9233	8817	88
2	$\frac{1}{16}$	0.817	1.67	0.55	9254	7416	89
2	$\frac{1}{16}$	1.010	1.635	0.448	9381	7721	92.6
Solid end covers					9345	11,000	0

that study. All of the variables were not examined in detail; however, several suggestions for increasing the Q for style-2 plates are that (1) the ring should be located where the magnetic field has no z component, (2) the ring length E should be at least 0.500 in.; and (3) the ring thickness should be kept as large as possible, preferably at least $\frac{1}{16}$ in.

The cylindrical TE_{111} cavity is again analogous to its rectangular counterpart, i.e., it can be cut lengthwise and at the $\lambda/4$ point as indicated in Fig. 4-13c. Slot and hole locations also follow the pattern for the rectangular cavity, but the curved current flow lines will encounter more interference with straight slots in the ends of a cylindrical cavity.

(b) Materials and Surfaces. It is easy to specify the ideal material and surface for maximizing the cavity Q but it is difficult to select the best compromise for a particular experimental situation; consequently, this is a fruitful subject for witchcraft and the practices are many and varied. We will start with the ideal case, then consider some of the experimental factors responsible for compromises, and finally list some of the materials in use along with their advantages and disadvantages.

From the standpoint of maximum Q, very pure silver is the metal of choice for nonsuperconducting cavities because of its superior electrical conductivity throughout the temperature range of EPR experiments. With reference to Table 4-3, copper is a close second choice and gold a rather feeble third. The surface should be optically smooth, free from external impurities such as oxides, sulfates, waxes, and grits left from the polishing operation, and free from internal irregularities in crystal structure—either native or produced by work hardening during machining. These pure metals are difficult to machine and the surface is always disturbed in this operation; also the surfaces of Cu and Ag corrode readily when in contact with the air. Consequently, the nearly ideal cavity is seldom ever found and fortunately never required. At microwave frequencies electrical conductivity is largely a surface phenomenon; therefore, the characteristics that describe a surface require consideration, i.e., roughness, porosity, corrosion, composition, and resistivity. In Ref. V-11, von Baeyer considers these parameters in considerable detail, either directly or by reference. Recalling that $Q \sim (1/\rho)^{1/2}$, the other factors can easily dominate in a comparison of materials such as Ag and Cu where resistances are comparable. Roughness is a geometrical factor which increases the path length for current flow. When surface irregularities are small compared with the skin depth, this increase becomes negligible. In Ag and Cu at X-band or higher frequencies, this criterion imposes limits of a few microinches, e.g., at 1 kMc the skin depth for silver is about 100 μin. Unfortunately irregularities of 600 μin. can readily occur

Table 4-7

Effects of Treatment and Aging on the Surface Resistivity of three Cavity Materials (V-11)

Freq., kMc	Copper	r^a	Coin silver	r^a	Silver plating	r^a
1					Fresh silver plating with rhodium flash measured relative to measured value for Cu	0.83
3	Drawn wire, oxidized surface	1.19	Drawn rod, oxidized surface	1.08	Silver-plated brass guides	1.34
5	Drawn wire, oxidized surface	1.21	Drawn rod, oxidized surface	1.31		
7			Drawn waveguide, oxidized surface	1.29		
9	Commercial wire	1.135	Commercial alloy	1.16	Immediately after silver plating, depends on plating	1.37–2.27
	Immediately after electro polishing	1.02			Immediately after silver plating, depends on buffing	1.23–2.05
	18 weeks after electro-polishing	1.12			Immediately after silver plating on brass	1.58
	Aged out of doors 4½ months	1.41			Silver plated from cyanide bath	1.58
10	Normal drawn copper waveguide	1.102 to 1.120				
15	Drawn waveguide, oxidized surface	1.32	Drawn waveguide, oxidized surface	1.28	After aging, periodic reversing process	1.33
35	Drawn waveguide, oxidized surface	1.6	Drawn waveguide, oxidized surface	1.73	Few months after aging	up to 2.60
			Drawn waveguide, aged	1.65	After aging, periodic reverse process	1.74

^{a} $r = R_s'/R_s$ = measured value/theoretical value. Here $r = R_s'/R_s$ for copper where $R_s = (\mu\omega/2\sigma)^{1/2}$; σ = dc conductivity; μ = permeability; and $\omega = 2\pi f$.

in silver-plated surfaces, thereby nullifying the benefits of low resistivity. For this reason results obtained with ordinary silver plating are often very disappointing.

Reductions in Q resulting from surface corrosion and aging may be a matter of either roughening if the reaction products are good insulators or ohmic losses if the surface layer is a fair conductor. The corrosion products of Ag and Cu apparently are fair conductors; therefore, they increase the ohmic losses. When corrosion is removed, surface conductivity does not return completely to its initial value, probably because of roughness. Table 4-7 illustrates the properties of three surfaces, i.e., copper, coin silver, and silver plating at various frequencies and surface conditions (V-11). The ratio of measured-to-theoretical surface resistance increases with frequency and aging and is generally largest for the plated surface. Apparently the plating and buffing conditions have a pronounced effect.

Coatings such as a thin gold or rhodium flash can improve the aging characteristics of silver plate and DuPont clear lacquer can provide protection for pure copper with negligible losses to X-band frequencies. When cavities are plated, the substrate should meet the limitations on roughness and the coating should be of uniform thickness. Bussey has studied the effects of material and surface condition on what he calls Q depths and apparent resistivities (B-35). In materials where the permeability $\mu = \mu_0$, the Q depth is equal to the skin depth δ; therefore, the ideal surface has a minimum Q depth. Table 4-8 lists some of his results for a 9.2 kMc TE_{011}-mode cylindrical cavity where the test surface formed one end of the cavity. All final machining cuts were made with a diamond tool which produced less tearing and disturbance of the surface than conventional cutting tools. Annealing the copper changes the resistance about 1% and the presence of a 4 year old oxide film increases the skin depth about 3%. Silver plating produced a significant improvement on lossy materials such as brass and iron, but was ineffective over pure copper, apparently because the electrolytically deposited silver had a conductivity about 7% lower than bulk silver. Few laboratories sport silver cavities but oxygen-free high-purity copper (OFHC) is frequently used because it is almost as good as silver.

The most involved compromises in material are introduced by the use of external coils for high-frequency modulation. Here the skin depth must be thick enough at microwave frequencies to trap the internal cavity field, but thin enough at the modulation frequency to permit efficient modulation. Table 4-9 lists typical skin depths for several common microwave and modulation frequencies. Some other reasons for departing from solid Ag and Cu wall thicknesses are: (*1*) ease of construction; (*2*) corrosive

Table 4-8

Q Depths and Apparent Resistivities of Flat Cavity Ends of Various
Materials and Finishes (B-35)

Material	Finish, μin. (rms)	Q Depth, μin.[a]	Apparent resistivity, $\mu\Omega$ cm	dc Resistivity, $\mu\Omega$ cm
Electrolytic Cu	5	28.5	1.90	1.75
Same Cu deoxidized	6	27.6	1.79	1.75
Pb–Cu	15	30.3	2.15	1.76
Pb–Cu	22	31.2	2.28	1.76
Ag plated on brass or Cu	5–10	28.5	1.90	1.63[b]
Ag as above and diamond cut	6	28.2	1.86	1.63[b]
Ag plated on Invar	6	29.1	1.98	1.63[b]
Invar	3	560		81[b]

[a] Q depth = real part of $S^* = \delta_0$, the usual skin depth: $S^* = 2Z^*/\omega\mu_0$ where Z^* is the wall impedance.

[b] *Handbook of Chemistry and Physics*, 1965 values.

samples that would react with these metals, e.g., gas samples that fill the entire cavity for maximum sensitivity; (*3*) the low Q's obtained with other materials are completely adequate. Reasons *1* and *3* explain the prevalence of many brass cavities, frequently unplated. Brass is the butter of the machine shop; it machines easily and is readily assembled, both with soft and silver solders. In contrast soft Ag and Cu require care and patience in machining and a controlled atmosphere for good silver solder joints. Finally, most commercial *X*- and *Q*-band hardware is manufactured from brass. When brass cavities are made for high-precision *g*-value measurements, the brass should be checked for paramagnetic impurities which can distort the magnetic fields in the cavity (*6*).

The controlled-skin-depth cavities all involve a substrate which supplies the mechanical strength and a thin coating of silver or copper to control the electrical properties. Three general types of substrates are commonly encountered: (*1*) high-resistance metals; (*2*) inorganic dielectrics such as quartz, ceramics, and glasses; and (*3*) organic dielectrics, particularly the epoxy compounds. Suitable metal substrates will normally be the same metals selected for thermal isolation of low-temperature cavities (i.e., stainless steel and nickel silver). Here the chief advantage is ease of construction since only conventional machine shop and plating operations are involved. Disadvantages are loss of modulation power in the substrate,

Table 4-9
Skin Depths for Various Materials and Frequencies

Metal	ρ, $\mu\Omega$ cm[a]	\multicolumn{6}{c}{Skin depth δ in mils at}
		10^2 cps	10^3 cps	10^5 cps	10^6 cps	10^{10} cps	10^{11} cps
Silver	1.63	250	79	7.9	2.5	0.025	0.0079
Copper	1.72	260	82	8.2	2.6	0.026	0.0082
Gold	2.44	310	98	9.8	3.1	0.031	0.0098
Aluminum	2.65	320	102	10.2	3.2	0.032	0.010
Brass	7.00	520	166	16.6	5.2	0.052	0.017
Iron	10	630	198	19.8	6.3	0.063	0.020
Lead	22	930	293	29.3	9.3	0.093	0.029
German silver	33	1140	359	35.9	11.4	0.114	0.036
Monel	42	1280	405	40.5	12.8	0.128	0.041
Constanten	44	1320	415	41.5	13.2	0.132	0.042
Invar steel	81	1780	563	56.3	17.8	0.178	0.056
Climax	87	1850	583	58.3	18.5	0.185	0.058
Excello	92	1900	600	60.0	19.0	0.190	0.060
Nichrome	150	2420	766	76.6	24.2	0.24	0.077

[a] *Handbook of Chemistry and Physics*, 1965 values:

$$\delta = (\rho/\pi\mu f)^{1/2}$$

where $\mu = 4\pi \times 10^{-7}$ henry/meter.

and some sacrifice of rigidity because of the thin sections required, e.g., 304 Stainless Steel walls 0.018 in. thick have been used successfully with 100 kc modulation (F-10).

The inorganic dielectrics find extensive use in commercial cavities because high rigidity and precision can be achieved with essentially no attenuation of the modulation signal in the substrate. Fused quartz is favored where low thermal expansion is desirable; however, Pyrex, various alumina, magnesia, and zirconia ceramics, and natural talc* or soapstone are also in use. These materials exhibit excellent dimensional properties; therefore, when a highly conducting metal coating is obtained, the cavity Q value can be very close to the theoretical value. The problems with these materials usually involve the coatings and arrangements for attaching the ceramic parts to the rest of the system.

Organic dielectrics are readily formed into cavities either by casting or machining, and modulation field losses in the substrate are negligible. The main construction problem involves the conducting coating; thus,

* Talc is available as Grade A Lava from the American Lava Corp., Chattanooga, Tenn.

most of the folklore consists of formulas for good coatings. All of the plastics in use have substantial thermal-expansion coefficients so that the cavity frequency is sensitive to slight temperature changes.

(c) Tolerances. The literature contains numerous cavity designs and notes on construction but frighteningly little quantitative information about tolerances; consequently, the question of tolerances was raised in practically all laboratories visited during this survey. One answer was almost universal, namely, "We tell the machinist to do a careful job," but unfortunately, most instrumentalists do not measure quantitatively what this means in the finished cavity, particularly when the cavity was adequate for the experiment. Thus, there is no conversion factor to go from "a careful job" to fractions of an inch. Before giving some examples of cavities we will consider which dimensions require tolerances.

Usually the cavity length, diameter, etc. is not highly critical because it is seldom necessary to achieve a precise resonant frequency. Even if achieved, the presence of a sample in the cavity would alter the resonance frequency; consequently, adjustable cavities are always used where precise frequency control is required. Tolerances of about 2% λ_g are usually adequate for frequency purposes and these are easily achieved down to Q-band wavelengths. The dimensions requiring close control are the parallelism of opposing sides, the perpendicularity of intersecting walls, and the uniformity and circularity of cylinders. These geometrical considerations control the perfection of the mode pattern in the cavity and thus the obtainable Q. Cavity dimensions and the associated tolerances scale with the wavelength; therefore, high frequencies require the maximum precision. Table 4-10 lists some tolerances encountered in the manufacturing of cavity wavemeters, pertinent microwave components, and EPR cavities. Unfortunately, the most stringent tolerances cannot prevent field distortion when the sample and other paraphernalia are inserted into the cavity; therefore, some cavities are built with an adjustable end that can be moved to compensate for the affects of the sample on frequency and quality factor.

(d) Coupling and Matching. To achieve optimum usefulness a cavity must be coupled to the external circuit in such a fashion as to excite only the desired resonant mode and to achieve the desired power distribution. Mode control depends on the location of the coupling element while the power depends on the size of the coupling element, which may be an iris, loop, or probe. The coupling coefficient β given in Table 4-2 defines this power distribution (F-3), i.e.,

$$\beta = Q_0/Q_x = \frac{\text{power loss through the coupling to the outside}}{\text{power loss in the cavity}}$$

Table 4-10

Examples of Dimensions and Tolerances Encountered in the Construction of some Microwave Equipment

Item	Mode	Band desig- nation	Dimensions,[a] in.		Toler- ance, in.	Max. inner corner radius, in.	Cutoff fre- quency kMc	Ref.
Cylindri- cal cavity	TE_{11n}	Q	$D = 0.375$		$+0.0005$ -0.0000			M-12
	TE_{011} hybrid	Q	$D = 0.6607$	$L = 0.8584$				M-12
	TE_{011}	X	$D = 1.949$	$L = 2\frac{1}{32}$				M-12
	TE_{011}	S	$D = 6.140$	$L_{max} = 4.939$				M-12
	TE_{011}	X	$D = 1.905$	$L = 1.653$	0.001			T-2
Wave- guide	TE_{10}	S	$a = 2.840$	$b = 1.340$	± 0.005	$\frac{3}{64}$	2.080	b
	TE_{10}	X	$a = 0.900$	$b = 0.400$	± 0.003	$\frac{1}{32}$	6.560	b
	TE_{10}	K	$a = 0.420$	$b = 0.170$	± 0.0020	$\frac{1}{64}$	14.080	b
	TE_{10}	Q	$a = 0.224$	$b = 0.112$	± 0.0010	0.010	26.350	b
	TE_{10}	R	$a = 0.034$	$b = 0.0170$	± 0.0002	0.0015	173.290	b

[a] Letters correspond to dimensions in Fig. 4-1.
[b] Standard waveguide data, Narda Microwave corporation.

When $\beta > 1$, the cavity is overcoupled and the external losses predominate. When $\beta < 1$, the cavity is undercoupled and most of the power loss is due to the cavity. When $\beta = 1$, the cavity is critically coupled and the losses in the cavity equal the losses in the line; consequently, there is no reflection of microwave power at the coupling junction and the cavity is said to be "matched" to the waveguide line. First, we consider the location and type of coupling suitable for the rectangular TE_{10n} mode and the cylindrical TE_{101} and TE_{111} modes, then methods of suppressing unwanted modes, and finally suitable values for the coupling coefficient and methods of matching.

The common coupling elements are illustrated in Fig. 4-15 for a rectangular TE_{102} cavity, i.e., the iris hole and loop interacting with the magnetic field H, and the probe coupling to the electric field. In all cases the coupling is located at the appropriate field maximum and orientated so the field in the cavity and the element are parallel. Figure 4-16 shows various coupling positions and waveguide terminations suitable for coupling to the six equivalent positions in a rectangular TE_{102} cavity. A coaxial cable with a loop termination can always replace the waveguide and iris.

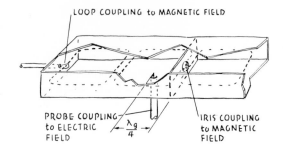

Fig. 4-15. Three methods of coupling rf field into a rectangular TE_{102} cavity.

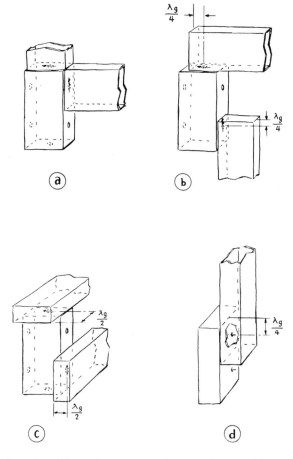

Fig. 4-16. Location of iris holes or antenna loops, and waveguide terminations for coupling to the magnetic field in a rectangular TE_{102} cavity: (a), (b), and (c). Arrangement (d) is for probe coupling to the electric field.

In the cylindrical TE_{011} mode the electric field is zero at all surfaces so coupling must be magnetic. Figure 4-17 shows coupling methods suitable for this mode. Best locations of the iris hole or coupling loop are at $0.48R$ on the ends or $\lambda_g/4$ along the z direction. The cylindrical TE_{111} mode can be coupled magnetically as shown in Fig. 4-18 at four positions analogous to the rectangular cavity. Similarly, electric field coupling is also possible.

Mode separation is a problem primarily in symmetrical cavities where degenerate modes such as the TE_{011} and TM_{111} exist. Figure 4-19 indicates several methods of discriminating against TM modes, including geometry of the coupling hole or loop, location of entrance and exit ports in transmission cavities, gaps in the conducting wall or lossy materials to interfere with the unwanted mode currents. The hole location and gap techniques are most commonly encountered. For the TE_{111} mode a wire loop over the iris hole gives the necessary asymmetry to establish the mode in the indicated orientation.

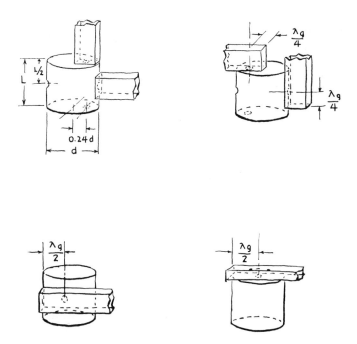

Fig. 4-17. Location of iris holes or antenna loops and waveguide terminations for coupling to the magnetic field in a cylindrical TE_{011} cavity. (After W-23.)

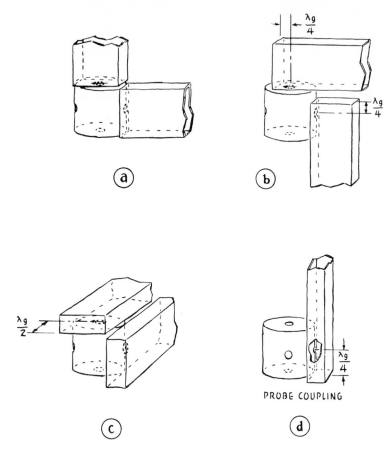

Fig. 4-18. Location of iris holes or antenna loops and waveguide terminations for coupling to the magnetic field of a cylindrical TE_{111} cavity: (a), (b), and (c). Arrangement (d) is for coupling to the electrical field.

A variety of practices prevail regarding the design of coupling elements; however, the cut-and-try method finds universal acceptance in determining the size. The difficulty in calculating the size of an iris hole or coupling loop in an ideal cavity becomes overpowering when irregularly shaped samples and supports are introduced into the cavity; consequently, the drill-and-file technique is the most expeditious. Most adjustments continue until the Feher (F-3) conditions for optimum coupling listed in Table 4-11 are satisfied by the standing wave ratio measured with the sample and all its associated containers in position. When it comes time to change the sample, present practitioners are equally divided between those who

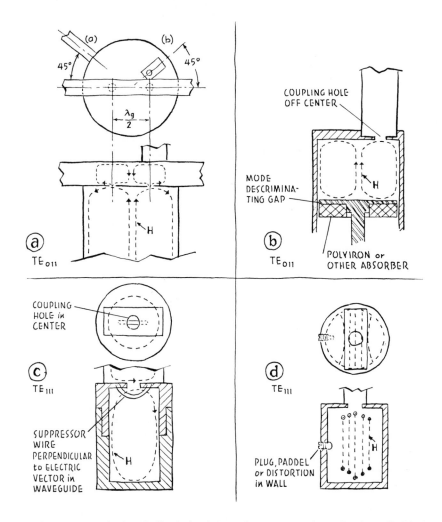

Fig. 4-19. Methods of discriminating against unwanted modes in cylindrical cavities. The two hole coupling arrangement at (a) feeds magnetic fields 180° out of phase into the cavity as indicated by the dotted lines. Therefore, only even modes, i.e., magnetic fields radiating out from the center, are excited. In this transmission cavity, locating the exit hole at 45° either on the end or side eliminates higher even modes so that only the TE_{011} mode appears. See Ref. B-16 for details. Figure 4-5 shows that the TM_{111} mode is degenerate with the TE_{011} mode. Arrangement (b) eliminates this TM_{111} mode by the gap which prevents radial current flow across the junction. As indicated in Fig. 4-8, this gap does not affect the TE_{011} mode. Arrangements (c) and (d) use protruding metal loops or posts to favor the orientation of the magnetic field, which cannot exist perpendicular to a good conductor. Slight departures from symmetry such as an elliptical cross section will also favor a particular orientation of the TE_{111} mode. The small size of the TE_{111} cavity eliminates all other modes so the procedures indicated at (c) and (d) are only to control orientation. [(a) after B-16; (b) after M-12; (c) after R-8.]

Table 4-11

Conditions for Coupling to Resonant Cavities for Maximum Output (F-3)

Type of cavity	Characteristics of the detecting element[a]	Coupling coefficient β	VSWR	Reflection coefficient $\Gamma = \dfrac{VSWR - 1}{VSWR + 1}$
Reflection	Square law	$R_0 n^2/r$ [b] $= 2 \pm \sqrt{3}$	3.74	0.58
Reflection	Linear	$R_0 n^2/r$ [b] $= 1$	1	0
Transmission	Square law	$\beta_1 = \beta_2 = R_0 n^2/r$	2	0.33
Transmission	Linear	$\beta_1 = \beta_2$ [c]	2.5	0.43

[a] Detector output proportional to incident power = square law. Detector output proportional to incident voltage = linear.

[b] The nomenclature comes from the equivalent circuit of a cavity where the coupling iris is represented as a transformer with turns ratio $1:n$. r = the cavity resistance and $R_0 n^2$ = the characteristic line resistance reflected onto the cavity side of the transformer.

[c] When $\beta_1 = \beta_2$, the transmission cavity cannot be overcoupled.

adjust the coupling element (the matched-cavity folk, MCF) and those who leave the element fixed and accept the loss in power through a transmission cavity or the increased reflection from a reflection cavity. This increased reflection can be balanced out in the magic T or circulator by introducing an equal reflection from the other arm of the bridge; therefore, we will call the second group the balanced-bridge folk (BBF). Neither group has a paramount advantage. When the samples are nearly the same, when the signal-to-noise ratio is large, and when the Rf power is adequate, both procedures yield the same results and the simplicity of the fixed coupling is attractive, particularly at cryogenic temperatures where the mechanics of adjusting the coupling become somewhat involved. Of course, when the dielectric properties of the sample change substantially the BBF have to change their coupling to avoid straying too far from the Feher conditions for maximum sensitivity; however, such changes are not numerous in many areas of research. The MCF trade extra design and construction effort at the outset for a little more ease of sample accommodation and perhaps a slight improvement in sensitivity in a reflection spectrometer. Because they are working with less reflected power, the MCF may encounter less noise of signal magnitude resulting from microphonic effects which vary the reflected power from positions between the cavity and the bridge. Table 4-12 shows some typical iris dimensions listed according to frequency and cavity type. The BBF are advised to start with a group of interchangeable irises bracketing the numbers in Table 4-12, or a smaller

Table 4-12
Examples of Iris Dimensions

Cavity	Mode	Band	Iris diam, in.	Thickness, in.	Ref.
Cylindrical	TE_{011}	X	$\frac{1}{4}$		T-1
	TE_{011}	X	0.250		M-12
	TE_{011}, hybrid	Q	0.1110		M-12
Square		K	0.110	0.020	37
Rectangular	TE_{10n}	X	$\frac{1}{4}$	0.010	15
	TE_{102}	X	0.19	0.010	H-6
	TE_{102}	X	$\sim\frac{1}{4}$		39
					40

fixed iris and a good file. Figure 4-20 will be of interest only to the MCF because it illustrates several matching devices. The inductive and capacitive tuners a and b are the simplest arrangements for room-temperature operation. With the conductive pin some type of loading, either by spring or jamb bushing, is advisable to insure the good electrical contact required for a smooth adjustment. Oversized screws work satisfactorily for awhile but soon the threads wear until poor contact and jerky electrical performance result. Arrangement c adjusts the size of the iris by a sliding leaf which must make good electrical contact along the edges where the currents are high. When the cavity and iris operate at cryogenic temperatures, the adjustments become a bit more involved and the cutoff waveguide system d is commonly used. Here the waveguide is reduced to cutoff dimensions by the metal inserts which are tapered to provide a smooth transition, thus minimizing reflections. A movable dielectric plug reduces the length of the incoming wave so that it can propagate through the reduced section, and the coupling varies according to the unfilled region. A relatively simple flexible cable arrangement adjusts the dielectric to the desired position. As a precaution against possible microphonic noise the dielectric should be spring loaded to avoid vibrations that would effectively modulate the coupling. Suitable low-loss dielectrics such as Teflon and polyethylene have large thermal expansion coefficients so that adequate clearance for motion at room temperature normally leads to a loose fit at low temperatures—thus the danger of microphonics.

(e) **Modulation.** The choice of modulation frequency is discussed in Section 3.3 in connection with spectrometer sensitivity. Here we consider only the design problems of providing the cavity with modulation coils.

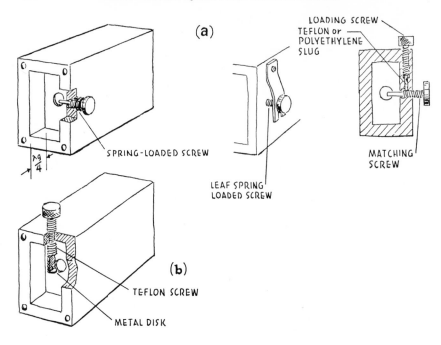

Fig. 4-20. Arrangements for matching cavities to the waveguide run: (*a*) inductive pin with three methods of loading the screw threads to insure good contact; (*b*) capacitive matching.

Three general arrangements cover the various designs currently encountered: (*1*) large coils wound on the magnet poles for low-frequency modulation up to about 500 cps; (*2*) small coils in the magnet gap or attached to the cavity for either low- or high-frequency modulation; and (*3*) coils inside the cavity for high-frequency modulation. Relative advantages of the three systems are compared in Table 4-13. Obviously, all the factors are not of equal weight, e.g., the available space frequently determines the choice without further consideration; however, barring such a limitation the first arrangement is slightly more convenient for low frequencies and the second arrangement is preferable for high frequencies. Figure 4-21 illustrates several methods of constructing and supporting coils on the magnet poles and subsequent cavity styles include methods of supporting coils on the cavity. Since the magnetic field is proportional to the ampere turns, wire size and turns can be traded to match the impedance of the power supply.

As indicated in Table 4-13 internal modulation is attractive from the standpoint of cavity simplicity and space requirements. The modulation

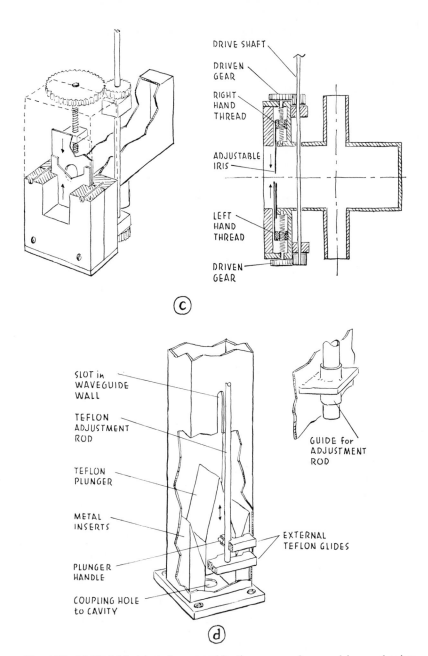

Fig. 4-20. (*c*) Variable iris hole—a combination gear and screw drive mechanism slides the movable iris plates back and forth to control the hole size (25); (*d*) beyond cutoff variable coupler. A Teflon plunger inserted into the reduced section of the waveguide brings the guide above cutoff and permits a reasonably good match between guide and cavity. [(*d*) After G-10 and 4.]

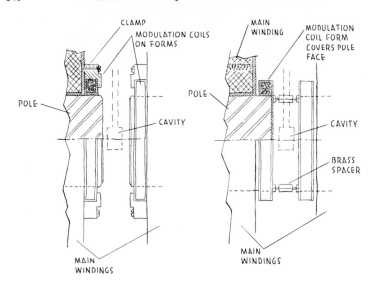

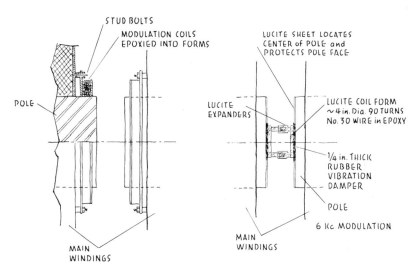

Fig. 4-21. Some methods of mounting low-frequency modulation coils on the magnet poles. Maximum modulation fields of 20–50 G are usually adequate (5,9, 27,28).

loops have been prepared by a variety of techniques ranging from judicious cuts in the cavity wall to form a modulating loop to a simple loop of wire at the electric nodal plane. Figure 4-22 shows the construction details and locations of several loop arrangements in cavities. Typically, the modula-

Table 4-13

Comparative Advantages of Modulation Coil Arrangements

Feature	Preferable for low-frequency modulation comparing 1 vs. 2[a]	Preferable for high-frequency modulation comparing 2 vs. 3[a]
Minimum space required in magnet gap	1	3
Most convenient for rotation of magnet or cavity	1 = 2	2 = 3
Largest area uniform modulating field	1	2
Minimum reduction in cavity Q	1 = 2	2
Largest magnitude of modulation field	1 = 2	2
Minimum limitation on cavity design	1 = 2	3
Minimum power requirements	2	2 $\cong$ 3
Minimum opportunity for microphonic noise	1	2

[a] 1 = modulation coils on magnet poles; 2 = modulation coils on cavity exterior; 3 = modulation coils on inside cavity.

tion field is limited to 5 or 6 G for a single loop carrying 2.5 or 2.7 A, respectively. Reported wire sizes range from 16 to 20 SWG (I-1,S-21). Effects on the cavity Q can be minimized by orienting the wires perpendicular to the E field or by locating the wires where $E = 0$. Two of the cavities described in Section 4.1.5 contain a pair of internal modulation coils arranged so that H_m can be rotated 90° by switching the external leads (see Fig. 4-30). These systems provide an effective component of H_m whenever H is rotated. In several laboratories the same power supply is used for both internal and external modulation coils. The impedance is matched with a simple stepdown transformer shown in Fig. 4-23 which plugs into the line between oscillator and cavity (S-21,31).

(f) Dielectrics in the Cavity. Dielectric materials frequently find themselves in the cavity either as samples or as containers and supports. Occasionally cavities are filled with dielectrics to permit the reduction of some crucial cavity dimensions. Regardless of the reason their presence effects the cavity performance in three ways: (*1*) the resonance wave length increases; (*2*) the cavity Q is reduced because all dielectrics have some loss at microwave frequencies; and (*3*) the field distribution is

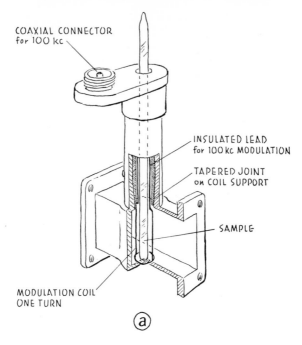

COAXIAL CONNECTOR
for 100 kc

INSULATED LEAD
for 100 kc MODULATION

TAPERED JOINT
on COIL SUPPORT

SAMPLE

MODULATION COIL
ONE TURN

(a)

Fig. 4-22. Construction details for internal single loop modulation coils: (a) free standing and (b) supported on an insulating form. [(a) from 21; (b) from 13.]

distorted unless the dielectric fills the entire cavity. When the dielectric fills the cavity, the new resonance wavelength $\lambda' = \lambda\sqrt{\epsilon}$, where λ is the empty cavity resonance and ϵ = the dielectric constant (M-12). By the principle of similitude all dimensions can be scaled down by $\sqrt{\epsilon}$ and the resonance wavelength will return to the original unfilled value. When such filling is used to reduce cavity size and a hole is left for the sample, the field strength in the hole is increased because of the difference in dielectric constants. This increase can offset the drop in H_1 from the reduction in Q. The same considerations apply to samples in dielectric containers such as quartz tubes where particular care must be exercised when quantitative measurements of spin concentration are involved. For example, Depireux (29) observed signal heights were increased by factors ranging from 2 to 3 when the samples were encased in quartz tubes. Methods of correcting for this container effect are discussed in the section on quantitative measurements. Water because of its extremely large dielectric constant is highly effective in distorting the field distribution. Table 4-14 lists the dielectric constant and loss tangent for dielectrics commonly encountered

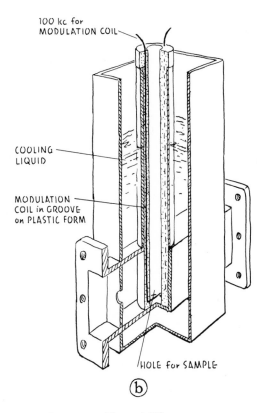

Figure 4-22b.

in EPR experiments. The dielectric constants can be used to determine permissible reductions in dimensions either for the cavities or for the waveguides feeding the cavities. A comparison of the loss tangent indicates the relative effect on Q for the various materials.

4.1.5 Construction

Choice of cavities to illustrate the book in general and this section in particular poses an interesting problem of selection. What criteria should be used to choose a few examples from the almost endless variety available? Possible bases are according to material, type of EPR experiment, or the laboratory where the cavity originated. This last point is an interesting thought, although not used. A school leaves many imprints on its students and their taste in spectrometers or cavities is frequently no exception. Here the examples are selected to illustrate the various design

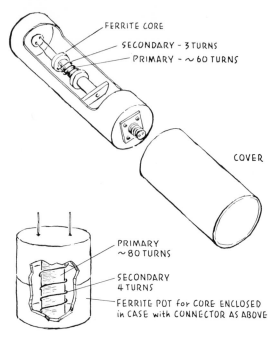

FERRITE CORE

SECONDARY - 3 TURNS

PRIMARY - ~ 60 TURNS

COVER

PRIMARY
~ 80 TURNS

SECONDARY
4 TURNS

FERRITE POT for CORE ENCLOSED
in CASE with CONNECTOR AS ABOVE

Fig. 4-23. Stepdown transformers for matching a single-turn modulation loop to 100-kc oscillators designed for use with multiturn external modulation coils. [(*a*) 31; (*b*) after S-21.]

considerations of the preceding sections, i.e., slots, cuts, holes, materials, and modulation. They are all working cavities and have been used at the laboratories indicated. No attempt is made at intercomparison because a yardstick such as Q has little meaning in view of the wide variety of compromises imposed by particular experiments; however, the strong design features are indicated. Some very characteristic designs have been left out because they are already widely described in the literature, e.g., the Oxford and Washington University transmission cavities.

(a) Examples of Cuts and Slots. Figure 4-24 shows several simple cavities machined from solid metal with joints located according to the prescription outlined in Fig. 4-13 for minimizing the interference with current flow in the cavity walls. Other features are:

1. Fixed coupling iris for the BBF.

2. Thick copper walls not suitable for external high-frequency modulation.

Table 4-14

Dielectric Properties of Materials Sometimes Encountered Inside Cavities
(All values of tan δ have been multiplied by 10^4)[a]

Material	Temp, °C		10^6	10^8	3×10^9	10^{10}	2.5×10^{10}
					Frequency, cps		
Fused quartz	25	ϵ'/ϵ_0	3.78	3.78	3.78	3.78	3.78
		tan δ	2	1	0.6	1	2.5
Pyrex	25	ϵ'/ϵ_0	4.84	4.84	4.82	4.80	4.65
		tan δ	36	30	54	98	90
Polyethylene	24	ϵ'/ϵ_0	2.25	2.25	2.25	2.25	2.24
		tan δ	<4		3	4	6.7
Polytetrafluoro-	22	ϵ'/ϵ_0	2.1	2.1	2.1	2.08	2.08
ethylene (Teflon)		tan δ	<2	<2	1.5	3.7	6
Polystyrene	25	ϵ'/ϵ_0	2.56	2.55	2.55	2.54	2.54
		tan δ	0.7	<1	3.3	4.3	12
Epoxy	25	ϵ'/ϵ_0	3.62–4.4	3.35–3.7	3.09–3.2	3.01–3.1	
		tan δ	190–770	340–1300	270–460	220–390	
Nylon 610	25	ϵ'/ϵ_0	3.14	3.0	2.84		2.73
		tan δ	218	200	117		105
Lucite	23	ϵ'/ϵ_0	2.63	2.58	2.58	2.57	2.57
		tan δ	145	67	51.3	49	32
Water, conductivity	25	ϵ'/ϵ_0	78.2	78	76.7	55	34
		tan δ	400	50	1570	5400	2650
Water, 0.5 molal	25	ϵ'/ϵ_0				69	51
solution of NaCl		tan δ				39,000	6300
Steak, bottom	25	ϵ'/ϵ_0	197		40	30	15
round		tan δ	610,000		3000	3700	4000
Apiezon wax "W"	22	ϵ'/ϵ_0	2.63		2.62		
		tan δ	25		16		
Caresin wax	25	ϵ'/ϵ_0	2.3	2.3	2.25	2.24	
(white)		tan δ	4	4	4.6	6.5	
Silicone oil	22	ϵ'/ϵ_0	2.26		2.20	2.19	2.13
DC500		tan δ	<3		14.5	30	60
Pliobond M-190-C	24	ϵ'/ϵ_0	6.3	4.0	3.76		
		tan δ	2000	1000	740		
LiF	25	ϵ'/ϵ_0	9.00			9.00	
		tan δ	<2			1.8	
KBr	25	ϵ'/ϵ_0	4.90			4.90	
		tan δ	<2			2.3	
Liquid helium	−269	ϵ'/ϵ_0	1.025	1.025	1.025		

[a] Reference: *Tables of Dielectric Materials*, Volume IV, Technical Report 57, Laboratory for Insulation Research, M.I.T., Jan. 1953.

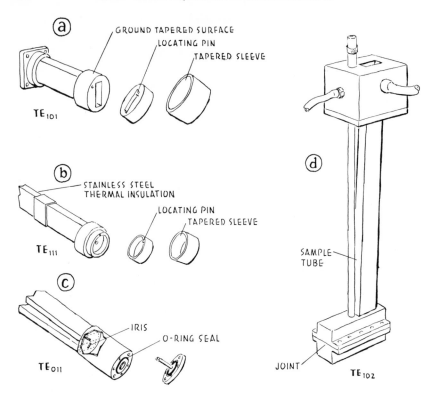

Fig. 4-24. Examples of cavities cut to avoid interference with the current flow in the walls. Cavities *a*, *b*, and *c* are used in liquid Helium and *d* is used in liquid nitrogen. Cavities *a* and *b* are cut at the midsection and are held together by the tapered sleeve which is coated with siliconegrease to seal out the cryogenic liquid. Cavity *c* is a transmission cavity; the rest are reflection cavities. [(*a*) and (*b*) from Ref. 27; (*c*) from 20; (*d*) from 23.]

3. Provisions for maximum heat transfer by direct immersion of the cavity in the cooling bath. Joints are sealed with silicone grease, glycerine or Beckman Spinco Gaskets. The TE_{111} and TE_{011} cavities were used from 4.2 down to $1.3°K$.

4. In cavities *a*, *b*, and *c*, the sample is sealed into the cavity—an appropriate arrangement for relaxation-time measurements where extensive data is obtained on each sample. In cavity *d* samples are changed without opening the cavity, which is appropriate to the numerous samples generally encountered in free radical work.

Figure 4-25 contains four examples of the location and construction of illumination slots and access holes for minimum interference with currents in the walls. The venetian blind-type slots in cavity a are formed by soldering thin copper strips into slots in the side supports. These joints interrupt the currents flowing in the wall so that good electrical contacts are required, preferably silver solder. In cavity b the solder joints are eliminated by machining the slots in a single end piece; however, a low-resistance joint between this end piece and the cavity side walls is essential. As previously indicated, the cylindrical TE_{011} mode is ideal for slots and accessibility. Cavity c consists of annular disks locked into four slotted supporting posts. The disks occupy about one-half the thickness of the openings and electrical varnish insulates the disks from the supporting posts. Commercial cavities with slots similar to b and c are available from several manufacturers, as indicated in the Appendix. Cavity d is included here to illustrate a relatively unusual access hole arrangement, i.e., cavities a and b exhibit the common locations. Cavity d is for experiments requiring the utmost uniformity in the magnetic field H. Here the needle shaped samples located with their axis parallel to H experience the minimum magnetic field variation.

Other features of these four cavities are:

1. Cavities a and b have mechanisms for matching the cavities to the line at low temperatures for the MCF. Cavity a has a dielectric wedge moving in a "beyond cutoff" section of waveguide and b contains both an adjustable matching stub and dielectric pins for tuning the cavity frequency.

2. Cavity c has a large access opening accepting dewar tips or sample containers up to $\frac{1}{2}$ in. in diameter.

3. Cavities a, b, and d fit inside dewars for low-temperature operation. The location of the sample relative to the cooling liquid in a insures efficient cooling.

(b) Metallized Dielectric Cavities. The popularity of high-frequency modulation with external coils has resulted in numerous arrangements for achieving suitably thin metal walls. Dielectrics coated with conducting silver paints, chemically deposited Ag, electroplated Ag and Cu, cemented foils, and cemented wires have all been used with varying degrees of success. Many dielectrics meet the electrical requirements of low loss at 100 kc; therefore, the main problem is a uniform high-conductivity coating. Some cavities have only dielectric structural members; others are a combination of metal and dielectric. Two general classes of dielectrics are involved: (*1*) inorganic ceramics, glasses, and quartz, which are difficult to fabricate but are dimensionally very stable; and (*2*) organic polymers, which are easy to fabricate by machining or casting but have high thermal expansion coefficients, thereby complicating their use over

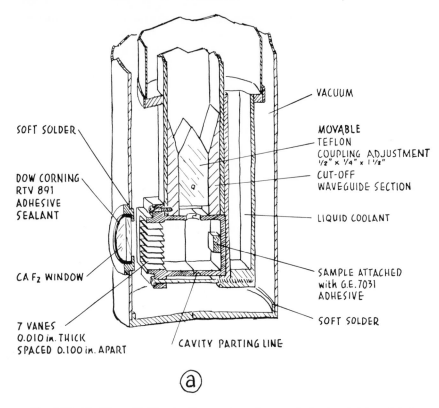

SOFT SOLDER

DOW CORNING
RTV 891
ADHESIVE
SEALANT

CA F₂ WINDOW

7 VANES
0.010 in. THICK
SPACED 0.100 in. APART

VACUUM

MOVABLE
TEFLON
COUPLING ADJUSTMENT
½" × ¼" × 1½"

CUT-OFF
WAVEGUIDE SECTION

LIQUID COOLANT

SAMPLE ATTACHED
with G.E. 7031
ADHESIVE

SOFT SOLDER

CAVITY PARTING LINE

(a)

Fig. 4-25. Cavities with illumination ports and access holes located to minimize interference with currents flowing in the cavity walls. [(a) After K-15; (b) from Ref. 30; (c) from 38; (d) from 29.]

extended temperature ranges. Furthermore, these organic materials limit the coating process to modest temperatures.

Figure 4-26 contains four examples of inorganic dielectric construction involving quartz, fired lava, and ceramic walls. Cylindrical TE_{011} cavities a and b are sections of quartz tubing ground to close tolerances and coated with conducting Ag paint, a on the inside in the usual manner and b on the outside so the coating will not be attacked when the cavity is used with corrosive vapors. Quartz has the advantages of low thermal expansion, high mechanical rigidity, and for type b designs a low electrical loss; however, shaping the cavity may be difficult with the tools frequently available. The lava chamber c offers the stability of quartz and a fairly low thermal expansion along with ease of fabrication. This natural rock has a hardness of about 1 on the Mohs scale and can be machined with

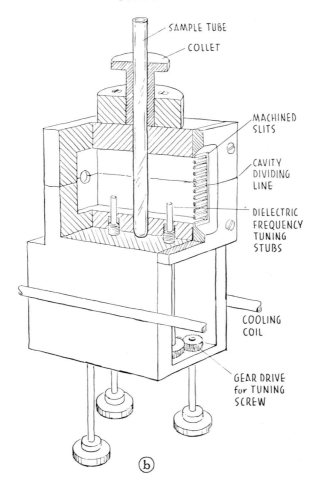

SAMPLE TUBE

COLLET

MACHINED SLITS

CAVITY DIVIDING LINE

DIELECTRIC FREQUENCY TUNING STUBS

COOLING COIL

GEAR DRIVE for TUNING SCREW

ⓑ

Figure 4-25*b*.

ordinary metal working tools. After firing the hardness is about 6. Expansion during firing according to a schedule of 150°C/hr heating rate, 45 min cure at 1100°C, and cooling in the furnace with the power off is about 2%; consequently, an allowance for the expansion is not normally required in machining, e.g., threads cut with a standard tap will accept the screws after firing. Inhomogeneities which cause warping or cracking during firing and porosity which can lead to nonuniform silver coatings are the principal disadvantages of lava. Cavity *d* combines metals and ceramics using the dielectric only under the modulation coils. Here the conducting

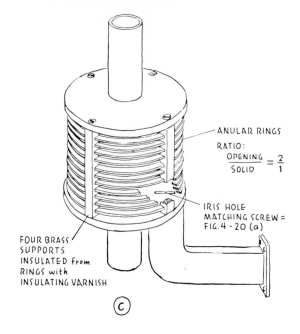

ANULAR RINGS

RATIO:
$$\frac{\text{OPENING}}{\text{SOLID}} = \frac{2}{1}$$

IRIS HOLE
MATCHING SCREW =
FIG. 4 - 20 (a)

FOUR BRASS
SUPPORTS
INSULATED from
RINGS with
INSULATING VARNISH

(c)

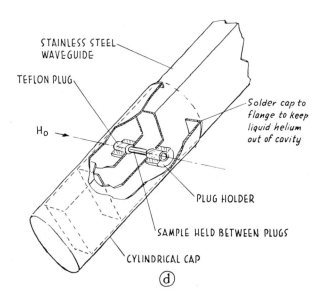

STAINLESS STEEL
WAVEGUIDE

TEFLON PLUG

H_0 →

Solder cap to
flange to keep
liquid helium
out of cavity

PLUG HOLDER

SAMPLE HELD BETWEEN PLUGS

CYLINDRICAL CAP

(d)

Figure 4-25c and d.

layer is a sheet of silver foil glued to the ceramic support with Epoxy cement. This foil construction and the printed circuit board scheme of Fig. 7.6-7a avoid the danger of mediocre electrical conductivity inherent in painted or plated films. "Fine" silver is available in thickness down to 0.001 in. from precious metal suppliers. Other features of the cavities in Fig. 4-26 are:

1. Cavity a has a groove etched through the silver coating to form a helical coil. Although the coil is used to generate the megacycle field for an ENDOR experiment the groove also improves the efficiency of high-frequency modulation. For example, Ref. C-19 reports that solid metal walls only one-tenth the thickness of the skin depth will attenuate the amplitude of a 100 kc modulation signal by more than 70%; however, wire wound cavities or plated cavities with a spiral groove provide very little attenuation. In cavity a the spiral was etched with nitric acid after the pattern had been cut in a wax coating over the metal. Cavity a is tunable at liquid helium temperatures by a gear driving the threaded bottom. A can soldered to the top plate with rose metal encloses the cavity and keeps out the liquid.

2. Cavity b was cooled by submersion in a cooling bath contained in a rectangular polystyrene foam bucket.

3. Cavity d is similar in general design and construction to commercially available dual-sample cavities except for the cooling loops that keep the cavity from heating up when high-temperature samples are measured. Quartz dewar tubes, through the sample ports, permit the samples to be heated to 500°C with hot air.

Figure 4-27 illustrates three methods of constructing plastic cavities of varying degrees of complexity: (1) rectangular cavity a is machined from solid blocks of plastic then polished, cleaned, and chemically silvered; (2) rectangular cavity b is cast to the finished dimensions and chemically silvered; (3) cylindrical cavity c is molded with the silver walls in place.

Some precautions observed in preparing these epoxy cavities are as follows:

Silvering the Cavity a. (1) Polish surfaces to be silvered with Al_2O_3–stearic acid Lucite polish.*

(2) Clean by soaking in a hot alkaline cleaning solution† for 1 min; acid dip 20–30 sec in one part HNO_3, four parts H_2SO_4, and four parts distilled water all by volume.

(3) Silver in a bath of 60 ml of $0.3M$ $AgNO_3$ and 7.0 ml of $2.0M$

---

* 1403 Plascor white high luster, manufactured by United Laboratories Co., Linden, New Jersey.
† Brass cleaner by Enthone Inc., New Haven, Conn.

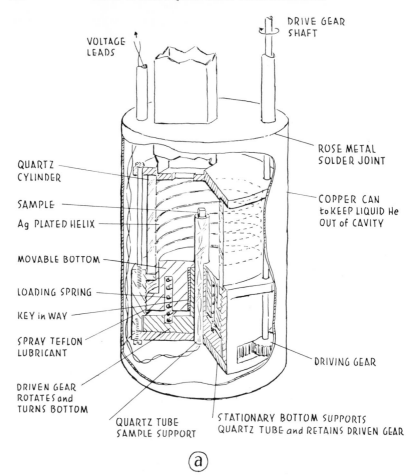

Fig. 4-26. (*a*) Tunable TE_{101} cylindrical cavity with quartz walls silvered on the inside. The spiral groove makes a Ag helix that can be used in an ENDOR experiment (leads not shown). Voltage leads permit application of electric field to sample for studies of such field effects on the energy levels. The cavity is matched to the waveguide with an arrangement similar to Fig. 4-20*d* (3).

KOH to which NH_4OH is very slowly added until the precipitate just disappears. Place cavity pieces inside surfaces down in this bath, add 12 ml of reducing solution, stir gently and allow to stand for 5 min.

(*4*) Rinse the cavity in running water and immediately apply the second and third coats in fresh silvering solutions without allowing the coating to dry. After the third coating rinse thoroughly in distilled water and dry in air. The reducing solution consists of 90 g/liter sucrose, and 3 ml/liter

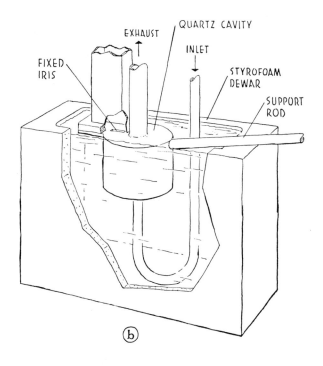

EXHAUST

QUARTZ CAVITY

INLET

FIXED IRIS

STYROFOAM DEWAR

SUPPORT ROD

(b)

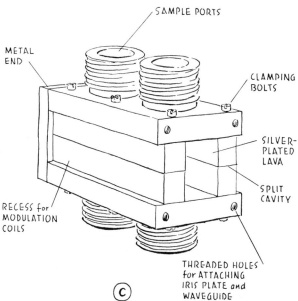

SAMPLE PORTS

METAL END

CLAMPING BOLTS

SILVER-PLATED LAVA

SPLIT CAVITY

RECESS for MODULATION COILS

THREADED HOLES for ATTACHING IRIS PLATE and WAVEGUIDE

(c)

Fig. 4-26. (b) Quartz cylindrical TE_{101} cavity for corrosive gases, silvered on the outside (4); (c) Fired lava TE_{102} cavity metallized on the inside with a coating of fired-on silver paint covered with silver plate. At high temperatures this cavity is more likely to crack than type d (39).

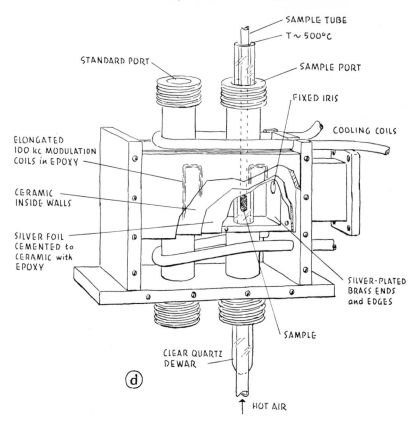

Fig. 4-26. (*d*) TE$_{102}$ cavity used in measurements on alkali metals. Exit air temperature of 500°C determines vapor pressure and requires some cooling of cavity, i.e. the cooling coils; elongated modulation coils gave no troublesome cross modulation. Ceramic side walls can be lava or another ceramic. Two possible coatings are Ag paint + Ag plate or Ag foil (39).

85% HNO$_3$ freshly made up and boiled together for 5 min. The second silvering system is prepared while the first coating is being applied.

Molding the Cavity b. (*1*) Taper the core and round the corners where indicated to facilitate removing the casting. These rounded corners also aid in cleaning and silvering the cavity.

(*2*) Polish all metal parts to a high luster and coat thoroughly with a mold release agent.

(*3*) By evacuation remove air trapped in the resin during mixing prior to casting in the mold. The container should be considerably oversized to avoid overflow during this evacuation.

(*4*) Thermal expansion can be reduced by using French chalk as a filler, e.g., filler-to-resin ratio 8:10 by weight (17).

Casting a Silver Helix in a Cylindrical Cavity c. (*1*) For X- and K-band cavities the aluminum mandril is electroplated with a 0.010 in. thick layer of silver. The spiral groove is 0.005 in. wide, extends through the silver into the aluminum, and has a pitch of 12 threads per inch.

(*2*) To insure a good bond between the epoxy resin and the silver, the silver is scrubbed with an abrasive powder, e.g., pumice, to remove any surface film and to provide a rough surface. A small amount of ground Vicor glass mixed into the epoxy was found to improve the bond.

(*3*) The Teflon mold releases readily from the epoxy* after the cure, in this case 16 hr at 170°F.

(*4*) Finally, the aluminum mandril is dissolved in a bath of concentrated NaOH.

(*5*) End plates can be attached with cement or mechanically since no electrical contact is required for the TE_{011} mode.

(c) Special Cavities. In this section we consider a few additional cavities that are noteworthy for extreme temperatures, pressures or sample flexibility. A typical example is described and others described in the literature are given references in tables.

Cavities for High-Temperature EPR Measurements. Figure 4-28 describes an X-band rectangular TE_{102} cavity used for measurements up to 1200°C. Specimens are electrically heated by platinum heating elements while water cooling keeps the cavity near room temperature. Construction details and performance are as follows:

(*1*) Cavity joints at the flange, end, and brass heater tube supports are silver soldered but the $\frac{1}{8}$ in. o.d. copper tubing cooling coils are attached with soft solder.

(*2*) Quartz heater tubes of 4 or 5 mm o.d. with a 0.5 mm wall are convenient although the size is not critical. The heating element consists of platinum paste strips $\frac{1}{16}$ in. wide bonded on opposite sides of the quartz tube except at the ends, which were completely coated. (Hanovia liquid platinum Paste No. 6082 was applied with a fine camel's hair brush and dried in air to between 650 and 680°C.) At room temperature the resistance

---

* Various epoxy resins have been used, e.g., Araldite CT200 with HT901 hardner, and Stycast 3050.

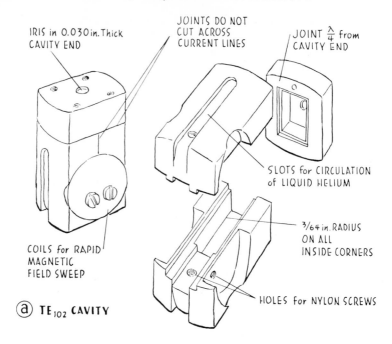

IRIS in 0.030in.Thick CAVITY END

JOINTS DO NOT CUT ACROSS CURRENT LINES

JOINT $\frac{\lambda}{4}$ from CAVITY END

SLOTS for CIRCULATION of LIQUID HELIUM

$^3/_{64}$ in. RADIUS ON ALL INSIDE CORNERS

COILS for RAPID MAGNETIC FIELD SWEEP

(a) TE$_{102}$ CAVITY

HOLES for NYLON SCREWS

Fig. 4-27. Three types of metallized plastic cavities suitable for operation at cyrogenic temperatures when cooled slowly. (a) Rectangular X-band TE$_{102}$ cavity machined from Hysol 6000 C-8 cast epoxy resin and chemically silvered. Three-piece construction with rounded interior corners simplifies machining and silvering. (Courtesy C-12.)

is between 5 and 10 Ω. When the planes of the platinum strip are located perpendicular to the electric field vector (as indicated), the cavity Q equals the empty cavity value.

(3) A water flow of 200 cm^3/min holds the cavity at room temperature during the maximum operating temperature of 1200°C.

(4) To avoid modulating the magnetic field, a well-filtered dc supply is used for the heater, e.g., 2 A at 30 V heated samples to about 1000°C.

(5) The temperature stability with time depends on the stability of the dc supply. With a regulated supply variations of only a few hundredths of a degree are obtained. Spacially the temperature gradient over the central $\frac{3}{4}$ in. of sample tube was less than 10°C at 800°C. Other high-temperature cavities are listed in Table 4-15.

Sample Changers for Cavities at Liquid Helium Temperatures. Numerous low-temperature cavities are illustrated throughout the book; however, most arrangements do not permit repeated sample changes at the low

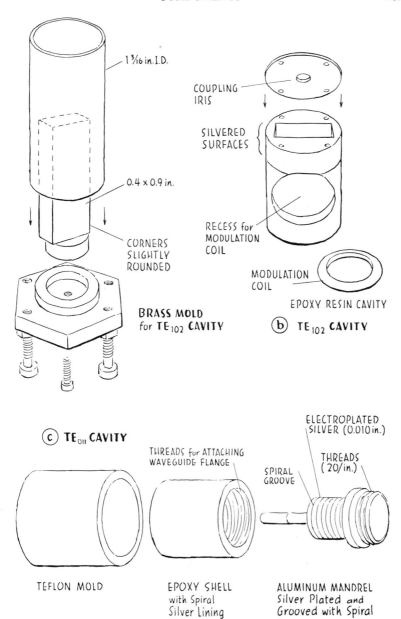

1 3/16 in. I.D.

COUPLING
IRIS

SILVERED
SURFACES

0.4 x 0.9 in.

RECESS for
MODULATION
COIL

CORNERS
SLIGHTLY
ROUNDED

MODULATION
COIL

BRASS MOLD
for TE$_{102}$ CAVITY

EPOXY RESIN CAVITY

(b) TE$_{102}$ CAVITY

(c) TE$_{011}$ CAVITY

THREADS for ATTACHING
WAVEGUIDE FLANGE

ELECTROPLATED
SILVER (0.010 in.)

SPIRAL
GROOVE

THREADS
(20/in.)

TEFLON MOLD

EPOXY SHELL
with Spiral
Silver Lining

ALUMINUM MANDREL
Silver Plated and
Grooved with Spiral

Fig. 4-27. (b) One-piece cast rectangular TE$_{102}$ cavity and the three-piece mold. The silver coating can be applied as described for (a). (Courtesy F-4.) (c) Cylindrical K-band cavity with band and groove silver lining construction, aluminum mandril, and Teflon mold. (Courtesy C-19.)

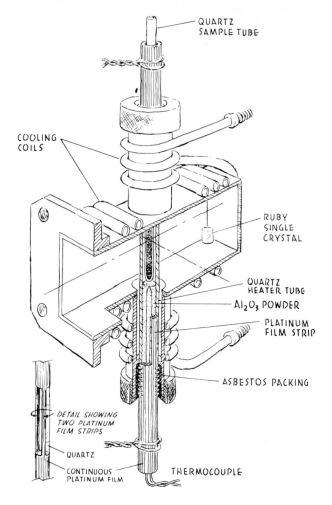

Fig. 4-28. Microwave cavity for high-temperature electron spin resonance measurements. (Courtesy S-11.)

pressures involved in the cavity of Fig. 4-29 (E-1). A TE_{011} cylindrical cavity is illustrated; however, the sample changing technique will work also with rectangular cavities. The object is to change samples without admitting air which can freeze and block further sample manipulations. Samples are inserted and removed in a Teflon capsule which screws into a brass plug soldered to a thin-walled stainless steel tube handle. The two O-ring seals and the plug valve exclude air during operations as follows.

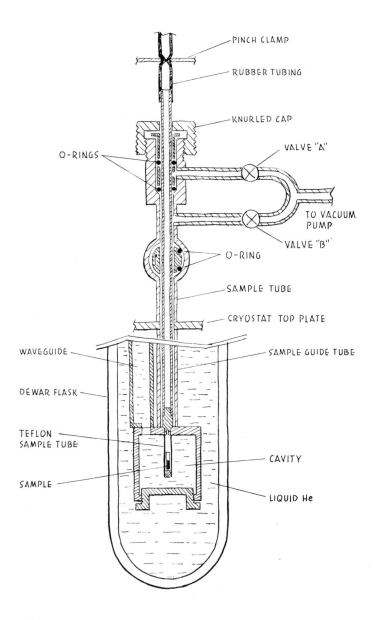

Fig. 4-29. Air lock for changing samples in a low-temperature electron spin resonance cavity. (Courtesy E-9.)

Table 4-15

Cavities for High-Temperature EPR Measurements

Cavity geometry	Frequency	Mode	Heater type	Temperature range, °C	Ref.
Rectangular	X band	TE_{102}	External oven	25–500	P-13
Cylindrical	20 kMc	TE_{011}	External oven	25–600	W-27
Rectangular	X band	TE_{104}	Internal hot air	25–250	M-13
Rectangular	X band	TE_{102}	External heater	25–1000	V-4

Loading. With valves a, b, and the plug valve closed, insert the sample tube through the two O-rings, then open valves a and b to evacuate the air. Next close b, open the plug valve and lower sample to surface of liquid helium, allow the sample to cool for a few minutes, and then insert into cavity until the brass locating plug seats on the cavity top. Sample contact with the liquid surface was determined visually by rippling of the surface.

Unloading. With valve a open, raise the sample to clear the plug valve, close the plug valve and valve a, then complete the extraction.

The two O-rings with the interstitial pumpouts were necessary to avoid air leaks during the rod motion. The helium loss from a slow (10 min) sample change was about 20 cm^3, i.e., about an order of magnitude less than that for samples plunged immediately into the helium bath. If the joint between tube and brass plug leaks, the rubber tubing and pinch clamp valve permits the gas to escape. Table 4-16 lists references for other low-temperature cavities.

Table 4-16

Low-Temperature EPR Cavities

Cavity geometry	Frequency	Mode	Temp, °K	Special features	Ref.
Rectangular	K band	TE_{101}	0.48	Continuously cycled He^3 operation	A-1
Rectangular	X band	TE_{101}	~1.3	Multiple samples changed without opening dewar	O-1
Rectangular	X band	TE_{101}	~4	Illumination slits also adjustable coupling to E field	M-4

Multiple-Wavelength Cavities. Several techniques involving multiple-wavelength cavities have already been mentioned, e.g., measurements of the splitting factor and radical concentration by comparison to a standard located at a second field maximum and modulated with a second pair of coils. Also, these long cavities are favored by some for use with lossy samples such as aqueous solutions or biological specimens where the extra length provides a method of reducing the filling factor when it is inconvenient to reduce the actual sample size. The pros and cons of this technique are discussed in Section 7.7; here we consider only the construction features of several cavities. Figure 4-30 shows three rectangular cavities operating in the TE_{10n} mode where n ranges from 4 to 10. Cavity *a* is slit along the median plane for minimum interference with the current flowing in the cavity walls. The method of aligning the two halves with the split studs which also support the modulation coils is unique. Actually the studs have a slight taper so the pressure squeezing the two halves together increased as the coils were screwed into position. This cavity was used for measurements of radical concentration by locating a standard at one coil position and the unknown at the other. With low-frequency modulation, some problem of cross modulation was encountered, particularly when samples with strong and weak signals were compared, i.e., the coils at position *1* modulated the sample at position *2* and vice versa. A cavity of style *b* also encountered cross modulation difficulties when the length was $4\lambda/2$, however, the $5\lambda/2$ cavity pictured functioned satisfactorily. Presumably, the field from these internal coils does not extend as far as the low-frequency field from the coils in cavity *a*. Additional features of cavity *b* are sufficient room for spacial adjustment of the sample tubes to permit locating the sample at the maximum of the H_1 field and a Teflon tuning screw to adjust the frequency of the cavity. Cavity *c* is designed for detecting free radicals in a thick sample of water, i.e., 1 mm as compared with the optimum of about 0.25 mm for a TE_{102} cavity. Internal modulation coils consisting of 8 turns each of No. 36 enamel-covered copper wire were driven at 455 kc. A maximum modulation field of 50 G was achieved; however, the associated power dissipation in the cavity raised the sample temperature about 10°C. Normally the heating was avoided by blowing cold gas into the cavity (C-20). This cavity also has a dielectric paddle for tuning the frequency.

Dielectric Cavities and Slow-Wave Structures. Two other approaches to the problems of accessibility and lossy samples are (*1*) the dielectric cavity of Fig. 4-31 and (*2*) the slow-wave structures of Fig. 4-32. Dielectric cavities require a material with a sizable dielectric constant (ϵ) and a low loss factor ($\tan \delta$) in order to confine the rf field efficiently in the sample

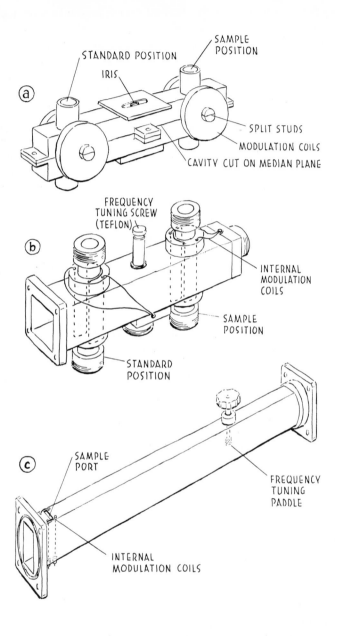

Fig. 4-30. Rectangular TE_{10n} cavities where n is as large as 10 for cavity (c). Cavities (a) and (b) have access ports for multiple samples. [(a) 23; (b) 32; (c) after C-20.]

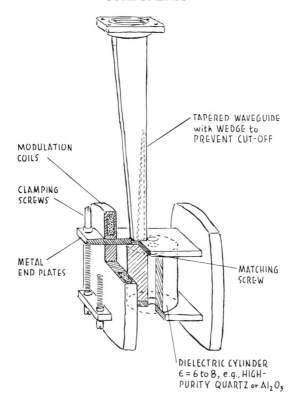

TAPERED WAVEGUIDE
with WEDGE to
PREVENT CUT-OFF

MODULATION
COILS

CLAMPING
SCREWS

METAL
END PLATES

MATCHING
SCREW

DIELECTRIC CYLINDER
$\epsilon = 6$ to 8, e.g., HIGH-
PURITY QUARTZ or Al_2O_3

Fig. 4-31. Commercial *X*-band dielectric cavity. (Courtesy 43.)

region. Quartz and Aluminum oxide have been used but a larger ϵ would be preferable. The chief advantage of these cavities is convenience in modulating with high frequencies and if the dielectric is transparent, sample illumination. Slow-wave structures are also convenient for modulation and illumination. In addition these structures can be immersed in large liquid samples for monitoring or process control purposes. As mentioned in Section 3.5.2(a) the Q achieved with these structures is usually lower than that for metal cavities; however, the structures may be more convenient to use with lossy samples.

Cavities for High-Pressure Experiments. EPR experiments involving high pressures as one of the variables have followed two general approaches: (*1*) uniform loading on all surfaces of the sample by hydraulic pressure generated with Bridgman-Type equipment (3) or (*2*) unilateral compression with pistons and anvils. In the first case the resonant chamber and the

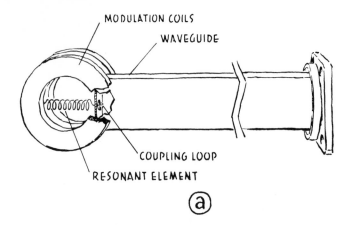

Fig. 4-32. *X*-band slow-wave structures suitable for operation over a range of frequencies. The open structure permits ready access to the sample. [(*a*) Commercial structure, courtesy of 43; (*b*) 17.]

power leads must withstand the high pressures while in the second arrangements analogous to the squeeze cavities of Section 7.2.3 are applicable when provided with sturdier pistons. Reference P-12 contains a good description of both systems along with numerous references to the original papers.

4.1.6   Testing Cavities

Many cavities go directly from shop to spectrometer without stopping at a test bench for a check on the Q or a determination of the required iris size, and as long as adequate spectra are obtained, the cavity designer and builder need have no inferiority complex because of a low Q. However, it is desirable to know ones tools, particularly if an increase in Q means success or failure in the experiment. Consequently, we describe several circuits for measuring cavity Q and for determining the coupling. Reference W-24 lists the following four general methods for measuring the cavity Q based on various properties of resonant circuits.

1. Half-power point method: i.e., Eq. 4-6 and a measurement of the bandwidth between half-power points.

2. Phase or impedance method. At the half-power points the resistive and reactive components are equal and the phase of the current shifts 45° from the current at resonance; therefore, standing wave ratio measurements as a function of frequency when interpreted with an impedance chart can yield the half-power points and frequencies.

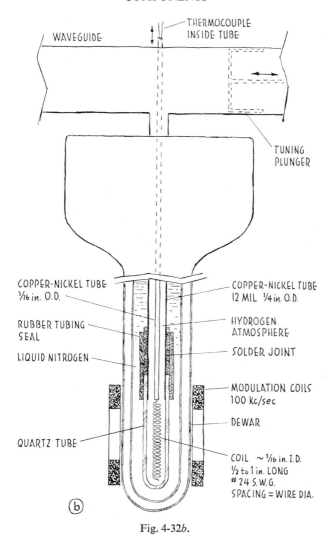

Fig. 4-32*b*.

3. Time decay or ringing method: This is a pulse technique where Q is determined from the decay of energy in a cavity after excitation by the pulse.

4. Deflection point method: At the two inflection points on a resonance curve, the curve is approximately a straight line and at those frequencies the cavity behaves approximately like a linear circuit element. These frequencies can be determined by modulation techniques that are sensitive to the linearity of the circuit element, i.e., harmonic generation.

The first technique is used most frequently so we will limit our discussion to several modifications of the half-power method.

(a) Direct Power Measurements on the Transmission Cavity. Figure 4-33 is a schematic diagram of the test circuit with typical values indicated for the components and an insert showing the quantities to be measured in relation to the resonant curve.

Measuring Procedure. (*1*) Adjust frequency to f_0 and tune cavity and crystal until usable signal a is obtained with attenuator *1* set at a calibration point, e.g., 10 db.

(*2*) Determine signal level corresponding to half-power points b by increasing the attenuation 3 db, e.g., to 13 db.

(*3*) Reset the attenuator at 10 db, and find frequencies f_1 and f_2 by varying the frequency until the signal equals b.

(*4*) Check the signal generator for constant power output over the range from f_1 to f_2. If the variation is less than 5%, no correction is needed; otherwise find the corrected value for up to about 25% variation; b_1 corrected $= (a_1/a)b$.

(b) Direct Power Measurements on the Reflection Cavity. Figure 4-34 shows the circuit diagram and nomenclature for the following procedure:

(*1*) Tune to the resonant frequency f_0 (minimum reflected power) and adjust attenuator *2* to give a convenient reference reading, i.e., *1* at f_0.

(*2*) Completely detune the generator (to position *2*) and adjust calibrated attenuator to restore reference reading, i.e., to point *3*.

(*3*) Locate the calibrated attenuator setting in column *D* of Table 4-17 and read out decibel level in one of the following columns, e.g., the

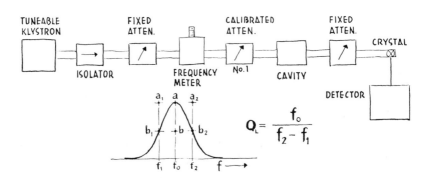

Fig. 4-33. Test circuit for measuring Q_L for a transmission cavity by the half-power point method. (After W-24.)

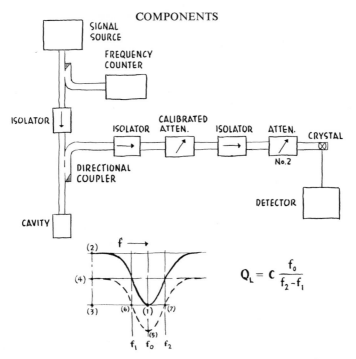

Fig. 4-34. Circuit for measuring Q_L for a reflection cavity by the half-power point method. (After G-18.)

0.5 column is better for low Q valves while the 1 column is best for high Q cavities.

(4) Set the calibrated attenuator at the tabulated value and adjust attenuator 2 to restore the reference value at point 3.

(5) Turn the calibrated attenuator to zero to get to point 4, restore resonance point 5, and vary the frequency until points 6 at f_1 and 7 at f_2 are found where the detector returns to its reference signal level.

(6) Calculate $Q_L = Cf_0/(f_2 - f_1)$ where C = constant from the appropriate column of the table.

(7) Again the power level of the generator should be checked over the frequency range f_1 to f_2.

(c) Sweep Generator Method (Transmission Cavity). Figure 4-35 shows the circuit diagram and appropriate oscilloscope patterns.

(1) Adjust the klystron frequency until a resonant pattern appears on the oscilloscope with the cavity resonance frequency f_0 about in the middle of the frequency range swept by the saw tooth sweep.

(2) With the calibrated attenuator set at 10 db determine the signal height a.

Table

Attenuator Settings for Measuring the Q of an Absorption

D	C=0.5 A	C=1.0 A	D	C=0.5 A	C=1.0 A	D	C=0.5 A	C=1.0 A
4.02	2.865	1.561	5.02	3.450	1.822	6.02	3.979	2.041
4.04	2.877	1.566	5.04	3.461	1.827	6.04	3.989	2.045
4.06	2.889	1.572	5.06	3.473	1.831	6.06	3.999	2.049
4.08	2.902	1.578	5.08	3.484	1.836	6.08	4.009	2.053
4.10	2.914	1.583	5.10	3.495	1.841	6.10	4.019	2.057
4.12	2.926	1.589	5.12	3.506	1.846	6.12	4.029	2.061
4.14	2.938	1.594	5.14	3.517	1.850	6.14	4.039	2.065
4.16	2.950	1.600	5.16	3.528	1.855	6.16	4.049	2.069
4.18	2.962	1.605	5.18	3.539	1.860	6.18	4.058	2.073
4.20	2.974	1.611	5.20	3.550	1.864	6.20	4.068	2.076
4.22	2.986	1.616	5.22	3.561	1.869	6.22	4.078	2.080
4.24	2.998	1.622	5.24	3.572	1.873	6.24	4.088	2.084
4.26	3.010	1.627	5.26	3.582	1.878	6.26	4.097	2.088
4.28	3.022	1.633	5.28	3.593	1.883	6.28	4.107	2.092
4.30	3.034	1.638	5.30	3.604	1.887	6.30	4.117	2.096
4.32	3.046	1.644	5.32	3.615	1.892	6.32	4.127	2.099
4.34	3.058	1.649	5.34	3.626	1.896	6.34	4.136	2.103
4.36	3.070	1.654	5.36	3.637	1.901	6.36	4.146	2.107
4.38	3.082	1.660	5.38	3.647	1.905	6.38	4.155	2.111
4.40	3.094	1.665	5.40	3.658	1.910	6.40	4.165	2.114
4.42	3.106	1.670	5.42	3.669	1.914	6.42	4.175	2.118
4.44	3.118	1.676	5.44	3.679	1.919	6.44	4.184	2.122
4.46	3.129	1.681	5.46	3.690	1.923	6.46	4.194	2.126
4.48	3.141	1.686	5.48	3.701	1.928	6.48	4.203	2.129
4.50	3.153	1.692	5.50	3.711	1.932	6.50	4.212	2.133
4.52	3.165	1.697	5.52	3.722	1.936	6.52	4.222	2.137
4.54	3.176	1.702	5.54	3.732	1.941	6.54	4.231	2.140
4.56	3.188	1.707	5.56	3.743	1.945	6.56	4.241	2.144
4.58	3.200	1.712	5.58	3.754	1.949	6.58	4.250	2.147
4.60	3.211	1.717	5.60	3.764	1.954	6.60	4.259	2.151
4.62	3.223	1.723	5.62	3.774	1.958	6.62	4.269	2.155
4.64	3.234	1.728	5.64	3.785	1.962	6.64	4.278	2.158
4.66	3.246	1.733	5.66	3.795	1.967	6.66	4.287	2.162
4.68	3.258	1.738	5.68	3.806	1.971	6.68	4.297	2.165
4.70	3.269	1.743	5.70	3.816	1.975	6.70	4.306	2.169
4.72	3.281	1.748	5.72	3.826	1.979	6.72	4.315	2.172
4.74	3.292	1.753	5.74	3.837	1.984	6.74	4.324	2.176
4.76	3.304	1.758	5.76	3.847	1.988	6.76	4.333	2.179
4.78	3.315	1.763	5.78	3.857	1.992	6.78	4.343	2.183
4.80	3.326	1.768	5.80	3.868	1.996	6.80	4.352	2.186
4.82	3.338	1.773	5.82	3.878	2.000	6.82	4.361	2.190
4.84	3.349	1.778	5.84	3.888	2.004	6.84	4.370	2.193
4.86	3.360	1.783	5.86	3.898	2.009	6.86	4.379	2.197
4.88	3.372	1.788	5.88	3.909	2.013	6.88	4.388	2.200
4.90	3.383	1.793	5.90	3.919	2.017	6.90	4.397	2.203
4.92	3.394	1.798	5.92	3.929	2.021	6.92	4.406	2.207
4.94	3.406	1.802	5.94	3.939	2.025	6.94	4.415	2.210
4.96	3.417	1.807	5.96	3.949	2.029	6.96	4.424	2.214
4.98	3.428	1.812	5.98	3.959	2.033	6.98	4.433	2.217
5.00	3.439	1.817	6.00	3.969	2.037	7.00	4.442	2.220

[a] Footnote additional values of A can be calculated from

$$A = 10 \log \frac{1 + C^2}{10^{-(D/10)} + C^2}$$

4-17

Cavity by the direct Power Method of Fig. 4-34 (Courtesy B-36)[a]

D	C=0.5 A	C=1.0 A	D	C=0.5 A	C=1.0 A	D	C=0.5 A	C=1.0 A
7.02	4.450	2.224	8.02	4.865	2.374	9.02	5.225	2.498
7.04	4.459	2.227	8.04	4.873	2.377	9.04	5.232	2.500
7.06	4.468	2.230	8.06	4.880	2.380	9.06	5.238	2.502
7.08	4.477	2.233	8.08	4.888	2.382	9.08	5.245	2.504
7.10	4.486	2.237	8.10	4.896	2.385	9.10	5.252	2.506
7.12	4.494	2.240	8.12	4.903	2.388	9.12	5.258	2.509
7.14	4.503	2.243	8.14	4.911	2.390	9.14	5.265	2.511
7.16	4.512	2.246	8.16	4.919	2.393	9.16	5.271	2.513
7.18	4.521	2.250	8.18	4.926	2.396	9.18	5.278	2.515
7.20	4.529	2.253	8.20	4.934	2.398	9.20	5.284	2.517
7.22	4.538	2.256	8.22	4.941	2.401	9.22	5.291	2.519
7.24	4.546	2.259	8.24	4.949	2.403	9.24	5.297	2.522
7.26	4.555	2.262	8.26	4.956	2.406	9.26	5.304	2.524
7.28	4.564	2.266	8.28	4.964	2.409	9.28	5.310	2.526
7.30	4.572	2.269	8.30	4.971	2.411	9.30	5.317	2.528
7.32	4.581	2.272	8.32	4.979	2.414	9.32	5.323	2.530
7.34	4.589	2.275	8.34	4.986	2.416	9.34	5.329	2.532
7.36	4.598	2.278	8.36	4.993	2.419	9.36	5.336	2.534
7.38	4.606	2.281	8.38	5.001	2.421	9.38	5.342	2.536
7.40	4.615	2.284	8.40	5.008	2.424	9.40	5.348	2.538
7.42	4.623	2.287	8.42	5.015	2.426	9.42	5.355	2.540
7.44	4.631	2.290	8.44	5.023	2.429	9.44	5.361	2.542
7.46	4.640	2.293	8.46	5.030	2.432	9.46	5.367	2.544
7.48	4.648	2.296	8.48	5.037	2.434	9.48	5.373	2.546
7.50	4.656	2.299	8.50	5.045	2.436	9.50	5.380	2.548
7.52	4.665	2.302	8.52	5.052	2.439	9.52	5.386	2.550
7.54	4.673	2.305	8.54	5.059	2.441	9.54	5.392	2.552
7.56	4.681	2.308	8.56	5.066	2.444	9.56	5.398	2.554
7.58	4.689	2.311	8.58	5.073	2.446	9.58	5.404	2.556
7.60	4.698	2.314	8.60	5.080	2.449	9.60	5.410	2.558
7.62	4.706	2.317	8.62	5.087	2.451	9.62	5.416	2.560
7.64	4.714	2.320	8.64	5.095	2.454	9.64	5.422	2.562
7.66	4.722	2.323	8.66	5.102	2.456	9.66	5.429	2.564
7.68	4.730	2.326	8.68	5.109	2.458	9.68	5.435	2.566
7.70	4.738	2.329	8.70	5.116	2.461	9.70	5.441	2.568
7.72	4.747	2.332	8.72	5.123	2.463	9.72	5.447	2.570
7.74	4.755	2.335	8.74	5.130	2.465	9.74	5.453	2.572
7.76	4.763	2.338	8.76	5.137	2.468	9.76	5.458	2.574
7.78	4.771	2.341	8.78	5.144	2.470	9.78	5.464	2.576
7.80	4.779	2.343	8.80	5.150	2.473	9.80	5.470	2.578
7.82	4.787	2.346	8.82	5.157	2.475	9.82	5.476	2.580
7.84	4.795	2.349	8.84	5.164	2.477	9.84	5.482	2.582
7.86	4.802	2.352	8.86	5.171	2.479	9.86	5.488	2.583
7.88	4.810	2.355	8.88	5.178	2.482	9.88	5.494	2.585
7.90	4.818	2.358	8.90	5.185	2.484	9.90	5.500	2.587
7.92	4.826	2.360	8.92	5.192	2.486	9.92	5.505	2.589
7.94	4.834	2.363	8.94	5.198	2.489	9.94	5.511	2.591
7.96	4.842	2.366	8.96	5.205	2.491	9.96	5.517	2.593
7.98	4.850	2.369	8.98	5.212	2.493	9.98	5.523	2.595
8.00	4.857	2.371	9.00	5.218	2.495	10.00	5.528	2.596

If the absorption of the resonator amounts to less than 1 db, it may be advisable to eliminate the inaccuracy involved in readjusting the detector sensitivity. In this case, step 4 could be eliminated, and, in step 5, the calibrated attenuator set to D minus the value read out of the table in step 3. This amounts to carrying an offset in the calibrated attenuator.

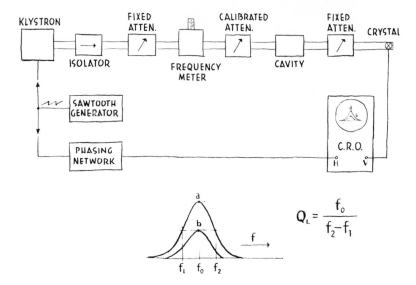

$$Q_L = \frac{f_0}{f_2 - f_1}$$

Fig. 4-35. Circuit for measuring Q_L for a transmission cavity by the sweep generator method. (After W-24.)

(3) Increase attenuation 3 db, i.e., to 13 db and determine the height b corresponding to the half-power point.

(4) Return the attenuator to 10 db and measure f_0, f_1, and f_2 by the dip marker produced by the frequency meter. As before, $Q = f_0/(f_2 - f_1)$.

(d) Marker Generator Method (Reflection Cavity). Figure 4-36 shows the circuit diagram and pertinent scope presentations.

(1) With the scope connected to crystal detector position 1 and the frequency of klystron No. 1, modulated with a saw tooth sweep, adjust the klystron frequency and the iris until resonance is centered on the sweep and the cavity is matched as at b. Adjust the signal to a convenient level with attenuator 2.

(2) Add 3 db attenuation with the calibrated attenuator to obtain the signal level at the half-power points, then remove the 3 db.

(3) Adjust the frequency of klystron No. 2 and the setting of attenuator 3 until a pip is visible at f_0; then adjust the frequency and amplitude of the sine wave generator modulating klystron 2 until side band pips appear at the half power level as at c. Observe the modulating frequency f_m.

(4) Move the scope pickup to crystal detector No. 2 and measure the frequency of klystron No. 2. The steady horizontal scope trace rises or falls abruptly when the wave meter is tuned to the resonant frequency.

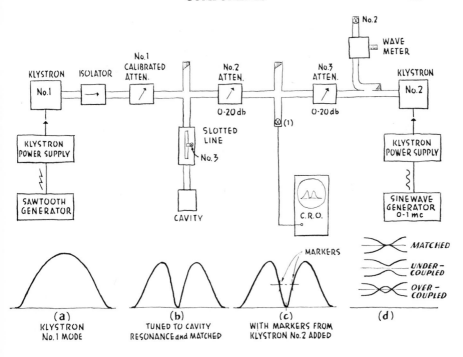

Fig. 4-36. Circuit for measuring Q_L by the marker generator method and for matching the cavity to the waveguide (44).

This bridge is also convenient for determining the iris size to match the cavity.

a. Mount the cavity on the slotted line and attach the scope input to the pickup in the slotted line.

b. If the probe is moved back and forth rapidly in the slotted line, the scope pattern will appear as at *d.* When the cavity is matched to the line the dip and peak will just touch as indicated. A gap or overlap means undercoupled or overcoupled, respectively.

4.2 MAGNETS

Three types of magnets are encountered in EPR experiments: (*1*) the air core solenoids of low-frequency spectrometers, (*2*) the iron core magnets used in the microwave region, and (*3*) superconducting solenoids suitable for extremely high-field requirements.

Types (*1*) and (*3*) are relatively rare so most of these remarks apply to iron core magnets. Even the most ardent believers in home-built spectrometers resist the impulse to build iron magnets; therefore, this section is primarily concerned with features to be considered in selecting and installing commercial magnets. A few tailor-made units continue in service such as the 60 some year old battery powered Du Bois type magnet at the Zeeman laboratory (25) and the ultra parallel pole magnet at the University of Nottingham (16) but even here the construction was by industrial concerns. Now manufacturers offer a variety of pole sizes, geometries, gap spacings, and power supplies sufficient for essentially all EPR requirements. In selecting a magnet, the EPR conditions for distortionless resonance establish the minimum pole and gap geometry but beyond this point considerations of convenience, flexibility, and economics often determine the size selected.

4.2.1   Magnet Types

(a) Air Core Solenoids. Typical solenoids for low-field measurements accommodate cavities like the ones illustrated in Fig. 6.3-7 and 7.5-20 where the field requirements are about 100–200 G for the free-electron g value when $v = 300$ and 600 Mc, respectively. For example, the solenoid in Fig. 7.5-20a is 2 in. i.d. and 10 in. long; it can be operated air cooled over a range of about 100 G around the central value. If a modulation coil is wound coaxially with the main field coil, the form should be either a dielectric or a slit metal sleeve which cannot accommodate induced circulating currents. A winding such as Fig. 7.3-7 contains a modulation coil 9 in. long centered on the sample, a main field winding 18 in. in length, and trim field coils 5 in. long at each end of the solenoid. Proper adjustment of the trim coils generate a larger uniform field at the sample location than is obtained with a simple solenoid. Although low-frequency spectrometers are selected for other reasons, the solenoid offers several desirable features: (1) the field is directly related to the current in the windings; (2) air cooling is adequate for most experiments; and (3) the solenoid cost is negligible.

(b) Iron Core Magnets. For rigidity and stability of alignment these magnets normally have a rectangular yoke so the mounts usually hold the yoke at some angle, e.g., 45°, to facilitate inserting and removing samples and cavities. Pole diameters commonly range from 4 to 15 in. and both tapered and cylindrical geometries are available. Gaps between poles range from about $\frac{1}{2}$ in. to several inches. Typical fields with gaps adequate for EPR work range up to 5 or 6 kG for 4 in. diameter poles and 13–18 kG with 12 and 15 in. diameter poles. At X- and Q-band frequencies the free electron resonance occurs at about 3.5 and 12.5 kG, respectively. Fields up to about 50 kG can be obtained with tapered pole tips; however, the high magnetizing currents and small working volume severely limit their convenience and usefulness.

(c) **Superconducting Solenoids.** Low has used this type of magnet (6) in studying very high field transitions. These solenoids provide appreciable volumes for the experiment and the power expenditure is relatively low. Some typical examples are fields up to 60 kG, uniform to better than 0.2% over a $\frac{3}{4}$ in. spherical volume inside a 2 in. i.d. Nb 25% Zr coil. With Nb_3–Sn windings fields up to 100 kG have been produced in a 1 in. i.d. coil. Once started, the currents in a superconducting coil continue to circulate free from fluctuations in the power lines that disturb other electromagnets; consequently, superconducting solenoids exhibit extremely high field stability over long time periods. In this mode of operation the solenoid is analogous to a permanent magnet so provisions to find resonance require either a variable frequency spectrometer or auxiliary sweep coils. This inconvenience coupled with the complexities of refrigeration will probably limit superconducting magnets to the very high field region for some time to come.

4.2.2 Magnet Characteristics

The characteristics of electromagnets important to EPR are: (1) spacial uniformity of the field over the sample volume; (2) temporal stability during the measurement; and (3) linearity of the sweep while traversing a resonance line. Fluctuations in (1) and (2) introduce line broadening, and nonlinear sweep distorts both the line splitting and shape. Minimum values of the uniform field volume are set by the largest sample and the minimum linewidth anticipated. For example, solid samples in X-band cavities have an effective length of about 1 in. and linewidths in excess of 1 G; consequently, variations of 0.1 G over the center inch of the pole will not distort the spectrum from such materials. Commercial 6-in. magnets meet this requirement as indicated by the specifications in Appendix I. In the discussion of high-resolution spectroscopy, Section 3.4, dilute-solution liquid samples were encountered with line widths down to about 17 mG and the measurement times extended up to 15 hr. If the field uniformity is maintained, an order of magnitude below the line width such specimens require a field uniform to about 3 ppm over the sample volume. Such spectra have been recorded with carefully adjusted 12 in. diameter poles but as the specifications in the Appendix indicate this uniformity is not normally available over a 1 in. diameter. Similar homogeneity requirements in NMR spectroscopy lead to the introduction of spinning samples and pole face shim coils.

Gap widths are determined by the size of the cavities, and the associated dewars or temperature control apparatus. The fringing distortion in the field at the edge of the pole caps increases with the ratio of gap width to pole diameter. "Rose" or ring shims can counteract some of this fringe distortion; however, it is necessary to keep the gap width-to-pole diameter ratio within limits if reasonable homogeneity is to be maintained. Squires suggests a ratio of 1:4 as about optimum for a compromise between access and distortion (S-21).

In addition to pole diameter and gap width, the homogeneity is effected by the uniformity of the pole cap material, the flatness of the caps, and their parallelism. Careful selection, treatment, and testing minimize field distortions resulting from inhomogeneities in the pole caps. Typical commercial grinding tolerances hold cylindrical pole caps flat to within a few microns. Probably the optimum parallelism was achieved by Standley (16) who used poles held apart by three sections of a quartz optical flat mounted in the gap.

Stability specifications for commercial spectrometers are quoted for various tests and times ranging up to 15 and 30 min. For most materials such times are adequate; however, in high-resolution EPR 15–30 hr may be required. Quoted stabilities in the range of 1 part in 10^5 or 10^6 for the magnet current are adequate even for high-resolution EPR.

Linearity of the field sweep is probably more of a convenience than a necessity since the magnetic field can be measured and the spectrum adjusted accordingly. Most of the existing spectrometers have a linear current sweep so saturation and hysteresis effects in the iron distort the sweep linearity. With the modest fields and linewidths encountered in most radical spectra, the distortion is negligible at the X band. The newer control systems are based on a Hall plate or other sensors which measure the magnetic field; consequently, these devices provide a linear sweep over large field variations.

After considering the factors which determine the minimum acceptable magnet for the job, it becomes a matter of convenience and economics in going to larger pole diameters and gap spacings. Large gaps offer flexibility in the choice of external dewars and cylindrical cavities so where versatility is an important factor, 9–12 in. poles deserve serious consideration.

4.2.3 Magnet Mounts

Selection of a magnet mount depends on the experimental ritual. For example some spectroscopists take the microwave bridge and cavity to the magnet while others move the magnet. Also some rotate the sample alone or sample plus cavity while others rotate the magnet when measuring sample orientation effects. Moving the magnet can be justified when it is used with several spectrometers or when the dewar's piping and other paraphernalia are more troublesome or dangerous to move than the magnet. In most laboratories the ratio of inertia to convenience prescribes a stationary magnet where translation is in question; when it comes to rotation, however, the majority select a rotating magnet and a stationary cavity. Commercial accessories are available for rotating samples or magnets; however, the third alternative, a rotating cavity, appears to have received little attention. With complex dewar and plumbing systems the rotating magnet probably offers the maximum flexibility and convenience —for a price.

CHAPTER V

General Techniques

In Section 2.5 various methods were described for determining such important EPR parameters as the splitting factor g, the fine structure constants D and E, the hf coefficients $A_\perp$ and $A_\parallel$, etc. These computations assumed the availability of certain experimental information, particularly the frequency and magnetic field strength at resonance. This chapter is concerned with the measurements of frequency, field strength, spin concentrations, and other experimental parameters needed for evaluating and interpreting a spectrum. As is usually the case relative measurements are the simplest and frequently a comparison to a well-established species is both adequate and expedient. At other times the need for quantitative results requires the use of yardsticks and standards. Therefore, this section will embrace some techniques in both of these categories. In addition, this chapter contains various miscellaneous recipes covering the sealing wax and string aspects of EPR, cements, seals, tapes, dielectrics, dewars, lubricants, etc.

5.1 FREQUENCY MEASUREMENTS

Normally the frequencies encountered in EPR spectroscopy fall within the range from about 300 to 40,000 Mc. Translated to free air wavelengths this range extends from about 100 cm to 7.5 mm. Dimensionally these lengths are convenient for measurement; therefore, the frequency can either be measured directly or it can be computed from the wavelength. In the first case the fundamental yardstick is time, which ultimately goes back to determinations at a government observatory and in the second case the basic unit is the international meter. In this range wavelengths are normally simpler and cheaper to measure than frequencies; however, frequencies can be measured with greater accuracy; therefore, rough measurements are usually based on wavelengths while the most precise determinations are direct frequency comparisons. Table 5-1 lists three of these techniques and the accuracies typically obtained.

Some of the factors effecting the accuracy of these techniques are considered in the following paragraphs along with experimental precautions.

Table 5-1

Typical Accuracies of Frequency Measurement Techniques

Method	Accuracy
Slotted line wavelength	$\pm 0.1-5\%$
Resonant cavity wavemeter	$\pm 0.05-0.01\%$
Crystal-controlled frequency meter	± 1 part in 10^6-10^7

5.1.1 Slotted Line Techniques

Figure 5-1 shows the dimensions to be measured and a typical arrangement for attaching the slotted line to the EPR spectrometer. The properties of slotted lines, their design, and their construction are considered in detail in Ref. M-12 and Fig. 5-2 shows the general features of several commercial units. Slotted lines are available for most of the standard waveguide sizes listed in Table 3-1. Coaxial lines or parallel planes with center conductor are used at the lower frequencies, e.g., 300–4000 Mc. Waveguide sections are physically more convenient for the G through P bands and this range can be measured with a single probe carriage plus a series of six interchangeable waveguide sections. At higher frequencies several factors combine to limit the accuracy of a slotted line. First, it becomes increasingly difficult to maintain the accuracy of the length measurements. Second, it becomes more difficult to fulfill such basic assumptions as (1) the line is uniform and lossless and (2) the presence of the

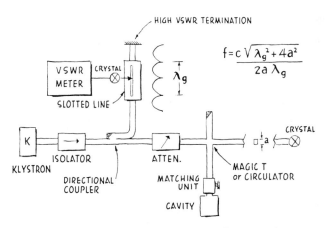

Fig. 5-1. Arrangement for determining spectrometer frequency from measurements with a slotted line: all dimensions a and wavelength λ_g are indicated. c = the velocity of light = 3×10^{10} cm/sec if a and λ_g are measured in centimeters.

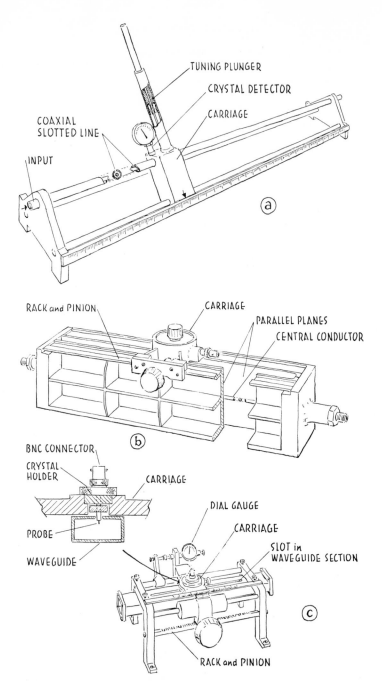

Fig. 5-2. Typical commercial slotted lines: (*a*) coaxial line useful in the 300–600 Mc range; (*b*) a coaxial line suitable for 500–400 Mc range; (*c*) slotted waveguide section. A series of waveguides permit coverage from 3.9 to 18 kMc.

probe does not seriously modify the electromagnetic field. For example, in a commercial slotted line at 600 Mc the linear scale can be read to 0.1 mm, or about 1 part in 5000 or 0.02%. In contrast a slotted line for the Q band with a linear resolution of 0.01 mm indicates 1 part in 1000 or 0.1% for a 30-kMc wave. When the other factors contributing to the accuracy are considered, wavelength measurements are frequently no better than 0.1 to 0.5%. Other factors effecting the accuracy are: (*1*) the magnitude of the voltage standing wave ratio; (*2*) the amount of probe insertion; (*3*) the relative harmonic content of the power source; and (*4*) imperfections in the slotted line. In order to achieve a maximum resolution, λ_g is measured between minima as indicated in Fig. 5-1 in preference to the maxima, which are poorly resolved. Searching should commence with the probe retracted to avoid damage to the crystal. After a minimum is located, the sensitivity of the detector system can be increased to give a full scale reading for high sensitivity. A still better procedure is to calculate the minimum from points of equal signal strength measured on each side of the minimum. Usually the simple crystal detector is monitored with a microammeter or VSWR meter; however, more elaborate detection arrangements can be used for a higher sensitivity, e.g., an audio-modulated klystron locked to an audio amplifier detector or a superheterodyne detector (W-24).

5.1.2 Resonant Cavity Wavemeters

Cavity wavemeters are constructed for various degrees of accuracy; however, as indicated in Table 5-1 they generally permit an order of magnitude improvement over the slotted lines. When the approximate wavelength is known, cavities are as easy to use as a slotted line. Most commercial wavemeters are constructed to avoid spurious modes within the designated frequency range; however, frequencies outside the normal range can excite such modes so as a safety precaution it is desirable to know the approximate frequency. Because of their inherently high Q values, the cylindrical TE_{01n} modes are preferred for wavemeters. Usually they are attached to the spectrometer by a directional coupler as was used for the slotted line. Some factors effecting the accuracy of cavity wavemeters are:

1. Temperature: expansion of the metal changes the cavity size.

2. Humidity: the high dielectric constant of water alters the resonance frequency.

3. Imperfections and backlash in the drive screw.

4. An external load which reduces the cavity Q and thus the sharpness of resonance.

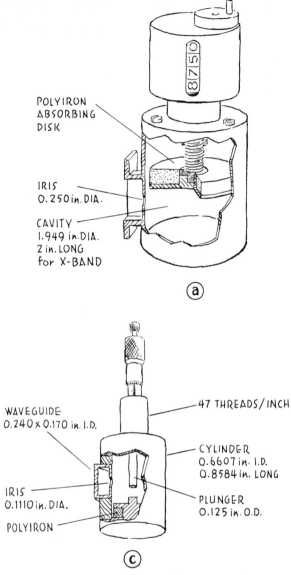

POLYIRON
ABSORBING
DISK

IRIS
0.250 in. DIA.

CAVITY
1.949 in. DIA.
2 in. LONG
for X-BAND

(a)

WAVEGUIDE
0.240 x 0.170 in. I.D.

47 THREADS/INCH

CYLINDER
0.6607 in. I.D.
0.8584 in. LONG

IRIS
0.1110 in. DIA.

PLUNGER
0.125 in. O.D.

POLYIRON

(c)

Fig. 5-3. Most wavemeters are circular cylindrical geometry for ease and precision of manufacture; however, rectangular and coaxial geometries are available. Mechanically the TE_{011} mode (a) is the simplest since no electrical contact is involved with the moving plunger. The lack of contact plus the polyiron absorber suppress unwanted modes. TE_{111} mode cavities (b) are fairly popular because the small cavity size provides good mode discrimination. At high frequencies, e.g., above 20 kMc, hybrid cavities where only part of the end wall moves (c) are sometimes used to permit finer tuning than is convenient with arrangements (a) or (b). Cavity (c) is for the 24 kMc region. All the cavities can be arranged for reflection single port, transmission (double iris) or absorption measurements. [(a) and (c) after M-12.]

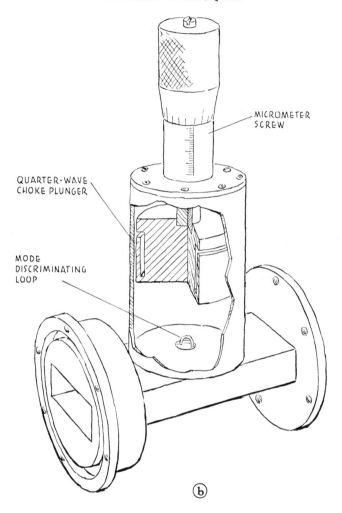

QUARTER-WAVE
CHOKE PLUNGER

MICROMETER
SCREW

MODE
DISCRIMINATING
LOOP

(b)

Figure 5-3b.

To minimize the first two effects the standard conditions used by the National Bureau of Standards in calculating cavities are a temperature of 25°C and a relative humidity of 60%. In some instruments the cavity body is made of Invar to minimize thermal expansion errors. Other instruments are supplied with temperature correction curves. Two general classes of meters are available: (1) general purpose or search cavities and (2) precision or standard meters. The first type usually covers a broader frequency range with a modest Q and an accuracy of about 0.01–1%. These cavities are open to the air and the correction for relative humidity may go as high as 0.06%. Precision meters are hermetically sealed and filled with inert gas to avoid a change in the dielectric properties of the gas. Accuracies of 0.005% are achieved and frequency differences can be measured to 0.001% (W-24). As with the slotted lines the higher accuracies are achieved with the longer wavelengths. For example, in one style of general purpose meter the quoted accuracies are 0.065, 0.08, and 0.12% for J-, X-, and R-band wavemeters, respectively. Figure 5-3 shows the appearance and construction of various cavity wavemeters.

5.1.3 Frequency Meters

The techniques for direct measurements of frequency are highly developed and permit some of the most precise measurements performed by man. Stable oscillators provide the basis for such measurements and they are commercially available, e.g., quartz crystal-controlled frequency standards have a stability of better than ± 5 parts in 10^{10} per 24 hr. With this stability the accuracy of frequency measurements depends on how well the oscillator can be calibrated. Thus, the calibration procedure provides the basis for classifying frequency standards. Primary standards are stable crystal oscillators that have been checked against time signals from government observatories such as those broadcast over Station WWV. Accuracies as high as one part in 10^7 are available from primary standards (W-24). Secondary standards are the second-generation, stable, crystal-controlled oscillators calibrated by comparison with a primary standard. The frequency of the crystal oscillators in these standards is usually in the 50 kc to 1 Mc range; therefore, they are not suitable for direct comparison with spectrometer frequencies in the 300 Mc to 40 kMc range. Microwave frequency standards use harmonics from a primary or secondary standard to establish a precise reference frequency (W-24). Figure 5-4 shows a typical circuit arrangement for comparing the spectrometer frequency to a secondary standard. The tunable oscillator generates a stable signal in the 100–200 Mc range which is fed into a harmonic generator for conversion to a microwave signal to match the unknown frequency coming from the spectrometer. These two signals beat against each other in the crystal mixer and the oscilloscope indicates when the frequencies match. Part of the signal from the oscillator goes to the counter which has been calibrated against a primary or secondary standard and is now ready to measure the fundamental frequency; therefore, the unknown frequency equals the product of the fundamental frequency and the harmonic number. All of the components in the dotted box come together in commercial transfer oscillators. Accuracy is largely controlled by the counter and its calibration. The overall accuracy should be at least

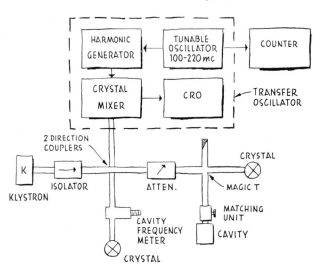

Fig. 5-4. Circuit arrangement for frequency measurements by comparison to a secondary frequency standard built into the counter.

an order of magnitude better than for the best cavity wavemeter; therefore, this is the preferred technique for precision frequency determinations. While commercial equipment is convenient to use, a knowledge of the approximate spectrometer frequency will minimize the search through the various harmonics. Stability comes with thermal equilibrium; consequently, the usual precautions in warming up the standard are in order.

Another method of determining the frequency was mentioned in Section 3.3.2, namely, locking of the klystron to a crystal oscillator so that the frequency is both fixed and known at all times. This system has been used on several home-built spectrometers (3,19) and is also available commercially. Stabilities of a few parts in 10^7 are available (11). A commercial oscillator synchronizer* contains the essential components necessary to control the klystron.

5.2 MAGNETIC FIELD MEASUREMENTS

Four general techniques are in use for measuring the external field intensity: (1) induction or flip coils: (2) NMR gaussmeters, (3) EPR systems of known g, and (4) Hall plates. Methods 1 and 4 convert the problem of measuring the field into one of accurately measuring an

* Hewlett-Packard Dy 2650A.

induced voltage while the resonance methods involve frequency measurements and a well-established nuclear or electronic splitting factor. Various degrees of elegance and automation have been achieved ranging from simple one-point observations to automatic control of the field. Table 5-2 indicates field intensities and accuracies quoted for typical commercial equipment.

Table 5-2
Range and Accuracies of Some Commercial Gaussmeters

Method	Range of magnetic field, G	Accuracy	Mfg.[a]
Induction coil	0–100,000 in 8 ranges: 0–30, 0–100, 0–300, 0–10^3, 0–3 × 10^3, 0–3 × 10^4, 0–10^5	±0.5% of range	Alpha Scientific
NMR	300–150,000; nuclei H, 500–9000; Li, 8.5–23.6 × 10^3; D, 21.5–59 × 10^3	1 part in 10^5 or 10^6	Alpha Scientific
		1 part in 10^5	JEOL
Hall plates, InAs	0.1–20,000 in 22 ranges	1% + accuracy of reference magnet (about 1 to 1.5%)	RFL Labs
Field dial		Set field to ±1 G, 1 part in 10^5 repeatability, 0.02 G resolution	Varian

[a] See Appendix for locations.

5.2.1 Search Coils

The traditional method of measuring the magnetic field intensity involves a search coil arranged to cut the lines of force by an appropriate motion. Most commercial and home built units found in EPR applications have consisted of a synchronous motor rotating the coil in the magnetic field and an amplifier to strengthen and detect the generated ac potential. These systems offer the advantages of economy and first principle simplicity, e.g., search coils can be certified by the National Bureau of Standards. Although the accuracy as indicated in Table 5-2 is usually less than for the other methods, the simplicity, convenience, and freedom from temperature dependence make these coils practical for routine measurements. For example at Berkeley (34) magnets throughout the Physics Department were equipped with a standard design of flip coil and monitoring circuit which puts pips along the spectrum base line at uniform field intervals. Typical probes containing the rotating coils are about $\frac{1}{2}$ in. in diameter so there is seldom room for the probe to mount where it will cut the same flux passing through the sample.

5.2.2 NMR Gaussmeters

Nuclear magnetic resonance has become the preferred method for precision measurements of the magnetic field intensity. For X-band spectrometers the proton resonance occurs at frequencies convenient to measure by direct comparison to the primary or secondary frequency standards of Section 5.1.3. At higher magnetic fields other nuclei such as lithium and deuterium will resonate at convenient frequencies. Table 5-3

Table 5-3

Nuclei for NMR Gaussmeters, Typical Ranges and Sensitivities

Nuclei	Spin	Frequency range, Mc	Magnetic field range, kG	Relative sensitivity[a] (equal number of spins)	
				Constant ν	Constant H
H^1	$\frac{1}{2}$	2–39	0.5–9.2	1	1
Li^7 in LiCl	$\frac{3}{2}$	14–39	8.5–23.6	1.94	0.294
H^2	1	14–39	21.5–59	0.409	0.0096

[a] Alpha Scientific Laboratories, Inc., Berkeley, Calif.

shows the relation between resonant frequency and magnetic field strength for these materials and the range of magnetic fields covered in some commercial NMR gaussmeters. Recalling that the accuracies of primary and secondary frequency standards can be a few parts in 10^7, the field measurement can have a comparable accuracy, provided the nuclear spectroscopic splitting factor is as well known, the field is sufficiently homogeneous over the sample volume, and the spectrometer frequency stability permits full usage of the inherent accuracy of the frequency meter. Inhomogeneities and instabilities of these types will broaden the resonance lines and thus interfere with accurate measurements. Since the magnetic field is normally determined in order to obtain the electronic splitting factor, the procedure should be designed to minimize the in-homogeneities and instabilities that can alter H_0 between the nuclear and electron resonance measurements. If the expressions for electron and nuclear resonance are combined and solved for g_e in a common field H_0, the splitting factor becomes

$$g_e = (\beta_n/\beta_e g_n)\nu_e/\nu_n = K(\nu_e/\nu_n) \qquad (5\text{-}1)$$

Ideally ν_e and ν_n should be measured simultaneously in the same sample; then the electron and nuclear spins would be in the same magnetic field. Usually this ritual is impractical so it is necessary to carefully establish the relationship between the fields at the electron and nuclear probe positions by interchanging two identical nuclear probes between the two positions. As EPR theory developed, more precise values of g_e were required and the coefficient K has been determined with an increasing accuracy until now $K = (3.0419971 \pm 0.0000005) \times 10^{-3}$ (S-6). A few years ago g_n estab-lished the accuracy limit for determining g_e; now magnetic field stability and uniformity are becoming the limiting factors.

The degree of complexity and automation in NMR gaussmeters varies substantially from one laboratory to another, ranging from a simple manually tuned oscillator monitored with an oscilloscope to systems where the oscillator is locked to the proton resonance throughout the magnetic field sweep and where the oscillator frequency is automatically measured and recorded on the EPR spectra at periodic intervals. Figure 5-5 illustrates four of these gaussmeters in block diagram form. Con-struction details for the probe and complete circuit diagrams for the oscillator and amplifier of arrangement a are given in Refs. S-21 and I-2. In operation the marginal oscillator frequency is adjusted until the protons in the glycerine surrounding the tank coil experience NMR, thereby absorbing rf energy and modulating the amplitude of the signal fed to the amplifier and oscilloscope detector. Resonance can be detected by the drop in the level of the rf signal reaching the detecting scope or by modu-lating the magnetic field sufficiently to generate an absorption curve in the scope. At resonance the frequency is measured with a frequency counter and the field is calculated from $H = 2.3487 \times 10^2 \nu$ for H in gauss and ν in megacycles. The small probe described in Ref. S-21 is also suitable for mapping or checking the uniformity of the field in the magnet gap. As indicated on the recorder system b provides a central resonance line and two precisely spaced side bands suitable for measuring hf splitting. The operation is different from a in two major respects. First, the frequency is controlled by a crystal oscillator driving the marginal oscillator through the frequency divider so that the frequency stability is established by the crystal. Second, the 80 cps modulation of the rf power generates the two side-band resonances and permits phase-sensitive detection. Arrangements *a* and *b* are available commercially.*

Arrangement *c* is an automatic method for measuring the field and calibrating the EPR spectrum (H-16). Again, the marginal oscillator frequency is crystal controlled but now there are 11 quartz crystals mounted on the turret of a commercially available television tuner so that the field can be determined at 11 frequencies 18 G apart. In operation the protons are modulated with a sinusoidal field which is sufficient to swing the instantaneous magnetic field H through resonance, when H is within about 1 G of H_0. As the steady field is swept, resonance will occur for a band of field strengths where $H_0 = H - H_m \cos \omega t$ and two resonances will occur on each cycle. These resonances will be equally spaced only when resonance occurs at the point where $\cos \omega t = 0$. At all other values of H the lines will be paired as indicated in the insert. The second amplifier and flip-flop circuits convert the absorptive signals into strong sharp pulses which enter a gating circuit controlled by the 87 c modulator. When the pulses are equally spaced and in proper phase with the modulating signal, the pulses will be transmitted through to a solenoid activating the marker pin, and the turret advance motor. Consequently, after each NMR has been recorded, the oscillator is automatically switched to the next frequency. In the unit described in Ref. H-16 the frequency interval between successive crystals was 75.9 ± 0.1 kc/sec which made the calibration points fall 17.83 G apart. A similar system (13) was ultimately relieved of the automatic switching feature when it was observed that student spectroscopists generally stood by watching the switching operation; therefore, before building an automatic system be sure the planned use saves more time and effort than construction expends. Arrangement *d* (F-10) is an automatic recording gaussmeter which permits continuous monitoring of the magnetic field. Here the oscillator is locked to the NMR frequency in the usual way with a phase-sensitive detector operating at the modulation frequency of 105 cps feeding an unfiltered output signal to an electronic integrator which provides both filtering and amplification. The resulting signal controls the rf oscillator frequency via a voltage variable capacitor in the oscillator tank circuit. This arrangement will maintain automatic frequency control for scanning rates up to at least 400 G/min. At selected intervals the EPR spectrum is indexed and the NMR frequency is measured with the frequency counter and printed. During the counting period which was typically (0.1 sec) the maximum NMR frequency excursion was about 0.05 kc/sec or about 0.01 G out of 3000 G. The same counter in consort with the transfer oscillator monitors

* Alpha Scientific produces a gaussmeter similar to *a*, and *b* is manufactured by Japan Electron Optics Laboratory.

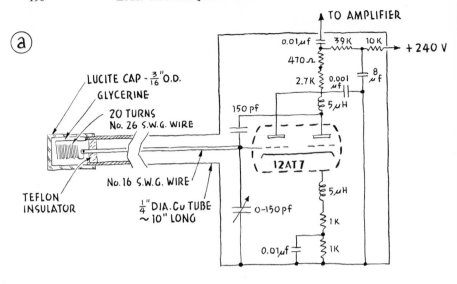

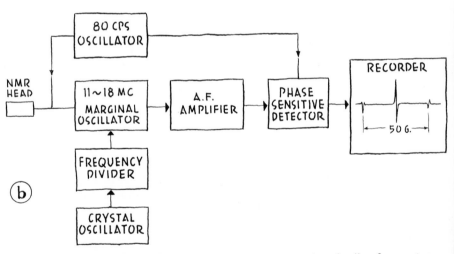

Fig. 5-5. Proton resonance gaussmeters: (*a*) construction details of a proton NMR head and an associated marginal oscillator suitable for frequencies near 15 Mc/sec. The construction follows Ref. S-21; however, similar oscillators and probes are described in Refs. I-2 and I-3. The variable capacitor (0–150 pF) controls the frequency. Diagram (*b*) shows the components involved in one of the commercial gaussmeters based on the marginal oscillator-NMR head arrangement. Additional features include a known frequency and sidebands on the proton resonance absorption to provide an accurate gauge for hf splitting measurements (JEOL JESS-FC-1).

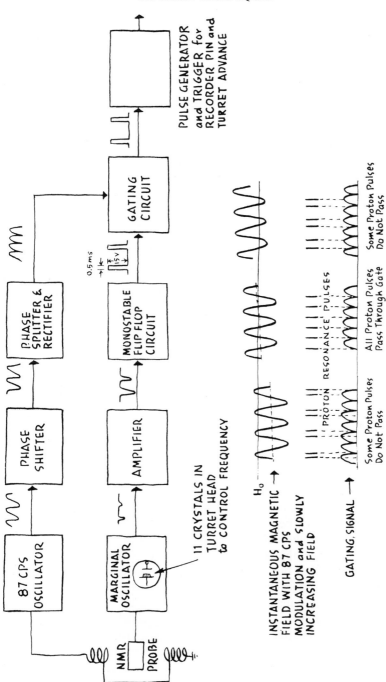

Fig. 5-5. (c) Circuit automatically marks the recorder output at 18 G intervals (H-16).

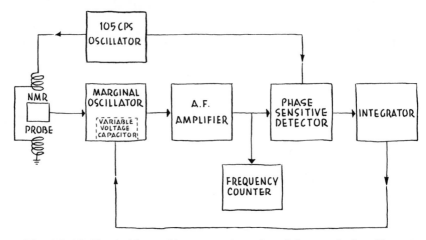

Fig. 5-5. (*d*) Circuit (*d*) provides automatic tuning of the marginal oscillator to maintain the frequency on resonance throughout the magnetic field sweep. The frequency as monitored with the frequency counter can be recorded at any selected time (F-10).

the microwave frequency. When this system was used to measure g values, the principal error resulted from inhomogeneities in the magnetic field over the sample volume, i.e., a 1–6 cm^3 sample and 6 in. diameter pole faces. An estimated error of about 0.1 G would produce an error of 0.00007 in the splitting factor.

5.2.3 Hall Plates

Gaussmeters with Hall probe sensing elements are commercially available both for magnetic field measurements and for magnet field control. Figure 5-6 illustrates the operation and pertinent parameters of the probe. When the current I passes through the Hall plate, the magnetic field displaces the charge carriers as indicated so a Hall voltage V develops which is proportional to both I and H, i.e., $V \sim RIH/t$ where R is the Hall coefficient and t = thickness. If the current is held constant, V is proportional to H, thus providing an appropriate indication of the magnetic field strength. A typical commercial unit contains a stable 3 kc oscillator to supply the constant current so the resulting ac Hall voltage can be filtered to discriminate against noise. The signal is then amplified, rectified, and detected in a meter circuit. Small size is a prominent advantage of the Hall probe. Since the Hall voltage is inversely proportional to the plate thickness, thin samples are in order, e.g., one commercial probe is

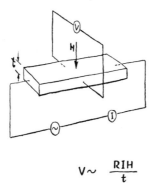

$$V \sim \frac{RIH}{t}$$

Fig. 5-6. Schematic representation of a Hall plate as used to measure the magnetic field H.

0.025 in. thick, $\frac{1}{8}$ in. wide, and $\frac{3}{16}$ in. long. In contrast to NMR and the induction technique which are insensitive to the temperature the Hall effect has a substantial temperature coefficient; consequently, precise measurements require either control or calibration at the measuring temperature. Control involves some type of thermostat arrangement which adds both bulk and cost to the probe, thus compromising the prominent advantage. The other alternative, "on-the-spot calibration," is performed through the use of reference magnets which are available with fields covering the 200–10,000 G range.* Typical accuracies are about 1% plus the accuracy of the reference magnet.

The next step toward automation is to couple one of the field measuring techniques to a programmer and a regulator to provide magnetic field control. Several commercial field control systems of this type† use a Hall probe as the field measuring component. According to the specifications fields can be set to ± 1 G with a repeatability of one part in 10^5 and a resolution of ± 0.02 G.

5.2.4 EPR Gaussmeters

If a sample of known g value is available, the resonance condition $h\nu = g\beta H$ can be used to calculate the magnetic field strength from a measurement of the resonant frequency or vice versa. This technique was considered briefly in Section 2.5.1 in the comparison method of measuring g values. Here we list a few problems and precautions to be observed in exercising the ritual. The utility of the technique depends

---

* Radio Frequency Laboratories, Inc., Boonton, N.J.
† Fieldial, Varian Associates, Palo Alto, Calif., Digital Field Control, Alpha Scientific Laboratories, Berkeley, Calif.

strongly on the spin systems under study and their compatibility with systems whose well-established g values make them suitable for standards. Other desirable characteristics in the standard are known hyperfine splittings and lines that are near but do not interfere with the unknown spectra. In considering several variations of the measuring procedure, Hyde (H-28) notes that the comparison technique is usually more useful for measuring g values and the hfs of free radicals than for transition elements or systems with large angular momenta. Several procedures are possible including superposition, exchange, and dual modulation. When the standard and unknown spectra do not interfere, the simplest procedure is to make a simultaneous measurement with two spin systems located so that they will encounter the same magnetic field. When the spectra overlap sufficiently to interfere with locating the crossover point on a derivative curve, an adjustment of the intensity or a change of standard may resolve the lines; 1% accuracy in measuring fields differing by several gauss is possible by the superposition method (H-28). In the exchange technique, the standard is substituted for the unknown on successive runs; consequently, any shift in the resonance frequency or hystereses in the magnet between runs introduces errors in absolute field measurements; however, the procedure is completely satisfactory for measuring field intervals as required to determine hf splittings. Finally, the dual cavity purchases the advantages of superposition for interfering systems at the expense of some additional electronics, i.e., separate modulation coils and frequencies for the standard and the unknown. In the system reported by Hyde (H-28,L-12) the sample modulated at 100 kc and the standard at 400 c were mounted one wavelength apart, in a rectangular TE_{104} cavity similar to the arrangement of Fig. 4-30. After the signals have passed through the crystal detector, filter circuits separate the two signals so they can be independently amplified, phase-sensitive detected, and displayed on a two channel recorder. Once set up, this technique is useful for measuring the magnetic field, splitting factors, hf splittings, and spin concentration. Usually the magnetic field will be slightly different at the two cavity positions; therefore, it is necessary to determine this difference by a measurement on identical samples located in the two positions. Of course this calibration must be repeated each time the cavity is moved with respect to the magnet poles.

5.3   QUANTITATIVE MEASUREMENTS OF SPIN CONCENTRATIONS

In Ref. H-28 Hyde concludes that "of all the measurements one can make with EPR equipment, the determination of absolute spin concentrations is the most difficult." In concept the problem is straightforward since, in the customary behavior of absorption spectroscopy, EPR follows the general rule that the area under the absorption curve is proportional to the number of absorbers; however, in execution, the required control or measurement of many parameters places stringent requirements on the spectrometer's stability and the spectroscopist's patience. Two general approaches have been tried: (1) "the absolute" where spin concentrations are calculated from the spectrometer parameters and the relation between spin concentration and the magnetic susceptibility and (2) "comparison" where unknowns are measured relative to standards of known spin concentration. By far the largest number of EPR practitioners adhere to the comparison methods and with good justification; nevertheless, a few remarks about the absolute approach are important in order to emphasize the parameters that require attention in both procedures.

5.3.1   Absolute Determinations

The procedure outlined here follows Ref. Y-2; however, similar information is available in Refs. F-3 and I-2. Starting with an expression for the reflection coefficient of a reflection cavity containing a paramagnetic sample

$$\Gamma = \Gamma_0 + [8\pi Q\eta\beta/(1 + \beta)^2]\chi'' - j[8\pi Q\eta\beta/(1 + \beta)^2]\chi' \quad (5\text{-}2)$$

and simplifying for operation near the critical coupling point $\beta \approx 1$ with the spectrometer tuned to χ'' at resonance Yariv and Gordon (Y-2) find

$$\Gamma_{\text{res}} = \Gamma_0 + 2\pi Q\eta\chi''_{\text{max}} \quad (5\text{-}3)$$

where Γ_{res} = reflection coefficient at resonance, $\Gamma_0 = (\beta - 1)/(\beta + 1) = $ reflection coefficient far off resonance, $\beta = $ cavity Q/external $Q = Q/Q_x$, and $\eta = $ the filling factor. Combining Eq. 5-3 with a conventional expression for the absorptive component of the susceptibility

$$\chi''_{\text{max}} = \frac{N_0\beta g_\perp{}^2 h\nu_0(S + M)(S - M + 1)}{2kT\Delta H g_\parallel(2S + 1)} \quad (5\text{-}4)$$

and substituting $N = N_0V_s$, $\eta = aV_s$, and $(k/\pi\beta h) = 7.08 \times 10^{29}$ gives

$$N = 7.08 \times 10^{29}\left(\frac{T\Delta H g_\parallel}{Qav_0g_\perp{}^2}\right)\frac{(2S + 1)}{(S + M)(S - M + 1)}(\Gamma_{\text{res}} - \Gamma_0) \quad (5\text{-}5)$$

where $N = $ the total number of spins

$a = $ proportionality constant, cm^{-3}

$V_s = $ sample volume

$\Delta H = $ the width of a Lorentzian curve at half-maximum, gauss

$\nu_0 = $ the resonance frequency

S and $M = $ the quantum numbers for the transition

$T = $ the absolute temperature which is high enough so that $h\nu \ll kT$

$g_\parallel \cong g_\perp$ obtains when the H_0 is along the crystal symmetry axis.

Q, v_0, and ΔH are measured by methods already described; S and M are known if the transition has been identified and two methods are suggested for obtaining $(\Gamma_{res} - \Gamma_0)$. The reflection coefficients can be obtained from $\Gamma = (\text{VSWR} - 1)/(\text{VSWR} + 1)$ by measuring the voltage standing wave ratio VSWR at resonance, and off resonance.

In a second procedure the reflection coefficients are determined from the ratio reflected power/incident power. The cavity is mismatched to produce total reflection and thus an indication of the incident power. Then series attenuation is introduced until the detected power level is the same as observed for the matched cavity both on and off resonance. The reflection coefficient in decibels is equal to the inserted attenuation.

Assuming the cavity Q remains fixed, Eq. 5-5 requires the knowledge of seven parameters in order to compute the number of spins. Sometimes g, ΔH, and T are known for the material so it may be possible to escape with only four measured quantities. If the number of measurements does not drive one to a comparison technique, the fact that many experimental spectra do not have a conveniently determined line shape, i.e., not Lorentzian or even gaussian, may lead to this alternate path.

5.3.2 Comparison Techniques

Hyde has divided the problem of quantitative measurements by the comparison method into three parts: (*1*) finding a suitable standard or reference material, (*2*) calibrating the standard, and (*3*) comparing the unknown to the standard (H-28). To deal with the standards problem, many spectroscopists resort to two kinds of standards, primary and secondary. The principal prerequisite for the primary standards is accuracy. These standards can be inconvenient to use and moderately unstable but when necessary it must be possible to calibrate the spin concentration accurately. Conversely, the working standards should be extremely stable and convenience is highly desirable. Hyde lists four desirable properties which are applicable to both primary and secondary standards.

1. A linewidth close to that of the unknown resonant system. Several sets of standards are required to cover the anticipated spectra since EPR linewidths extend over a range of four decades.

2. A spin concentration near that of the unknown resonant system. Since measurable spin concentrations may range over nine orders of magnitude, again several standards may be required.

3. Stability both with time and temperature. The number of spins, the linewidth, and the g value should all remain stable.

4. A short relaxation time T_1 in order to avoid rf power saturation.

In addition, the standards and samples should have similar dielectric losses so the perturbations in the rf field will be the same for both spin systems (H-4).

Table 5-4 lists some of the primary standard materials and the calibration techniques used in determining the spin concentration.

Table 5-4

Primary Standard Materials

Material	Calibration technique	Line-width, G	Remarks	Ref.
DPPH	Optical absorption coefficient = 0.95 × 10^{13}; weighing and diluting; weighing and titration	1.9	See Section 7.5.2 sensitive to preparation technique, storage atmosphere and light	H-28 29 32
$CuSO_4 \cdot 5H_2O$	Weighing		Use fresh, very blue, single crystal to be sure all the waters of hydration are present	H-28
$MnSO_4 \cdot H_2O$				S-10
O_2	From pressure, volume, and temperature			4 38
F centers in LiF	Optical absorption	65		H-8 32
KCL	Optical absorption	50		H-28
KBr	Optical absorption	150		H-28
Peroxylamine	Titration			H-28
Protons in H_2O	NMR		Compare EPR sample of identical shape and size to NMR water sample varying only the magnetic fields.	H-28
Vanadyl Etioporphyrin(I)	Dissolved in petroleum distillate free from trace metals			S-1

Table 5-5

Comparative Measurements on the Absolute Number of ESR Centers[a]

(H-8,B-23)

Laboratory and Investigator	Type of spectrometer[b]	Reference system[c]	Spins per g × 10^{18} in irradiated sucrose[d]		
			0.5	1.0	2.0
Karlsruhe, Germany					
Köhnlein, W.	9450 Mc/sec	DPPH			
Müller, A.	100 kc/sec	$CuSO_4 \cdot 5H_2O$	0.355	0.66	1.2
	TE_{105}, refl	F centers in LiF			
Stockholm, Sweden					
Ehrenberg, A.	9600 Mc/sec				
Ehrenberg, L.	100 kc/sec	NO titration	0.355	0.64	1.22
Löfroth, G.	TE_{102}, refl				
Uppsala, Sweden					
Lund, A.	9500 Mc/sec	$[(C_2H_5)_2NCS_2]Cu$			
Vänngård, T.	100 kc/sec	in benzene	0.393	0.77	1.38
	TE_{102}, refl				
Utrecht, Holland					
ten Bosch, J. J.	8900 Mc/sec	DPPH			
Braams, R.	100 kc/sec		0.6	1.0	2.0
	TE_{102}, refl	MnS in ZnS			
Frankfurt, Germany					
Redhardt, A.	9525 Mc/sec				
Pohlit, H.	30 c/sec	DPPH	0.56	1.0	2.0
	TE_{102}, refl				
Oak Ridge, USA					
Randolph, M. L.	9400 Mc/sec				
	13 c/sec	DPPH	0.51	0.95	1.86
	TE_{011}, trans				
Oslo, Norway					
Henriksen, T.	9200 Mc/sec				
	110 kc/sec	DPPH	0.55	0.98	2.02
	TE_{102}, trans				

[a] This table was presented at the Second International Congress of Radiation Research, Harrogate, August 5–11, 1962.

[b] The first figure is the microwave frequency, the second is the modulation frequency, and the third describes the type of the resonance cavity. Refl denotes reflection cavity and trans transmission cavity.

[c] DPPH: Purified diphenylpicrylhyrazyl contains about 0.95 unpaired spins per molecule.

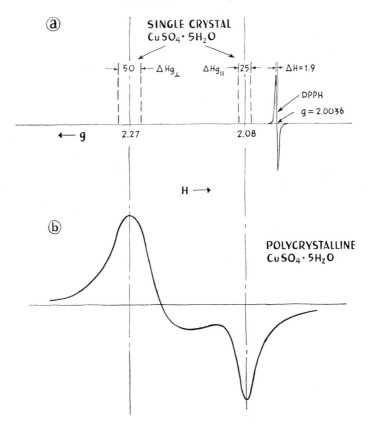

Fig. 5-7. (*a*) Linewidths and *g* values compared to DPPH for EPR in single $CuSO_4 \cdot 5H_2O$ at two orientations in the magnetic field. In the $g_\perp$ orientation there is no interference between the two standards (B-1). (*b*) Spectrum of polycrystalline $CuSO_4 \cdot 5H_2O$ exhibiting two principal *g* values. All measurements at room temperature. [(*b*) courtesy K-11.]

and illustrates a point noted by Feher that the *g* values differ sufficiently to permit simultaneous use of both standards (F-3). Figure 5-8 shows several simple mounting arrangements for dual standards. A side benefit from such combination standards is the check provided on their stability. Widely differing materials should lose their unpaired spins at different rates so a change in the relative signal amplitude indicates that one of the standards has started to drift.

The various single-crystal standards in Table 5-4 offer a selection of hf structures and linewidths; however, the spectra are dependent on orientation in the magnetic field. Figure 5-9 shows the spectra for some of these

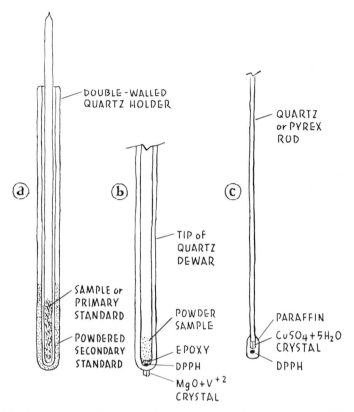

Fig. 5-8. Arrangements for supporting two noninterfering standards. [(a) from Ref. 36; b and c from Ref. 39.]

materials. Several spectroscopists have used the F centers in alkali halide crystals for yardsticks, KCl, KBr (H-28) and LiF (32). The number of spins were determined by optical absorption measurements and Eq. 7.3-3. Here the main error stems from uncertainties in the oscillator strength f which has always been difficult to determine precisely. Early evaluations of f were based on titrations of dissolved additively colored crystals. Interestingly, some of the recent oscillator strengths have been obtained from EPR measurements in conjunction with some other primary standard. Since F centers are photosensitive only additively colored crystals have the stability required for a standard (see Section 7.3).

Oxygen, O_2, offers several advantages as a primary standard. The number of molecules, i.e., spins, can be determined quite accurately from measurements of pressure, volume, and temperature. Also the problems

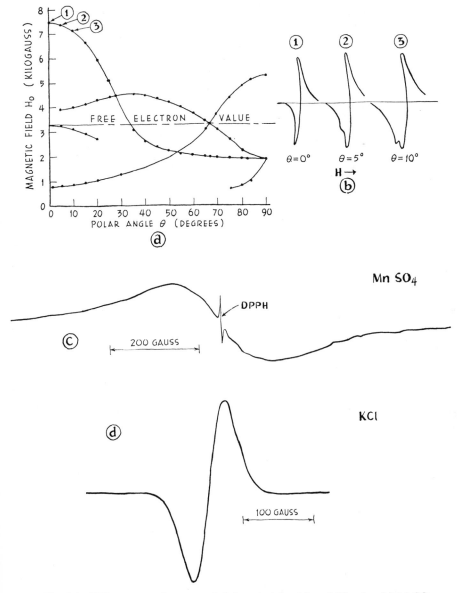

Fig. 5-9. EPR spectra of some yardstick materials: (a) and (b) ruby, (c) MnSO₄, and (d) KCL, where (a) shows the position dependence of the absorption lines in Ruby on the orientation of the magnetic field and (b) indicates some of the line shape variations. When compared with free radicals such as DPPH, an orientation should be selected to put the ruby lines well away from the free electron value. Other F-center EPR spectra are given in Fig. 7.3-7. [(a) and (b) after G-3; (c) after K-5.]

of dilution and filling factor are easily handled. Oxygen is used both as a primary standard to calibrate solid spin systems in terms of equivalent oxygen atoms (4) and as a working standard particularly in EPR studies of gases. Tinkham and Strandberg did the classic work that provides the basis for quantitative measurements (T-4). They resolved 120 hf lines with X-band and 78 lines with S-band spectrometers. Also they calculated and measured the intensities of the lines and measured the frequency and field strength so that g values can be calculated. Most practitioners compare the absorption of the unknown gas to one of the most prominent O_2 absorption lines, preferably while holding as many of the experimental parameters constant as possible. Assuming the absence of rf saturation the expression for the number of spins as derived in Refs. K-17 and W-15 becomes

$$N_u = C_1 \left(\frac{2kT}{h\nu_0\eta\beta}\right) \int_0^\infty \chi_u'' \, dH \tag{5-6}$$

where N_u = number of unknown spins, C is a constant, the terms in the bracket have their usual meaning, and the integral is the area under the absorption curve. When compared with the O_2 standard the ratio is

$$N_u/N_{O_2} = C_2 \left(\int_0^\infty \chi_u'' \, dH \Big/ \int_0^\infty \chi_{O_2}'' \, dH\right) \tag{5-7}$$

Table 5-7 lists values of C_1 for some of the common gases and Table 5-8 lists values of C_2 for a comparison of these gases to various prominent O_2 lines. The field values and intensities included in Table 5-8 will assist in locating these lines. Figure 6.1-2 shows a spectrum for molecular oxygen with some of the lines labeled. The lettering is the same as used in Ref. W-15 and has no significance other than a simple label. The possibility of determining the spin concentration from several O_2 lines immediately suggests the probability of dispersion in the results; however,

Table 5-7
Values of the Constant C_1 for the spectra of
Various Atoms at 300°K (W-15)

Atom	Spectral lines measured for area	C_1
Oxygen	Six-line composite	0.206
	Four-line composite	0.225
Nitrogen	One line of triplet	0.6
Hydrogen	One line of doublet	2

Table 5-8

Values of C_2 to be Used in Eq. 5-7 when Comparing Oxygen, Nitrogen, and Hydrogen Atom Spectra to Prominent Lines in the Oxygen Molecule Spectrum

Molecular oxygen line (Fig. 6.1-2)	g_{eff}	P, at 300°K	Magnetic field H, G[a]	Signal intensity measured	Signal intensity calculated	Oxygen 6-line composite	Nitrogen, one line of triplet	Hydrogen, one line of doublet
						$\times 10^{-3}$	$\times 10^{-3}$	$\times 10^{-2}$
C	1.40	0.741	5583.8	0.78	0.741	2.02	5.88	1.96
E	1.24	1.21	6087.5	1.34	1.21	3.71	10.8	3.61
F	1.01	1.50	6710.2	1.45	1.50	5.64	16.4	5.48
G	1.24	0.545	6509.3	0.57	0.545	1.67	4.88	1.63
J	1.20	1.39	8575.2	1.36	1.39	4.40	12.8	4.27
K	0.95	1.24	7254.3	1.15	1.24	4.96	14.4	4.82
B	1.31	0.37	5353.2	0.37	0.37	1.07	3.12	1.04

(Column groups: "Values for O_2 lines (T-4)" spans g_{eff} through Signal intensity calculated; "C_2 (W-15)" spans Oxygen 6-line composite through Hydrogen one line of doublet.)

[a] Spectrometer frequency = 9476.75 Mc/sec.

some indication of the reproducibility and reliability of the system is gained by comparing the integrated intensities of the various O_2 lines. Table 5-9 lists the theoretical integrated intensity ratios for some of the lines as computed from the expression (W-15)

$$I_1/I_2 = P_1(g_{eff})_2/P_2(g_{eff})_1 \qquad (5\text{-}8)$$

where the values of P and g_{eff} are listed in Table 5-8. Spectrometers, cavities, and the appropriate gas handling equipment are discussed in Chapter

Table 5-9

Comparison of Experimental and Theoretical Integrated Intensity Ratios for Various O_2 Lines (W-15)

Line pair	Theoretical	Experimental	Exptl./Theoretical
C/E	0.544	0.535	0.98
E/G	2.22	2.38	1.07
F/G	3.37	3.45	1.02
F/J	1.28	1.23	0.96
J/K	0.887	0.858	0.97
B/E	0.289	0.236	0.82
B/F	0.190	0.168	0.88
B/G	0.641	0.555	0.87

VI. Appropriate pressures are in the millimeter range and can be measured with a McLeod gauge. With O and O_2 in this pressure range rf saturation apparently is not a problem for powers less than 100 mW; however, saturation is observed at much lower power levels in some other gases, e.g., hydrogen and nitrogen atoms exhibit saturation at 0.1 mW (W-15).

5.3.3 Secondary Standards

The two main prerequisites for secondary standards are stability and reliable dilution. Much of the interest in anthracite coal standards originated in the search for highly stable spin systems. Presumably the spins in such geological materials have been on their way to equilibrium for eons so they should be rather stable by now. Furthermore, the coal could be ground and diluted uniformly to lower radical concentrations than DPPH. As discussed in Section 7.5 various charred carbohydrates and carbonaceous fuels with a similar single lined spectrum about 8 G wide are suitable as standards for use in free radical work. Reference H-28 reports the use of pitch derived from coal and diluted in a ball mill with powdered KCl; Ref. 32 used coal diluted with chalk, and Ref. H-17 describes in detail the preparation of charred dextrose standards. The radicals in these carbonaceous materials are sensitive to oxygen which causes line broadening as illustrated in Figure 7.5-6; consequently, the standards should be sealed in vacuum or an inert atmosphere.

Several groups advocate single-crystal Al_2O_3 containing an appropriate paramagnetic impurity as the secondary standard, e.g., Ref. S-10 uses synthetic ruby containing about 0.5% Cr^{+3} by weight and Ref. 20 uses Al_2O_3 containing copper. Singer (S-10) cemented the ruby into the cavity with the trigonal axis perpendicular to H_0 and found that at X-band frequencies the spectrum consisted of a strong line at about 5 kG and 3 peaks near 2 kG so that there was no interference with the usual radical spectra. Obviously, there are many possibilities for secondary standards and in many cases a well studied sample becomes a yardstick on the basis of expediency.

5.3.4 Calibration of Secondary Standards and Quantitative Measurements

Two general rituals are available, substitution or superposition, where, as the terms imply, the primary standard and the secondary under calibration are introduced into the cavity and measured either one at a time or simultaneously. Hyde has listed the hazards that plague the substitution method when there is an appreciable difference in the properties of the samples under comparison (H-28). Sample geometries, dielectric properties, and containers should be identical, otherwise it is difficult to determine precisely the filling factor and the distortion of the rf field. Preferably the interchange should not affect the cavity Q and match, otherwise these factors must be determined and introduced into the calibration as in the "absolute method." The substitution method has been used successfully where many essentially identical samples are involved. Normally, the superposition techniques are the most versatile and again there are two possibilities. When the EPR spectra do not interfere, the standards can be mounted at any of the sample positions in the cavity. When the spectra overlap significantly, a dual sample cavity offers the best approach. As described in connection with Fig. 4-30 various developments have eliminated the cross modulation interference so that well-behaved independent spectra are simultaneously obtained. Again it is desirable to use identical sample geometries, sample tubes, and dielectric constants to avoid the field distortion and filling factor problems. Furthermore, the calibration should be repeated with the standards interchanged to cancel out differences in the field modulation and rf field between the two sample positions. Hyde developed an expression for the ratio of spins when data is available for both standards in both positions

$$N_k/N_u = (M_{k_1} G_{u_2} M_{k_2} G_{u_1} / M_{u_2} G_{k_1} M_{u_1} G_{k_2})^{1/2} \qquad (5\text{-}9)$$

where M = the graphical first moment or the area under the absorption curve; G = the amplifier gain; and subscripts k and u refer to the known standard and unknown, respectively; and 1 and 2 are the two positions.

5.3.5 Obtaining the Number of Spins

When the standards have been selected and the spectra have been recorded, there are still several steps involved in finding the number of spins in the unknown. Collectively, the worldwide EPR community has expended considerable thought and effort in minimizing the time and exertion involved in these last steps. Since the number of spins are proportional to the area under the absorption curve and the spectrometers normally record the first derivative, the direct approach is to perform a double integration. First, we consider several cases where the double integral can be replaced by measurable quantities and then we look at methods of performing the integration. When identical spin species are being compared, the shape of the resonance curve remains constant so that the double integral is proportional to the amplitude of the absorption curve or the height "peak-to-peak" of the derivative. When the spectra are true Lorentzian or gaussian shapes, the areas are proportional to the product of the peak amplitude and the width at half maximum so that spectra with a common curve shape but different widths can be compared.

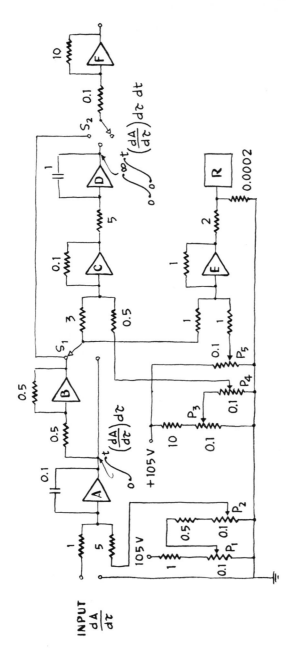

Fig. 5-10. Schematic circuit for analog computation of EPR spectra. Resistances are in megaohms and capacitances are in microfarads. Amplifier A integrates the input signals of less than 100 MV to give

$$\int_0^t \left(\frac{dA}{dt}\right) dt$$

Amplifier B shifts the phase 180° to accommodate both increasing and decreasing magnetic field scans. Amplifier C reduces the signal to a convenient level and D performs the second integration. With switches S_1 and S_2, as shown, the absorption curve signal goes to amplifier E which adds a base line value and feeds a 5 MV recording potentiometer R. A 100:1 multiplying amplifier F in conjunction with a sensitive voltmeter permits precise initial balancing of potentiometers P_1, P_2, P_3, and P_4 so that in the absence of a resonance signal the output will be zero. (Courtesy R-2.)

Unfortunately, most spectra are neither strictly Lorentzian nor gaussian in shape so that double integration is in order. Various rituals are currently in vogue for performing the integration. Initially, hand methods, such as counting squares, or graphical integration with an adding machine or planimeter sufficed but these methods were laborious and attention soon turned to automation. Both mechanical and electrical analog devices are adroit at integration so it is not surprising that soon a number of commercial and homemade integrators were wedded to EPR spectrometers. Under suitable conditions the results were quite satisfactory as illustrated by Figs. 5-10 and 5-11. The integrating circuit in Fig. 5-10 was used by Randolph (R-2) to obtain the spectra reproduced in Fig. 5-11 for radicals in irradiated glycyl–glycine. In many cases where quantitative measurements are desired, the sweep times are in the range of 10–30 min; therefore, extreme stability of both the spectrometer and the integrator is required. With large spin concentrations such as the 10^{18} value of Fig. 5-11 the signal overwhelms many of the sources of instability and excellent integrations are obtained. Unfortunately, many of the most interesting quantitative

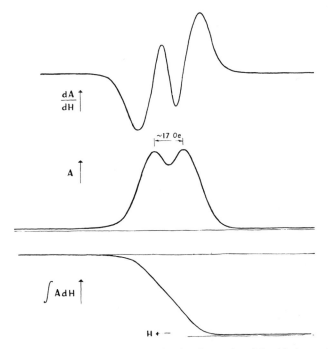

Fig.5-11. Simultaneous plots of the derivative, integral and double-integral curves for the EPR spectrum of gamma-irradiated glycyl–glycine; about 10^{18} resonant centers. (Courtesy R-2.)

measurements involve weak signals at the limits of spectrometer sensitivity. Under these circumstances the accompanying base-line drifts have been the undoing of numerous automatic integrators which now spend their time collecting dust while awaiting the appearance of a strong narrow signal. If all of the spectra are recorded as in Fig. 5-11, it is possible to correct for the drift but the time required to balance the integrator adequately and to make the corrections soon consumes all of the profits and it becomes just as easy to hand integrate a weak signal spectrum. Of course a shifting base line is a problem for any method of integration and extreme care is required in laying out the base line for manual integrations to avoid sizable errors. In the absence of other information most EPR practitioners assume the base line drifts at a constant rate so for a spectrum such as Fig. 5-12 the line would be drawn at an angle. After the first integration the absorption curve often fails to return exactly to zero at which time a triangular correction is applied, i.e., an area corresponding to the shaded triangle in Fig. 5-12 is either added or subtracted as required to make the curve close. This amounts to shifting the base line of the derivative curve by a constant amount which should be within the experimental uncertainty of the lines original location for reliable results.

Wyard (W-29) has outlined a numerical integration method for a desk calculator that is capable of doubly integrating a typical spectra in a few minutes. The method automatically corrects for a base-line drift of the constant rate variety. In terms of the nomenclature of Fig. 5-13 the ritual is as follows:

1. Divide the derivative spectrum into n intervals of length h, with an ordinate Y at the center of each interval.

2. The value of the absorption curve at the end of the pth interval is approximately

$$h \sum_{r=1}^{p} Y_r \tag{5-10}$$

3. The area A under the polygon is

$$A = \tfrac{1}{2}h^2 \sum_{r=1}^{n} (2n - 2r + 1)Y_r \tag{5-11}$$

4. The correction for constant base line drift is

$$(\tfrac{1}{2}nh^2) \sum_{r=1}^{n} Y_r \tag{5-12}$$

so the corrected area becomes

$$A = \tfrac{1}{2}h^2 \sum_{r=1}^{n} (n - 2r + 1)Y_r \tag{5-13}$$

If h is one-fourth of the linewidth, the average error is about 5%.

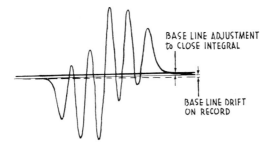

BASE LINE ADJUSTMENT
to CLOSE INTEGRAL

BASE LINE DRIFT
ON RECORD

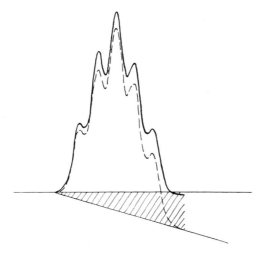

Fig. 5-12. Illustration of typical base line shift during recording of the derivative spectrum and effect of slight adjustment of base line to close the absorption curve.

Applying Eq. 5-13 to Fig. 5-13 the contribution to A from the Y_p term for $n = 18$ and $r = 6$ becomes $\frac{7}{2}h^2 Y_p$ which is the first moment of this segment about the midpoint of the spectrum. Since the other terms are also first moments, A becomes a numerical approximation to the first moment of the derivative spectrum.

Andrews (A-11), Burgess (B-34), and others have derived the equivalence between the area under the absorption curve and the first moment by direct integration and the moment method is extensively used both in numerical calculations and as a basis for the "moment balance." When the moments are taken with respect to the center of the spectrum, a constant drift of the base line produced no error (W-29). Figure 5-14 shows three types of

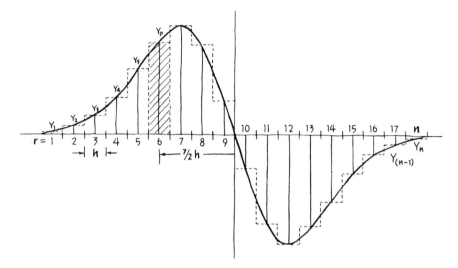

Fig. 5-13. Arrangement of spectrum for numerical integration by the Wyard method. The hystogram shows the area actually summed (W-30).

balances suitable for obtaining the first moments by weighing the spectra cut out of the recording paper. In arrangement a the spectrum is traced onto cardboard to provide additional weight. If an analytical balance is modified with an appropriate platform as in arrangements b or c, the sensitivity is adequate to permit direct measurements on cutouts from recorder paper. Variations in paper uniformity were found to effect the results by less than 2% (K-13). Reference K-13 also examined the error introduced by recording only a finite length of the spectrum. With Lorentzian curves the long tails can produce appreciable errors. For example, if ΔH is the derivative peak-to-peak width, a recording $15\Delta H$ long will enclose about 85% of the area under a Lorentzian curve as compared with essentially all of the area for a gaussian curve. Unfortunately open balances such as those of Fig. 5-14 are subject to complications from air currents, so some of the balance men are shifting to moment measurements with planimeters, which incidentally do not destroy the spectrum.

Others have automated the moment calculations through use of computers, e.g., curve readers have been connected to computers. More directly, spectra have been recorded in digital form suitable for direct input to a computer. Such mechanization is convenient when a large number of spectra are analyzed quantitatively. Finally for the laboratory that has everything, the spectrometer can be equipped with a digital output which is connected by a direct line to a time-sharing computer,

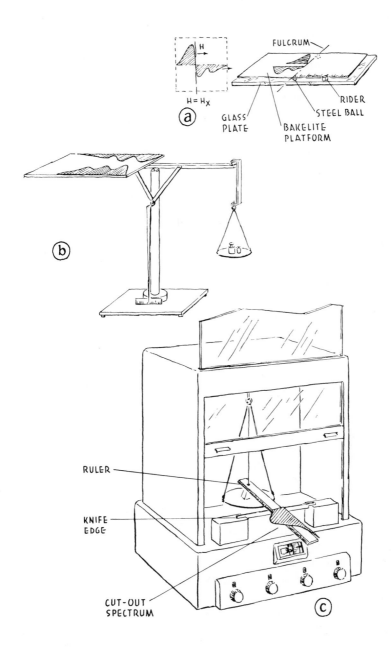

Fig. 5-14. Three balances arranged to measure the first moment of spectra cut out of recording paper. [(*a*) courtesy B-34; (*b*) after K-13; (*c*) 12.]

thus achieving the degree of automation sought in the automatic integrators previously discussed plus an ability to cope with a drifting base line. Once the spectrum is in the computer's memory, the base line can be adjusted at leisure to achieve the proper symmetry. While such an eloquent system is not justifiable for a few curves, it could be a convenient side benefit from spectrometers that have been coupled to computers in order to fit the hfs to theoretical spectra.

5.4   RELAXATION TIME MEASUREMENTS

The various methods of measuring relaxation times and the procedures for evaluating the data were introduced in Section 2.5.5; here we concentrate on the experimental problems, rituals, and equipment. Relaxation measurements have been made on a wide variety of spin systems, e.g., rare earth salts, copper Tutton salts, alkali metals, alkali metal–ammonia solutions, color centers, DPPH, and the importance of sample purity, temperature control, and spectrometer sensitivity depends strongly on the materials involved. The important experimental parameters involved in relaxation time studies are spin concentration, spin temperature, and the rf field used to disturb the spin distribution. Other factors usually of minor importance are spectrometer frequency, sample size and form, monitoring power, and other sample environmental parameters.

To obtain measurable relaxation times the paramagnetic species are diluted in a nonmagnetic host material as described in the various recipes of Chapters VI and VII. Typical dilutions are 1–5% rare earth or transition element ions in a compatible host crystal (L-1) and 10^{16} to 10^{17} color centers per cubic centimeter in irradiated alkali halide crystals (F-9). In all cases it is imperative to avoid the presence of paramagnetic impurities because they will interact with neighboring spin systems, thus introducing multiple relaxation processes and the accompanying complications of overlapping data that will have to be unraveled. Precise sample temperature control and measurement are vital because the relaxation mechanism is temperature dependent. Most relaxation measurements are conducted at cryogenic temperatures in the $1-77°K$ range because this is where the mechanism changes. Also the low temperatures lengthen the relaxation time and simplify the problem of adequate time resolution. Adequate sensitivity can become a problem when short relaxation times are involved or when the spin system is easily saturated. As the relaxation times become shorter, the bandwidth of the spectrometer electronics has to be widened to accommodate the signal and, of course, more noise comes through. Furthermore, most of the time-consuming techniques for recovering signal from noise are hampered by lack of time. The direct methods of measuring relaxation times involve disturbing the distribution of spins in the various energy levels and subsequently observing their return to thermal equilibrium. In order not to disturb the distribution appreciably during the observation period the EPR signal is measured at very low rf power levels, particularly for easily saturated spin systems.

5.4.1 Spectrometer Selections

Virtually all direct relaxation time measurements have been made with superheterodyne spectrometers which offer some definite advantages over the high-frequency modulated homodyne spectrometers that dominate the other areas of EPR spectroscopy. First, the short times involved usually preclude derivative measurements; therefore, a good signal-to-noise ratio is required when measuring the absorption curve directly. Second, after the spin distribution has been disturbed, the monitoring of the recovery period is performed at very low power levels, typically in the microwatt range where noise considerations favor the superheterodyne system. Third, most measurements are made at low temperatures where cavities are easier to construct without provisions for high-frequency modulation. Various cavities are in use: rectangular TE_{102}, and cylindrical TE_{011} and TE_{111}, both transmission and reflection coupled. Very short relaxation times limit the usable cavity Q, e.g., the maximum Q and minimum receiver band pass compatible with a time constant of 10^{-8} sec are about 500 and 30 Mc, respectively (K-3). Most systems feed the high powered signal to disturb the spins and the low powered monitoring signal through the same wave guide; however, the cavity in Figure 4-24c was used with separate waveguide feeds for the two rf powers. Both fixed and adjustable coupling systems are in use. When many samples involving host materials of the same dielectric properties are involved, the fixed iris hole is not only satisfactory but in the low-temperature arrangements, avoids the complications from microphonics and vacuum leaks that plague adjustable couplings. More versatile systems use a variable coupler such as that in Figure 4-20d. In all cases it is necessary to provide adequate isolation for the high-power pulse so that it will not overwhelm the monitoring detector and leave it prostrated while the signal goes by.

5.4.2 Saturation Recovery Techniques

As described in Section 2.5.5 the general process involves saturating the spin system with a high-powered rf pulse, then monitoring the return to equilibrium with a low-powered bridge. Variations in technique are concerned both with methods of generating and controlling the high-powered pulse and with the monitoring ritual. Figures 2-31 and 5-15 illustrate three

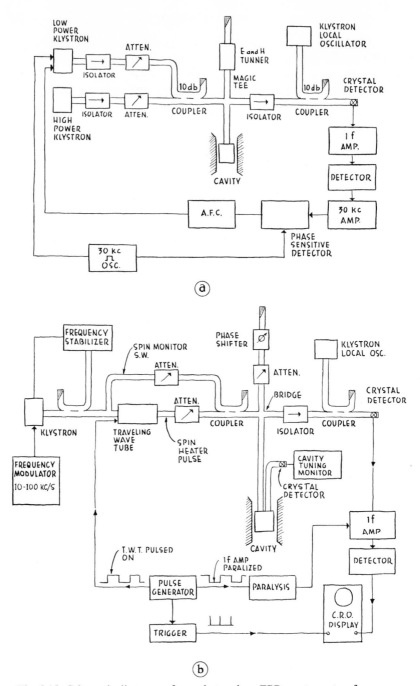

Fig. 5-15. Schematic diagrams of superheterodyne EPR spectrometers for measuring relaxation times by the saturation recovery technique. The methods for controlling the saturating or spin heater pulse are: (*a*) pulsing a high-power klystron; (*b*) pulsing a traveling wave tube.

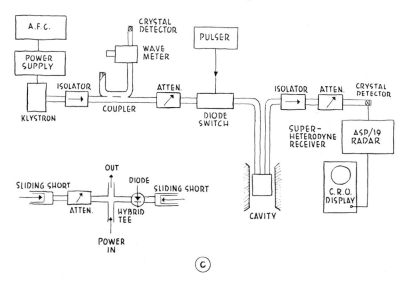

Fig. 5-15. (c) Pulsing a diode switch. [(a) 20; (b) after B-25; (c) after S-5.]

systems for controlling the high-powered pulse in superheterodyne spectrometers. In arrangement Fig. 5-15a the high-powered pulses are generated by a third klystron which is biased off while the two low-powered
klystrons monitor the recovery. Arrangement b contains a traveling wave
tube to control the length and intensity of the pulse. A bypass around the
traveling wave tube provides continuous power for monitoring the recovery. In arrangement c the rf pulse is formed by a germanium diode
switch* which also transmits the reduced power for monitoring. While
each of these systems has its own range of power levels and pulse dura-
tions, the operation is essentially the same as that illustrated in Fig.
5-16. The pulse generator activates the high-powered source for sufficient
time to saturate the spin system and at the same time paralyzes the IF
amplifier to avoid overloading the subsequent circuits. At the end of this
pulse, either immediately or after an appropriate delay, a timing pulse
triggers the oscilloscope to follow the recovery. In between the high-
power pulses the scope is triggered a second time at "comparison sweep"
to establish the signal level for the unperturbed system. If sufficient time
is allowed for complete recovery, the base line will remain unchanged on
successive pulses and will be equal to the value observed when the high-
power supply is turned off altogether (B-25). The power level, pulse duration, and relaxation periods are adjusted to provide reproducible recovery

* L4146 or L4136 in a Philco switch mount P901A.

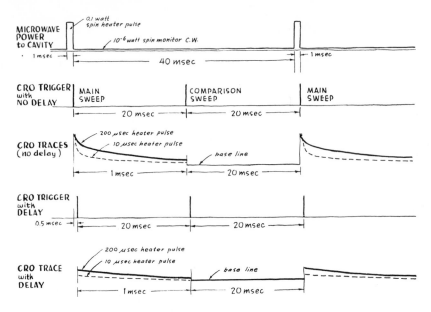

Fig. 5-16. Typical timing sequence used in observations on nickel fluosilicate. In each cycle after the saturation power pulse (spin heater) the cathode ray oscilloscope (CRO) is triggered once to show the decay trace, and once to provide a base line. Triggers may be delayed to show the decay after one or more half-lives. The time scale during the first part of the CRO trace is expanded to show the decay. When multiple relaxation processes lead to two or more decay periods, it may be possible to favor one of the processes by the length of the applied heater pulse as indicated by the superimposed CRO traces. Reference B-2 describes the diode switch in Fig. 5-15. Two crystals were used to cover the range from 8.8 to 60 kMc/sec. Sylvania IN419 from 8.8 to 18 kMc/sec and IN270 from 26 to 60 kMc/sec. (After B-25.)

curves. When several relaxation processes are in operation, the curve will represent the composite relaxation. Adjustments in the rf pulse duration may permit some resolution of the recovery rates by favoring one process over the other, as indicated by the dashed line. When a large number of measurements are in the offering it is a prudent idea to equip the oscilloscope with a calibrated adjustable exponential generator to control the x-axis sweep (L-1,M-8). If the relaxation is a single exponential process, the sweep time constant can be adjusted to produce a 45° line on the scope, thus directly measuring the relaxation time. Reference L-1 notes that higher accuracy and reproducibility are achieved with the exponential generator than with single shot photographs because the signal can be visually integrated over several seconds, thus increasing the signal-to-noise ratio. With arrangements b and c in Fig. 5-15 the klystron is locked either to a crystal-controlled frequency stabilizer or a cavity wavemeter; consequently, the frequency may be slightly off resonance for the sample cavity thereby permitting some of the real part of the susceptibility χ' to mix with the observations of the imaginary component, χ''. One procedure for checking the tuning throughout the recovery measurements is to modulate the klystron at a frequency which can complete 10 to 20 cycles during a relaxation half-life (B-14). Then if the amplitude is just sufficient to cover the resonance range, the presence of some χ' will be apparent as illustrated in Fig. 5-17 which shows a typical recovery curve obtained with a 10 kc modulation frequency.

Two monitoring procedures are illustrated: (a) low level in the ritual of Fig. 5-16, and (b) resaturation in Fig. 2-25. The properties of the spin system determine which procedure is most advantageous. When the power required to saturate the sample is large so that modest power levels can be used for monitoring without disturbing the spin system, the low level approach is adequate and preferable for short relaxation times, particularly when a number of measurements are to be superimposed in a time averaging

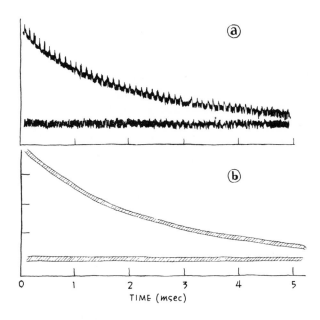

Fig. 5-17. (a) Decay curve for nickel fluosilicate with the klystron frequency modulated at 10 kc/sec to show the detuning effects of χ' changes. Minima correspond to on-tune settings and give χ'' values which are independent of χ' changes. When the χ' effect is small, the modulation is not required and a number of traces can be superposed as in (b). (Courtesy B-25.)

computer. Conversely, when long relaxation times are involved, the power required for saturation may be small and the monitoring power levels may be restricted to 10^{-8} W or less to avoid disturbing the spin system. Under such circumstances, the resaturation procedure of Fig. 2-25 simplifies the problem of obtaining a usable signal-to-noise ratio (B-2). In discussing the resaturation technique Baker and Ford describe three methods of pulsing the microwave power for both the initial saturation and the subsequent resaturation steps: (*1*) switching the rf power with the diode switch indicated in the insert of Fig. 5-15*c*; (*2*) switching the magnetic field through resonance, as demonstrated in Fig. 2-25; and (*3*) turning the klystron off during the relaxation period.

Switching the magnetic field is preferable when the relaxation time permits because the relaxation process can be studied as a function of field strength. Furthermore, establishing the spin system equilibrium at field strengths well above the resonance value enhances the concentration difference between energy levels. Some other characteristics of the systems described in Fig. 5-15 are listed in Table 5-10, including spectrometer parameters, power level, pulse length, and temperature. When the relaxation times are in the millisecond and longer range, the signal-to-noise ratio can be enhanced by using a time averaging computer to average a large number of recovery curves.

Table 5-10

Some Parameters of the Superheterodyne Spectrometers used to Measure Relaxation Times by the Saturation Recovery Technique

Parameter	Figure 5-15*a*	Figure 5-15*b*	Figure 5-15*c*
Rf pulse generator	Pulsed klystron	Pulsed traveling wave tube	Pulsed diode
Spectrometer frequency	X band	3.8–4.4 kMc	X band
Pulse power level (max. available watts)		1	~ 0.5
Monitoring power level (watts)		10^{-6}	10^{-8}–10^{-6}
Pulse length (sec)	Variable	10^{-3}–10^{-6}	10^{-1}–10^{-6}
Sample temperature ($^\circ$K)	1.2 up	1.8–4.2	1.4–5
Overall time response of system (sec)	$\sim 0.5 \times 10^{-6}$	$\sim 0.5 \times 10^{-6}$	$\sim 10^{-6}$
Repetition rate (per sec)		$2 \times 10^4 - \frac{1}{20}$	
Cavity		Rectangular TE_{011}	

In the examples described so far the magnetic field was set at H_0 throughout the measurement so that the oscilloscope displayed the peak of the absorption curve. When long relaxation times are involved, i.e., minutes, there is time to record the whole absorption curve. Thus, additional information may be available about the saturation process, e.g., the presence of hole burning.

The fourth arrangement, Fig. 2-31, is designed to push the lower limit for relaxation time measurements down to 10^{-8} sec. The principle has been described in Section 2.5.5. A backward wave oscillator supplies the rf power (100 W maximum) which can be modulated from 0 to 100% at frequencies ranging from 500 kc/sec to 30 Mc/sec. In order to pass the two sides bands resulting from this modulation the cavity Q is usually limited to about 10^{-3} (Fig. 2-31). As the modulation frequency increases, the signal induced in the pickup coil increases until the spins cannot relax between cycles then the signal approaches values as described in Fig. 2-32 for DPPH.

To insure adequate cooling some experimenters operate with liquid helium in the cavity directly in contact with the sample. Temperatures over the range from 1.2 to 5°K are controlled by evacuating or pressurizing the helium. A cartesian manostat will stabilize the pressure adequately (L-1).

5.4.3 Inversion Recovery

In the rapid passage technique the spectrometer considerations during the monitoring period are the same as for the saturation recovery method; however, the inversion process introduces a requirement for a fast magnetic sweep and a short rf pulse. For example, Castle et al. (C-3) used Helmholtz coils mounted on a dielectric cavity to provide a magnetic sweep of up to 120 G in times down to 20 μsec. A silvered epoxy resin cavity transmitted the rapid field sweeps without troublesome attenuation. Typically the temperature range starts about 1.5°K and may go to room temperature, the modulating power level ranges down to 10^{-8} W, and the pulse power may reach to 1–10 W for 50 μsec or so.

Figure 5-18 illustrates the sequence of events in this ritual. In line a the trace starts with the monitoring frequency locked to the cavity resonance and the magnetic field slightly below the resonant value H_0. A current pulse applied to the Helmholtz coils sweeps the spin system through resonance at 1 ascending and after an adjustable delay again at 2 descending. The monitoring scope records two absorption peaks, as shown on line b. To invert the spin distribution a short pulse of resonant frequency power is applied when the spin system passes through resonance, as indicated in line d. When the sweep returns at 2 the monitor signal will indicate the

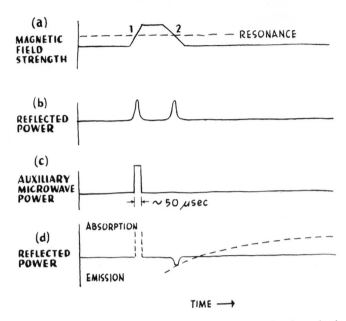

Fig. 5-18. Sequence of events in measuring relaxation times by the pulse inversion ritual. (Courtesy C-3.)

departure from equilibrium. Initially while the spin population is inverted, power is emitted; when the spin population in the two levels is equal (the saturation condition), the monitor signal is zero; finally at longer times an absorption curve returns as the system relaxes. The recovery curve indicated by the dotted line is obtained by varying the delay between pulse and monitor sweeps. Figure 5-19 is an oscilloscope trace of steps b and d superimposed.

Relaxation times longer than several seconds can be measured with a single pulse if the monitoring spectrometer can be swept back and forth through resonance to give a trace similar to Fig. 5-20. If the monitor signal is weak, it may be desirable to hold the spin system in a high magnetic field to increase the population difference in the energy levels before applying the inversion pulse, e.g., fields of 10 kG for "many" minutes lifted signals from F centers in KCl to a detectable level.

Inhomogeneous broadening can be detected by "hole" burning as indicated in Fig. 5-21, which shows monitoring spectra for two different delay times after the hole was created with a pulse that lasted part of the time required for the field sweep to pass through resonance. The hole disappeared with a time constant equal to that of the whole line (C-4). Table 5-11 lists a few spin systems and their range of relaxation times as determined by the rapid passage technique.

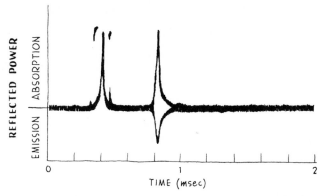

Fig. 5-19. Oscilloscope trace of lines *b* and *d* in Fig. 5-18. The two absorption peaks correspond to points *1* and *2* on line *b*. While the emission pulse indicates the spin, population is still inverted. (Courtesy C-3.)

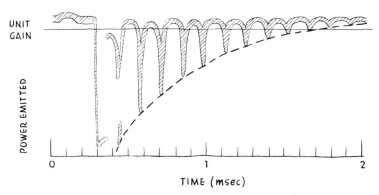

Fig. 5-20. Oscilloscope trace of a recovery curve following a single inversion pulse. Curve obtained by periodically monitoring the spin system. (Courtesy C-11.)

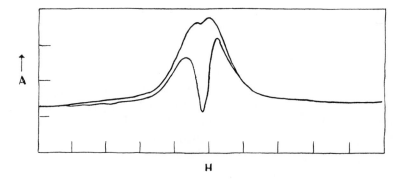

Fig. 5-21. Holes in the resonance line of E_1' centers in synthetic quartz at 27.3°K. The delay times for the two traces are 0.10 and 1.70 sec. The complete line has a $T_1 = 0.44$ sec at this temperature. (Courtesy C-4.)

Table 5-11

Examples of Relaxation Times Measured by the Rapid Passage Technique

Paramagnetic species	Temp, °K	T_1, sec	Ref.
E_1 center in synthetic quartz	1	10^3	C-4
	4.2	110	C-4
	77	0.013	C-4
E_2 center in synthetic quartz	1	29	C-4
	4.2	22	C-4
	77	0.017	C-4
A_1 center in synthetic quartz	2.1	0.1	C-4
Chromium doped $K_3Co(CN)^6$,	1.5	0.023	C-3
0.06% Cr:Co	4.2	0.0065	C-3
Chromium doped $K_3Co(CN)^6$,	1.5	0.013	C-3
0.5% Cr:Co			
Donors in silicon (antimony)	4.2	$T_s = 1$	C-5
Donors in silicon (phosphorus)	4.2	$T_s = 25$	C-5
Donors in silicon (arsenic)	4.2	$T_s = 100$	C-5

5.4.4   Free Precession, Free Induction, or Spin Echo

The pulse techniques developed by Hahn (H-1) and Carr and Purcell (C-2) permit direct measurements of both T_1 and T_2. Figure 5-22 shows two similar X-band spectrometers suitable for these techniques. They differ from the pulse spectrometers of Fig. 5-15 principally in the power-available and the short pulse times. Both instruments use pulsed magnetrons and the powers generated are 120 and 200 W in (a) and (b), respectively. In spectrometer b, which has a time constant of about 10^{-8} sec and a low Q cavity of about 500, this pulse produces an rf magnetic field H_1 of about 5 G (K-3). The superheterodyne receivers are protected during the high-power pulse either by (1) gating the local oscillator to detune it so the beat signal is well out of the amplifier frequency range, (2) activating high frequency microwave switches in front of the receiver, or (3) gating the receiver off directly.

The sequence of operation and the details of the various pulse procedures are conveniently explained with the vector diagrams of Fig. 5-23 following Ref. C-2. At equilibrium the total magnetic moment of a group of unpaired spins in a stationary magnetic field H_0 can be represented by the vector **M** aligned with H_0, i.e., the dotted vector in A. When an rf magnetic field, $2H_1$, satisfying the resonance criteria is applied perpendicular to H_0, the vector **M** will nutate through an angle θ while precessing as indicated. In time τ_ω, the angle of nutation $\theta = \gamma H_1 \tau_\omega$. Two angles are

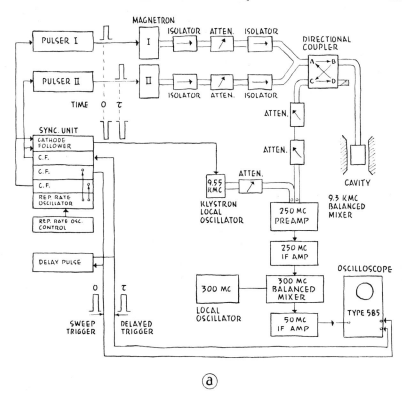

(a)

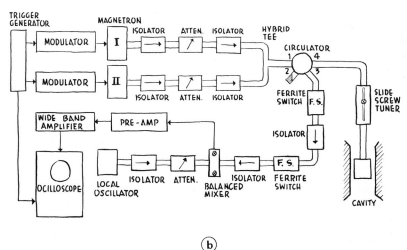

(b)

Fig. 5-22. Spectrometers for electron spin-echo measurements at the X-band frequency. [(a) courtesy R-6; (b) courtesy K-3.]

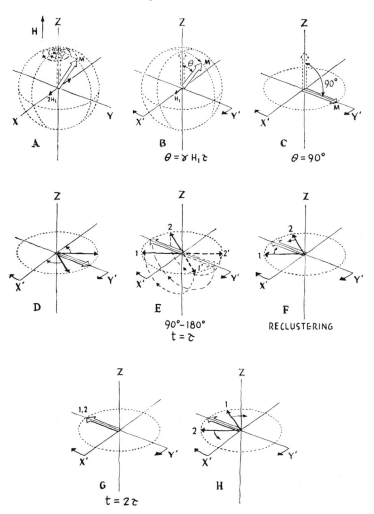

Fig. 5-23. The formation of an echo. Initially the net magnetic moment vector is in its equilibrium position (A) parallel to direction of the strong external field. Application of the rf field H_1 produces a combination precession and nutation of the net magnetic moment as viewed from the laboratory frame of reference. As viewed from the rotating frame of reference the magnetic moment appears (B) to rotate quickly about H_1. At the end of a 90° pulse the net magnetic moment is in the equatorial plane (C). During the relatively long period of time following the removal of H_1, the incremental moment vectors begin to fan out slowly (D). This is caused by the variations in H_z over the sample. At time $t = \tau$, the rf field H_1 is again applied. Again the moments (E) begin to rotate quickly about the direction of H_1. This time

of interest in these measurements: $\theta = 90°$ and $\theta = 180°$. When H is large, all the incremental moments that add to make **M** can be considered to rotate together as a single vector so for a 90° pulse from magnetron No. *1* the moments will arrive in the equatorial plane together as in C and the precession about Z will induce "free" induction signals in the cavity. As transverse relaxation (T_2) occurs, the incremental vectors will fan out as at D and the induction signal decays to zero as shown for four different spin systems in Fig. 5-24. If the dispersion of the vectors at D is entirely due to T_2 processes, T_2 can be computed from the decay of the free induction signal; however, it is usually safer to use the echo technique. In the 90°–180° pulse sequence (H-1), the 90° pulse is followed after a time interval τ by a $\theta = 180°$ pulse from magnetron No. *2* and all the incremental vectors rotate to a new position in the equatorial plane as indicated in Fig. 5-23E. Now the motion of the incremental vectors will cause them to recluster (F) so at the time 2τ they will be together again as at G and another signal called the echo will be induced in the cavity. The transverse relaxation coefficient T_2 is obtained from the decrease in the echo amplitude as a function of time, i.e., the time between the 90 and 180° pulses. Figure 5-25 illustrates the process with a series of 90°–180° pulses in which τ increases by a factor of 5 and the envelope of echo peaks generates the exponential decay curve governed by T_2. Figure 5-26 shows the oscilloscope traces for such a series of 90–180° pulses and echos for a potassium liquid ammonia spin system. Between each 90–180° sequence sufficient time must elapse for the spin system to return to thermal equilibrium. When spin diffusion is involved in addition to relaxation, the 90° free induction and 90–180° sequence lead to complex decay patterns; as a result, other pulse sequences have been evolved to cope with diffusion and to determine T_1. Carr and Purcell modified the 90–180° pulse to a series of 90–180–180°—180° which follows the decaying echos after one 90° pulse until the induced signal is no longer detectable. Figure 5-25b illustrates the echos resulting from 180° pulses applied at τ, 3τ, 5τ, etc. By an extension of the reasoning associated with Fig. 5-23 each 180°

H_1 is applied just long enough to satisfy the 180° pulse condition. This implies that at the end of the pulse all the incremental vectors are again in the equatorial plane. In the relatively long period of time following the removal of the rf field, the incremental vectors begin to recluster slowly (F). Because of the inverted relative positions following the 180° pulse and because each incremental vector continues to precess with its former frequency, the incremental vectors will be perfectly reclustered (G) at $t = 2\tau$. Thus maximum signal is induced in the pickup coil at $t = 2\tau$. This maximum signal, or echo, then begins to decay as the incremental vectors again fan out (H). While this example is for nuclear magnetic resonance, the explanation also applies to EPR. (Courtesy C-2.)

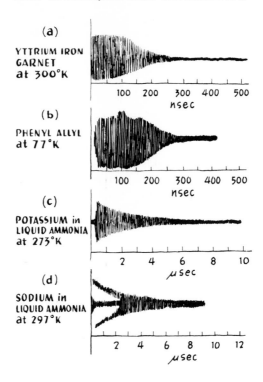

Fig. 5-24. Free induction signals following a 90° rf burst to align the magnetic moment in the equatorial plane (Fig. 5-23c). [(a), (b), and (c) made with the spectrometer in Fig. 5-22b, courtesy K-3; (d) courtesy B-22.]

pulse will lead to a reclustering of the remaining incremental vectors and the generation of another echo, etc. Sequences used to determine T_1 include (90°, θ, 90°), (90°, 90, 180°) (K-3), and (180–90°) pulses (C-2). The 180–90° sequence is particularly interesting because it leads to a null method of determining T_1. Referring to the reference system of Fig. 5-23 the 180° pulse inverts the total magnetic moment vector from the north pole to the south pole where the spin–lattice relaxation processes commence restoring the system to thermal equilibrium, i.e., **M** pointing north. If a strong 90° pulse is applied immediately after inversion, the excess south pointing spins will nutate to the equatorial plan and generate a free induction signal of maximum amplitude. As the time τ between the 180° and 90° pulse is increased, the excess spin population will be diminished and the amplitude of the free induction signal will decrease accordingly as shown in Fig. 5-27; when the spins are equally divided between the two

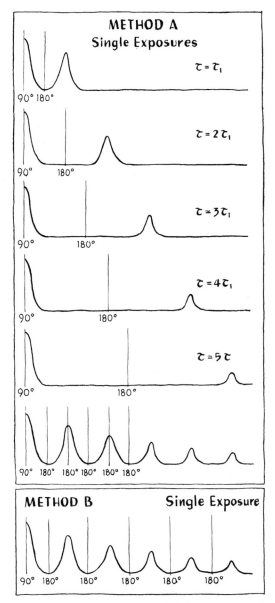

Fig. 5-25. Comparison of the two free precession methods for observing the decay time of the horizontal component of nuclear magnetic polarization. In method *A* the sample must return to its equilibrium condition each time an additional echo is to be observed. In method *B* the sample need only start from equilibrium once. The separate oscilloscope traces of method *A* are usually displayed superimposed in a multiple exposure picture. Only a single trace and hence a single exposure picture is required in method *B*. However, this latter method requires more than one 180° pulse. (Courtesy C-2.)

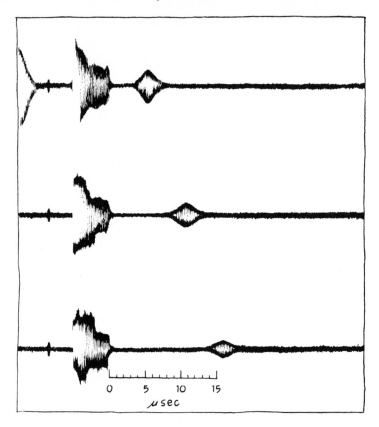

Fig. 5-26. Spin echoes for potassium in liquid ammonia, 273°K: T_2 decreased by
external field inhomogeneities, 1 μsec/div. (Courtesy K-3.)

energy states, i.e., at $M = 0$, the induction signal will be zero, i.e., at
τ_{null}. For τ larger than τ_{null} M will increase in the north direction and the
induction signal will build up to a maximum corresponding to the 90°
pulse applied to spins at thermal equilibrium; T_1 is found from the
expression $\tau_{null} = T_1 \ln 2$ (C-2). The spin system should be at thermal
equilibrium before commencing each 180–90° pulse sequence. Because of
the large power levels involved in the pulses, good thermal contact between
the sample and the temperature control medium is required to insure
reasonable control of the spin system temperature. In spectrometer a of
Fig. 5-22 the samples were cooled by direct contact with liquid helium in
the cavity. A Styrofoam bubble displacer filled the remainder of the cavity
to reduce the noise generated by bubbling helium.

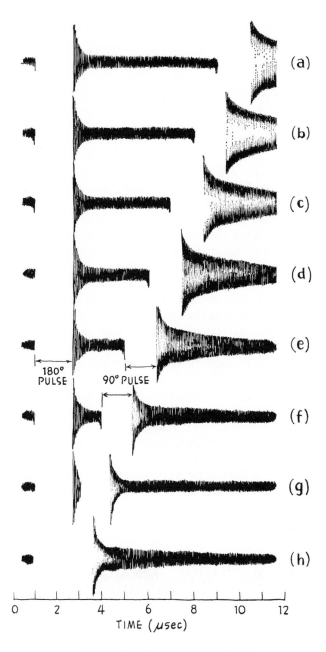

Fig. 5-27. Carr-Purcell (180–90°) sequence showing the longitudinal (T_1) relaxation process. In (a) the free induction signal following the 90° pulse is due to an $\mathbf{M}_z$ which is almost completely returned to equilibrium in the $+z$ direction. As the 90° burst is moved to the left [(b)–(f)], the available $\mathbf{M}_z$, and hence the free induction signal, first decreases to zero at (g) then begins to grow again (h). At (h) $\mathbf{M}_z$ is still in the $-z$ direction when it is flipped by the 90° burst. (Courtesy B-22.)

5.5 HIGH-RESOLUTION SPECTROSCOPY

We have already touched on the problems associated with high-resolution (HR) EPR in discussing the requirements for observing hfs and the spectrometer considerations in Sections 2.5.3 and 3.4, respectively. Briefly, the requirements are magnetically dilute spin systems, long relaxation times, low rf field intensities, and high spectrometer sensitivity, stability, and homogeneity. Here we are concerned primarily with samples that can meet these conditions and most of this section follows the remarks of Hausser (H-3,H-4). First, high-resolution EPR is restricted to solutions where rapid tumbling of the molecules can average out the anisotropic interactions, thereby eliminating this source of line broadening. Furthermore, solutions with low viscosities enhance the tumbling rate. Second, the intimate tie between relaxation times and linewidth requires attention to minimize the interactions responsible for relaxation.

1. A suitable spin system will have a very weak spin–orbit coupling. Since this coupling increases with atomic weight the best elements for HR spectra will be found in the first row of the periodic table.

2. The spin–spin interactions are reduced by diluting the spin system with a nonmagnetic solvent.

3. Molecular dipole interactions are minimized by eliminating dipolar impurities.

For example, oxygen is a well-known line broadener as illustrated in Fig. 6.2-12 where "air saturated" and "oxygen-free" spectra are compared for Wurster's blue. Third, HR spectroscopy has been most useful in dealing with spectra containing many lines spaced close together such as in Fig. 5-28 which contains a little over 300 hf lines in a 50 G span. Such proliferation of lines requires interactions with many magnetic nuclei, usually protons; therefore, the aromatic compounds are commonly

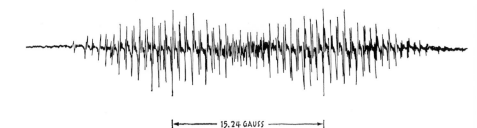

|←——————— 15.24 GAUSS ———————→|

Fig. 5-28. The first derivative of the absorption of a $5 \times 10^{-3}M$ solution of dimesitylmethyl in toluene at room temperature. (Courtesy C-9.)

Table 5-12

Examples of High-Resolution EPR Measurements

Radical	Solvent	Concentration moles/liter	Temp, °C	No. of hf lines (approx)	Splitting between milligauss	Ref.
1,3-Bisdiphenylene-allyl	CS_2	10^{-5}		> 400	60	H-3
Triphenylmethyl	Toluene	10^{-3}	−20 to −50	100		C-10
Dimesitylmethyl	Toluene	5×10^{-3}	room	300		C-9
Sodium naphthalene	THF[a]	$< 10^{-3}$	−80 to 45	25		
DPPH	THF	10^{-3}	room	> 100		T-7

[a] Tetrahydrofuran.

encountered in the high-resolution EPR literature because the benzene ring provides an excellent vehicle for coupling the unpaired electron to distant protons. A few examples of HR spectra are listed in Table 5-12 along with the radical concentration, solvent, between lines splitting, and temperature. Most of the concentrations are in the range from 10^{-3} to 10^{-5} mole/liter. The temperature is usually determined by trial, i.e., a compromise between viscosity, spin concentration, and temperature. Stability requirements are emphasized by the time required to record such spectra, e.g., about 15 hr for 400 lines (H-3).

5.6 SEALING WAX AND STRING

In the remainder of this chapter we turn to a variety of recipes that have been effective in discharging some of the mundane problems of EPR spectroscopy. No single item requires a greater deal of space so the subject matter will ramble in a manner analogous to the *Farmer's Almanac* or *Webster's Dictionary*.

5.6.1 Cements and Adhesives for Attaching Samples in the Cavity

Aside from sticking to the sample or the support the main prerequisite for a satisfactory cement is "no spins." Physically, the adhesives can be classed as rigid or pliable and chemically they are readily soluble or insoluble. When frequent sample changes or adjustments are required, the pliable-soluble cements are usually used while rigid-insoluble cements are preferable for permanent or very long-term mountings. Most single crystals are mounted with pliable-soluble glues such as:

1. Dow-Corning silicone stopcock grease (36,37).

2. Fishers Cello-Grease (35): Use where gravity will not pull the sample loose or as a safety measure tie sample in place with a fine nylon fishing line (16).

3. Apiezon-N (41), Apiezon-L (19).

Rigid soluble glues include:

4. Duco Cement (36).

5. Durofix or polystyrene type glue (20).

6. GE 7031 adhesive and insulating varnish (3).

7. Shellac (31).

Permanent bonds even repairs on broken crystal samples have been made with epoxy cements, e.g., Hysol C9-5062 (8).

5.6.2 Sample Supports

Such supports are required when samples are located in the center of a cavity such as the cylindrical TE_{011} or the rectangular TE_{102}. Most of the low-loss dielectrics are suitable from the dielectric standpoint; however, mechanical stability, thermal conductivity, and ease of fabrication and cleaning further restrict the choice. Favorite plastics are polystyrene (36), Teflon (35), and the preferred inorganic materials are quartz, sapphire, and Lucalox* (41). The plastics are adequate for most purposes, particularly Teflon which is easily cleaned. Many cements do not adhere well to Teflon so samples are usually attached mechanically or with one of the vacuum greases. When thermal conductivity is a factor, the inorganics are superior, particularly sapphire at liquid helium temperatures. Sapphire rods can be attached to metal dewar or cavity sections as in Fig. 7.5-8 by a solder joint that is vacuum tight. A layer of silver paint fired onto the sapphire followed with an electroplated coating of copper provide a satisfactory surface for soldering in a housekeeper type flange with 50–50 soft solder.

5.6.3 Seals to Keep Refrigerants Out of the Cavity

The procedures are quite varied, embracing the gamut of materials from rubber boots and ivory soap to indium O-rings. There is more latitude in the choice of materials than when mounting samples, provided the cement is excluded from the cavity. Again, the Silicone and Apiezon greases are most widely used for sealing tapered joints and flanges; however, two widely known homemade concoctions are also in use (7,17,19,20,22,25,27).

* Lucalox is a sintered material made of powdered sapphire by the General Electric Co.

1. Rubber Cement: ordinary Woolworth rubber cement is exposed in a dish until the solvent has evaporated, then 2 parts of rubber are mixed with one part kerosene by volume to form a fairly stiff cement (2,41).

2. Ivory Soap and glycerine: a 50:50 mixture by volume of Ivory Soap and glycerine produces a waxy, soapy solid that forms leak-tight seals for use down to 4°K. The mixture is heated to make it easy to apply (34).

Other flanges or joints have been sealed with indium O-rings or foil gaskets or soldered with woods metal (3). Glycerine has been used to seal rubber O-rings and bocts but the glycerine absorbs water and can spoil the Q if a little of it gets into the cavity. Several arrangements of boots, bags, and other membranes to keep refrigerants out of the cavity are shown in Fig. 5-29. The rubber boot *a* can be formed by dipping a glass

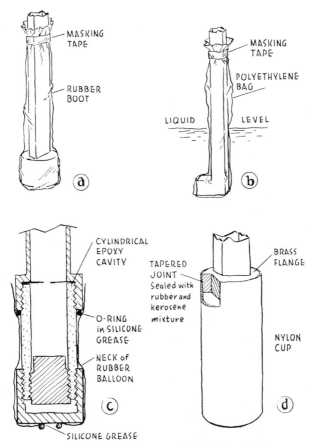

Fig. 5-29. Dielectric barriers to keep cryogenic liquids out of the cavities: (*a*) rubber boot (16); (*b*) polyethylene bag (22); (*c*) rubber balloon neck (17); (*d*) nylon cup (14).

tube mold in an air drying latex. To avoid pinholes, three layers should be applied by three separate dips (16). Rubber goods manufacturers can also produce the boots by the electrodeposition of neoprene latex on an aluminum mold. On short notice or whenever the bulk is not objectionable a polyethylene bag can be used as indicated in *b* (22). Arrangements *c* (17) and *d* (41) show a rubber sleeve barrier and a nylon cup, respectively. Nylon is superior to Teflon and polyethylene for submerging in liquid nitrogen because there is less trouble from creaking.

5.6.4   Microwave Windows and Detector Isolation

In the struggle to minimize noise and instrument drifts caused by ground loops or temperature changes involving the detector crystal or bolometer, some spectroscopists isolate and insulate the detector holder from the rest of the waveguide run with an insulating window. Windows of Mylar, polyethylene, mica, Teflon, or plastic electrical tape bolted between regular waveguide flanges with nylon screws provide electrical insulation and reduce air currents inside the waveguide that could effect the detector temperature. The soft plastic windows, particularly the electrical tape, are convenient for sealing off the waveguide section going into the low-temperature dewar thereby blocking the entry of condensable gases to the cavity. When the detector is a bolometer, a block of polystyrene foam around the outside of the detector holder will reduce the effects of room-temperature air changes.

5.6.5   Tapes

Modern pressure-sensitive tapes have replaced sealing wax and string as the "universal holders"; however, all tapes are not well-behaved at low temperatures, e.g., plastic electrical tape usually cracks because of the high expansion coefficient. Masking tape sticks to itself both in liquid nitrogen and helium but it will not always adhere to cold metal so the tape should be lapped on itself whenever possible. Adhesive tape, e.g., Johnson and Johnson, does stick to metal surfaces at $4°K$.

5.6.6   Gassy Liquid Helium Dewars

At certain temperatures helium can diffuse through Pyrex dewar walls sufficiently to ruin the insulating vacuum. The diffusion occurs only when the dewar is warming; therefore, it can be avoided by quickly removing the helium before the glass becomes warm. Two apparently successful rituals are to remove the gas by evacuation or to displace and boil off the helium by filling the dewar with liquid nitrogen.

5.6.7   Lubricant at Low Temperature

Teflon spray lubricant from a pressurized can has been used to $4°K$.

5.6.8 Dielectrics in Waveguide Runs

Waveguides have been filled with low-loss dielectrics to (*1*) permit reducing the cross-section to a convenient size for coupling onto the cavity or entering a small dewar and (*2*) provide rigidity in extremely thin-walled waveguides. Both polystyrene and quartz have been used for (*1*), and polystyrene foam is satisfactory for (*2*).

5.6.9 Protection for Magnet Poles

Plastic pole covers either thin films of polyethylene or sheets of Bakelite, Lucite, or other plastics will protect the poles from spilled materials and prevent magnetic particles from becoming attached to the surface.

CHAPTER VI

EPR of Gases and Liquids

While gases and liquids have been lumped together in one small chapter, the size of this chapter is not an indication of their importance but a reflection of the author's preoccupation with solids. Also the combination should not be interpreted to indicate a similarity between the technique and results of liquids and gases. Experimentally, gases and liquids are prone to exhibit numerous well-resolved hyperfine lines but in interpretation, radicals in liquids frequently bear a closer resemblance to their brethren in solids. The scope includes considerations of sample preparation, spectrometer selection, particularly the cavity, and examples of typical results. Gases are divided into stable paramagnetic molecules, reactive atoms, and radicals while liquids are classified according to the method of radical production.

6.1 GASES

Most reviewers of EPR in gases commence with the successful measurements on stable gases first reported by Beringer and Castle in 1949 (W-15) although a similar experiment on cesium vapor was described in 1946 (R-4). After the work in such stable paramagnetic molecules as NO, NO_2, and O_2, techniques were developed which extended observations to H, N, O, OH, SH, and other reactive species. Interest in the EPR of gases stems from two general areas: (*1*) the theory of coupling in molecules and (*2*) gas phase chemistry involving reactive intermediate radicals. In the first area, the spectra for paramagnetic molecules are generally more complicated than those for solids or liquids because the magnetic field does not uncouple the strong interaction between the magnetic moment of the unpaired electron and the angular momentum of the rotating molecule. Consequently, the rotational states lead to a wealth of absorption lines suitable for a detailed check of the molecular Zeeman effect theory (A-9,I-2). Details of the theory and the degree of agreement with experiment are available for specific molecules such as O_2 (T-4) and OH (R-1). From an experimental standpoint the complexity of the EPR spectrum will depend on the degree and characteristics of the coupling and therefore will vary from molecule to molecule. Usually molecules are discussed according to Hund's system of classification.* In terms of this classification the permanent gas molecules studied by EPR to date belong to the common cases, i.e., A or B or somewhere between these two. For example, nitric oxide (NO) is a good example of Case A where both L and S are coupled tightly to the molecular axis A. L couples electrostatically with the internuclear field and S has a strong spin orbit coupling with L. Nitrogen peroxide (NO_2) is an example of Case B where again L is strongly coupled to the molecular axis but S is coupled more strongly to the total orbital angular momentum N. Molecules such as O_2 and OH present a more complex case with couplings intermediate between A and B. In any event, a proper interpretation of the EPR spectrum requires a suitable theory and model for the molecule in question.

In the second area of interest, EPR exhibits two important characteristics pertinent to chemical kinetic studies of gas phase reactions: (*1*) The reactive intermediate species are observed without interference in the reaction and (*2*) the technique is amenable to quantitative measurements of reaction rates and diffusion coefficients.

6.1.1 Sample Preparation

The main experimental problems involve production of sufficient paramagnetic species for a good signal-to-noise ratio without losing resolution. With stable molecules such as O_2 the problem reduces to selecting the best pressure for the gas in the cavity, while with reactive species such as H, O, N, etc., both the details of production and the cavity pressure are involved. A few measurements have been made at pressures of 10–20 mm Hg or about 10^{17}–10^{18} molecules per cubic centimeter; however, at such pressures the lines are observably broadened. For example, Fig. 6.1-1 illustrates the line broadening for one of the O_2 lines over the pressure range from 5 to 20 mm Hg. At still higher pressures all

---

* Following Ref. T-5, Hund systematically described five ideal cases for coupling molecular angular momenta together using the following notations:

L = electronic orbital angular momentum

S = electronic spin angular momentum

N = total orbital angular momentum including rotation of molecule

O = orbital angular momentum due to nuclear motion (rotation of the molecule)

A = a vector along the molecular axis

Case A: $LA \gg LS$ or LO, i.e., L and S are strongly coupled to A and weakly coupled to N, $SA \gg SN$.

Case B: $LA \gg LS$ or LO, i.e., L is strongly coupled to A but S is coupled more strongly to N than to A, $SN \gg SA$.

The other three cases have not been observed with EPR: Case C, $LS \gg LA$; Case D, $LO \gg LA$; and Case E, L strongly coupled to S and their resultant coupled to O.

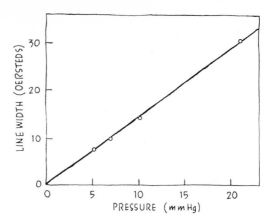

Fig. 6.1-1. Variation of width of line 5 in Fig. 6.1-2 with O_2 gas pressure at a temperature of 300°K. The ΔH values were determined using the measured intercept separations of second harmonic signal contours. (Courtesy B-9).

resolution is lost. Pressures of 0.1–1 mm Hg or about 10^{15}–10^{16} molecules per cubic centimeter are better for resolving the hf structure, provided the signal is acceptable. A convenient gas handling system will permit pressure adjustments for optimizing the signal and resolution. When reactive species are generated in an electrodeless discharge, adequate production may call for higher pressures than are optimum for the cavity. Two procedures have been used under these circumstances: (1) differential pumping to remove the excess molecules and (2) dilution with inert nonparamagnetic atoms such as helium and argon. These inert atoms perform a second function: they impede the diffusion of reactive species to the walls of the transport tube, thus increasing the possibility that the radicals will reach the cavity.

Sample purity is not a problem as long as the impurities are not paramagnetic, e.g., the technique of diluting the sample with inert atoms. Numerous measurements have been made with tank gases ranging from unspecified to 99.998% pure.

Sample temperature is connected to signal amplitude by the usual Boltzmann distribution of radicals populating the various energy levels. In addition, the relative amplitudes of the various absorption lines may change with temperature due to the temperature response of the molecular rotational states. In Fig. 6.1-2 where O_2 spectra at 300 and 85°K are compared, many lines are reduced in relative amplitude at the lower temperature. Measurements of strong well-resolved lines also showed that the linewidth increased as the temperature was lowered. The average increase for six prominent lines in O_2 was a factor of about 3 (B-9).

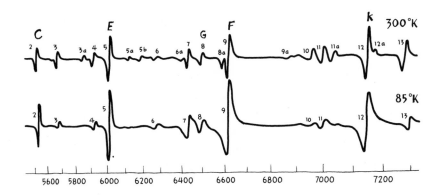

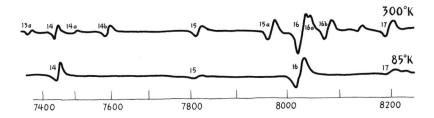

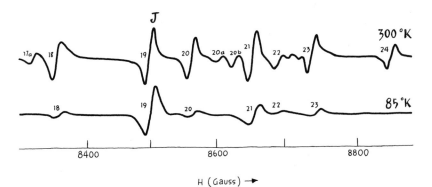

H (Gauss) →

Fig. 6.1-2. Effect of sample temperature on the EPR spectrum of O_2. The rotational states of O_2 can be identified by their marked temperature sensitivity. Sample pressure is 4.0 mm Hg, spectrometer frequency is 9360 Mc/sec, 8.5 Oe modulation amplitude at 300°K; 3.6 mm Hg and 4.2 Oe modulation at 85°K. (After B-9.)

With stable paramagnetic gases the arrangements for handling the sample can be quite flexible, ranging from sealed vials to flow-through systems. Figure 6.1-3 shows several systems suitable for stable samples where the designation "stable" is extended to include some radicals that exist only at high temperatures, e.g., alkali metal atoms. Arrangement a was used for both molecular and atomic oxygen. Oxygen atoms generated in the rf discharge cavity diffuse into the side tube where they are detected. Any system for reducing the pressure in the cavity to the 0.1 mm range should permit O_2 molecules from the air to exhibit their resonance. Arrangement b contains a quartz vial filled with N_2F_4 and sealed off so that the pressure is about 20–40 mm Hg at room temperature. Heating the sample in a commercial-type temperature control system between 345 and 435°K increases the equilibrium concentration of NF_2. Because of the high pressure and temperature only a single broad line is observed. Arrangement c is a high-temperature system used with the cavity of Fig. 4-26d to measure EPR of alkali metal atoms. Sealed off tubes are heated with air (up to 770°K) to generate free atoms for measurement. Pressure is controlled by the temperature of the tube outside the dewar. Purity is a problem; consequently, the alkali metal is initially brought in contact with the entire inner surface to act as a "getter," then the metal is returned to the bulb to establish the vapor pressure.

Atomic gas samples have been produced by a variety of techniques which vary principally in the source of energy used to generate the reactive species. In all cases the piping is arranged to sweep the radicals through the spectrometer cavity before the spins can become paired up again. The lifetime for these radicals can be translated to distance from the point of origin so lifetime measurements are made by moving either the source or the spectrometer cavity along the sample pipe. Figure 6.1-4 illustrates four techniques for generating free atoms: (a) the elementary electrical discharge method with a Woods tube; (b) the electrodeless discharge method where molecular bonds are ruptured by a high-frequency discharge in a cavity driven by a diathermy unit; (c) a high-temperature arc method; and (d) a method for sampling radicals produced by pyrolysis. Arrangement a was used in the initial experiments on atomic nitrogen, oxygen, and hydrogen. Tank nitrogen flows through a Woods tube attached to a relaxation oscillator which discharges about 8 times per second. Atoms are pumped out of the discharge tube and into the cavity for EPR detection. Normally with a 0.9-m long tube the available voltage was adequate to initiate a discharge but on occasions when the discharge did not occur, the addition of a little water vapor (introduced by bubbling the input nitrogen through a water bottle) would initiate regular discharges.

Electrodeless discharges similar to arrangement b have been selected for most of the recent experiments with atomic species (K-17,R-1,W-15). Gas flow rates and pressures are adjusted for optimum free atom production in the discharge resonator and for adequate resolution in the cavity; however, the permissible flexibility depends on the reactivity of the atoms. To prevent an excessive loss of atoms through recombination at the cavity walls, Dehmelt (D-4) suggests that the average transit time between the region of formation in the discharge and the measuring cavity should be less than half the time for an atom to diffuse to the wall, i.e.,

$$V = 40SD \qquad (6\text{-}1)$$

where V is the necessary pumping speed in cubic centimeters per second, S is the transit distance in centimeters, D is the diffusion constant in square centimeters per second, and the tube diameter has conveniently dropped out. Applying this criterion to an example of potassium atoms moving in an argon atmosphere, where $V = 6000$ cm^3/sec and $S = 6$ cm, he finds that $D = 25$ cm^2/sec. If atomic potassium diffuses in argon at a rate of 0.3 cm^2/sec at atmospheric pressure and room temperature, the minimum carrier pressure would be about 10 mm Hg. Actual temperatures and conditions may make this estimate too low; therefore, either higher pressures or preferably greater pumping speeds may be required for adequate resolution. When long-lived species are involved, e.g., OH radicals, a quartz tube, $1\frac{1}{2}$ m long with 1 cm i.d., can be inserted between the generator and the detector to establish a pressure differential. This separation introduces several other benefits. Interference between the discharge and the spectrometer circuits is reduced. Also free electrons from the discharge region will not enter the spectrometer cavity and establish a cyclotron resonance absorption band (R-1). Oxygen and hydrogen atoms have also been observed with separations of this length. The pressures used in Ref. R-1 are about 0.3 mm Hg in the discharge and 0.1 mm Hg or less in the cavity. Diathermy generators operating at 2450 Mc/sec and power levels of 100–125 W feed power into either a tapered, slotted, discharge section or a cylindrical resonant cavity to dissociate the gas. In reaction rate studies with arrangement b (Fig. 6.1-4) it is customary to vary the separation between the discharge region and the detecting cavity. Here two alternatives are available: (1) move the discharge or (2) move the spectrometer cavity. Both procedures have been used successfully; however, in most laboratories it is probably easier to move the discharge equipment than the spectrometer cavity and its magnet. The spectrometer cavity can be either cylindrical or rectangular, e.g., cylindrical TE$_{102}$ (R-1), TE$_{011}$ (K-17), or rectangular TE$_{102}$ (W-15). When

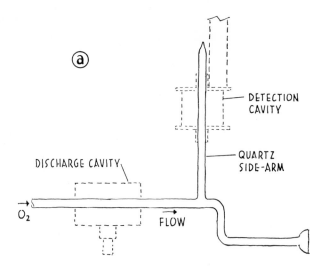

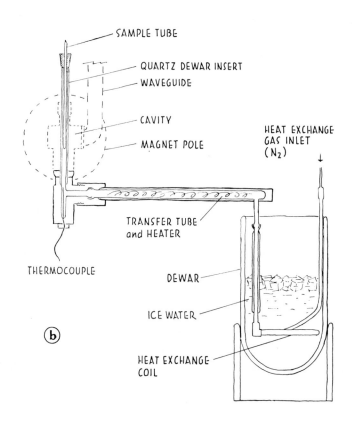

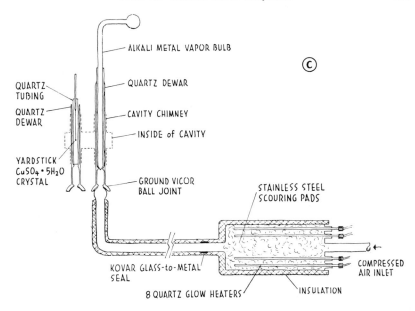

Fig. 6.1-3. (*a*) Side-arm method for observing the recombination of oxygen atoms. O_2 molecules dissociate in the discharge cavity and drift along the flow tube. The junction with the side arm serves as a constant concentration source of atomic oxygen which diffuses into the side arm. The concentration gradient of atomic oxygen, established along the arm as the atoms recombine, is measured with the detection cavity (after K-17). (*b*) Temperature control apparatus for varying the temperature of the sample over the range from 273 to 435°K (after P-9). (*c*) Simple heating apparatus for controlling sample temperatures up to 770°K (after M-13).

there is plenty of room, the cylindrical TE_{011} cavity offers the convenience of large end openings without much sacrifice in Q. Other items in arrangement *b* include vacuum gauges suitable for pressures in the millimeter range, flow meters, and side inlets. Wallace and Tierman vacuum gauges and thermocouple vacuum gauges permit continuous pressure readings while the precise McLeod gauge is best for quantitative measurements. Flow rates have been metered with calibrated orifices and capillary flow meters, but the orifices were preferred because of their faster response time. The side inlets have been used in a variety of procedures including sample dilution, the introduction of reacting components, and the introduction of metered amounts of a stable paramagnetic species such as O_2 which serves as a yardstick in quantitative measurements. Arrangement *c* (Fig. 6.1-4) is a "universal dissociator" used successfully in the measurement of atomic H, N, and ^{31}P (D-4). By subjecting samples to arc temperatures of up to about 6000°K, molecules are thermally decomposed into

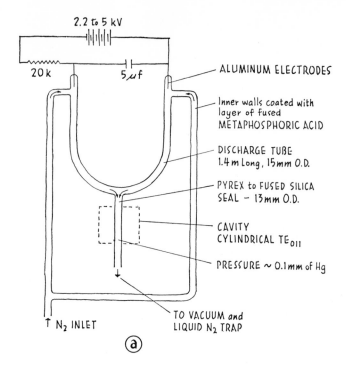

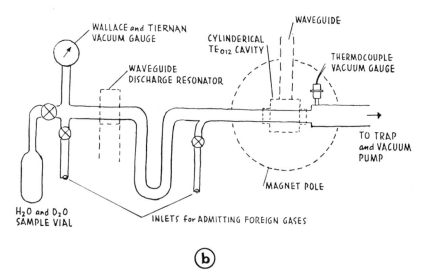

Fig. 6.1-4. Four arrangements for generating paramagnetic free atoms in the gas phase: (*a*) High-voltage electrical discharge in Woods tube generates free nitrogen atoms (B-11). (*b*) Diathermy unit driving waveguide discharge resonator generates radicals and free atoms in water vapor. Other molecules are admitted to the system through inlets located before and after the discharge cavity. (After R-1.)

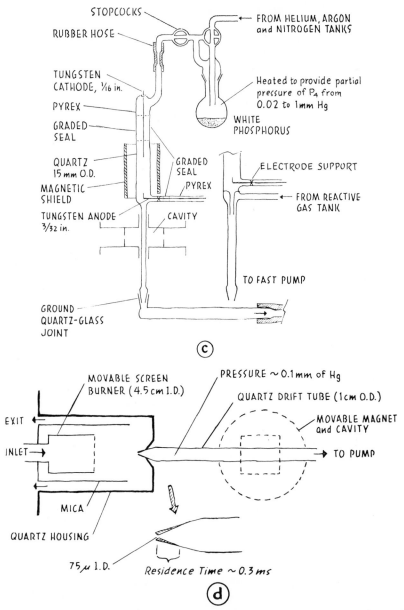

Fig. 6.1-4. (c) Universal dissociator employing helium–argon carrier gas. Gas and phosphorus vapor sweep through dissociator where the high temperature discharge generates free atoms; operating voltage, 130–250 V dc; current limited to <8 A, starting voltage, 800 V ac applied in series with dc until electrodes heat to about 3000°K and become thermionic emitters; warmup time about 1 min; a choke coil limits the alternating current to 4 A (courtesy D-4). (d) Radicals produced in the flame are sampled through the quartz orifice. Lifetimes are measured by varying the distance between the burner and the cavity (courtesy W-16).

Table 6.1-1

Typical Experimental Conditions for Observing Radicals in Gas Samples

Starting material	Cavity pressure, mm Hg	Method of generating radicals	Spectrometer type	Cavity	Observed radicals	Ref.
O_2						T-4
O_2, 99.5% pure	0.1	Microwave discharge	Similar to RH3-X	Cylindrical TE_{011}	O	K-17
				Cylindrical TM_{011}	O_2	B-9
H_2O–D_2O vapor	0.3 in generator 0.1 in cavity	Microwave discharge	RH1-X	Cylindrical TE_{102}	OH, OD, O, H, D	R-1
H_2O vapor + H_2S	0.4–0.6	Electrodeless discharge (diathermy machine)	RH1-X	Cylindrical TE_{011}	SH, SD SO	M-6
N_2F_4	20–40	Heat, 342–345°K	RH1-X	Rectangular TE_{102}	NF_2	P-9
Bi, Sb, As, ^{31}P		High-temperature arc	TH1-X	Rectangular TE_{102}	Atomic Bi, Sb, As, ^{31}P	D-4
C_2H_6–O_2 C_2H_4–O_2 C_2H_2–O_2	1.0	Flames	RH1-X	Rectangular TE_{102}	H, O	W-16

their atomic constituents. As used in the phosphorus experiment, a high direct-current arc (4–8 A) is established in the quartz tube between tungsten electrodes to decompose the phosphorus coming from the boiler. Starting the arc requires some assistance such as the discharge from a tesla coil and a warmup ac arc of about 4 A at 800 V (current limited by a choke coil). A helium–argon carrier gas was used in the arc because a pure helium arc overheated the quartz tube. Pressures at the arc covered a range from 40 to 200 mm Hg. By operating with a fast-flowing, high-pressure carrier gas system the loss of atoms through diffusion to the walls was not appreciable. Some typical measurements are 25 cm^2/sec for diffusion constants, a $\frac{1}{2}$ cm^2 tube cross-section, 6 cm from arc to cavity, and an optimum pressure of 10^{-1} to 10^{-2} mm Hg for the phosphorus vapor. Supposedly the method should be quite versatile for atoms with an S ground state. Unfortunately non-S ground states result in line broadening because the nonvanishing angular momentum provides a handle by which the total angular momentum can be turned over by collision with a carrier atom (D-4).

Arrangement d (Fig. 6.1-4) was used to measure oxygen and hydrogen atom profiles in flames generated by a C_2-hydrocarbon burning in oxygen. The sample probe remains stationary while the flames and the spectrometer cavity move. Various parts of the flame are sampled by moving the screen burner with respect to the probe. Details of the quartz probe are shown at the bottom of the figure. Rapid expansion of the gas passing through the probe's sonic throat quenches the reaction by decompression in a few microseconds and the associated cooling keeps the drift tube and the gas passing through the EPR cavity at near room temperature (W-16). The cavity is moved along the tube to measure the decay rate of the radicals. With a sampling pressure of 0.1 mm Hg, a 1-cm diameter drift tube, and a closest practical approach to the flame of about 23 cm, the loss of atoms between probe inlet and cavity was about 30–50%, due primarily to reactions at the walls. Concentrations of H and O atoms were measured quantitatively by comparison with O_2, which was essentially of constant concentration because it was present in a large excess.

A further indication of the materials and techniques involved in the EPR of gases is given by Table 6.1-1 which lists materials, pressures, type of apparatus, and some results for both stable and reactive radicals.

6.1.2 EPR Considerations

The main spectrometer problems are sensitivity and rf saturation of the spin system; however, heroic efforts are not required to obtain satisfactory spectra. Most of the existing data were obtained with commercial homodyne spectrometers and reflection cavities. All of the instruments and results described here are for X-band frequencies, which are adequate, particularly since spin concentration—not total spin measurements— is involved. Rf saturation limits the allowable power levels; consequently, spectrometer types TH2 and RH2 and RH3 are preferable because the bypass line or auxiliary automatic frequency control cavity permits low power operation in the sample cavity, e.g., Radford (R-1) used powers of less than 5 μW to avoid saturation and Westenberg and de Haas (W-15) observed saturation in H and N atoms in the vicinity of 0.1 mW. Interestingly when O_2 molecules or O atoms are measured or O_2 is present in the cavity with an easily saturated gas, no saturation is observed or the saturation threshold is substantially increased, e.g., an abundance of O_2 in with H or N atoms raised the saturation threshold above 10 mW (W-16). As already mentioned both rectangular and cylindrical cavities have been used successfully without comment regarding any particular advantages.

Molecular oxygen is the most reliable standard for quantitative measurements on gases because its characteristics are well established, the line shape is similar to the unknowns, and all gases will have the same filling factor.

6.1.3 Typical Results

Most of the experimental characteristics of the O_2 spectrum have been encountered in examples at the beginning of this section. In Ref. T-4 a total of 120 lines were observed at X-band frequencies and 26 lines were completely analyzed to confirm the theory of the molecular Zeeman effect. Figure 6.1-2 shows O_2 spectra of about 40 and 22 lines, respectively, obtained under various conditions of pressure, temperature, and sensitivity. Resonance conditions for some of the prominent lines used as yardsticks in quantitative measurements are listed in Table 5-8. Line shapes and the broadening due to high pressures and low temperatures are considered in some detail in Ref. B-9. The shape is Lorentzian, as illustrated in Fig. 6.1-5 by an enlargement of line 5 of Fig. 6.1-2. Line 5 is one of the wide lines; others range down to about 9 Oe under similar measuring conditions. Some spectral characteristics of other stable paramagnetic gasses are listed in Table 6.1-2, e.g., the spectrum of NO_2 goes from a triplet at 10 mm Hg pressure to a large number of partially resolved lines at 1 mm Hg pressure (A-9). Nitric oxide has a triplet fine structure which is further split by a triplet hyperfine interaction with the nitrogen nucleus.

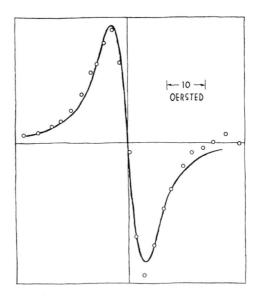

Fig. 6.1-5. Comparison of line 5 (points) of Fig. 6.1-2 with a Lorentzian line shape: ΔH, 14 Oe; temperature, 300°K; pressure, 10.1 mm Hg; modulation amplitude, 3.8 Oe. (Courtesy B-9.)

Table 6.1-2

Examples of EPR Characteristics of Some Paramagnetic Species in the Gaseous or Vapor Phase

Paramagnetic species	g Value	Number of observed lines	hf Splitting, G	Spectra shown in Fig.	Ref.
O_2		140		6.1-2	B-29
O_2		120			T-4
O	Lines a, b: 1.500971	2		6.1-8	
	Lines c, f: 1.500905	2		6.1-8	
	Lines d, e: 1.500904	2		6.1-8	K-17
		6			
^{14}N	2.002	3	3.8	6.1-7	U-2
^{15}N	2.002	2	5.3	6.1-7	U-2
NO_2		3			A-9
NO		3			A-9
SH		12	5.4	6.1-6	M-6
NF_2	2.010	1			P-9
Bi	1.65				D-4
Sb	1.967				D-4
As	1.994				D-4
^{31}P	2.0019	2			D-4
^{133}Cs		14			R-4

Electron spin resonance has been observed for several diatomic reactive species generated by electrical discharge methods, e.g., OH and OD (R-1) and SH and SD (M-6). Because of their high reactivity these species are relatively short lived and fair concentrations are required for detection. It is noted in Ref. B-12 that diatomic molecules with large electric dipole moments and suitable doubling of the Zeeman levels should be detectable by electric dipole EPR spectroscopy at considerably smaller concentrations than are required for conventional magnetic dipole EPR. Both types of transitions can be detected by filling the cavity with gas and arranging the orientation so that components of both the electric and magnetic rf field are perpendicular to the external magnetic field (M-6). Figure 6.1-6 shows such a spectrum for SH with the various transitions indicated in the associated energy level diagram. Transitions for the ground rotational state ($J = \frac{3}{2}$) leads to six lines which are split by hyperfine interactions with the hydrogen nucleus to yield the 12 lines shown. The indicated Zeeman splittings are about 190 G in contrast to 5.4 G for the hf inter-

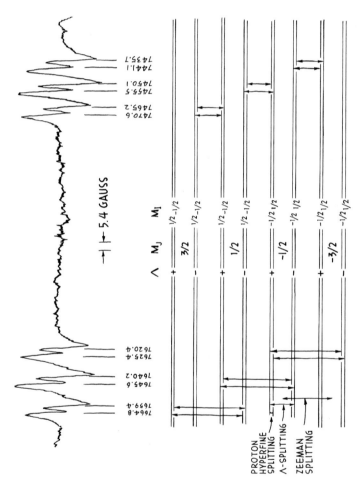

Fig. 6.1-6. Electric dipole EPR spectrum of SH radicals in the gaseous state and schematic representation of expected transitions between energy levels: spectrometer type RH1, 100 kc modulation; cylindrical TE_{011} cavity with a 35 cm³ quartz sample container. The sample H_2S is mixed into dissociated H_2O vapor at the entrance to the cavity; pressure, 0.4–0.6 mm Hg; H_2O is dissociated in the quartz inlet tube with an electrodeless discharge; spectrometer frequency, 8.850 kMc/sec. (Courtesy M-6.)

action (M-6). For the same rotational state in OH Radford (R-1) found a similar 12-line spectrum; however, the total width is about 2600 G in contrast to 230 G for SH.

Table 6.1-2 also lists characteristics for various reactive atomic radicals. In the nitrogen spectrum of Fig. 6.1-7 the hyperfine interaction leads to a spectrum of three prominent lines for the ^{14}N, $I = 1$, and two smaller but definite lines for ^{15}N, $I = \frac{1}{2}$. Although the small signals are not conducive to quantitative measurements, the relative amplitudes correspond approximately to the ratios calculated from the isotope abundances.

Atomic oxygen plays an important role in many high-temperature phenomena in air, e.g., discharges and flames; therefore, information about recombination rates and other reaction rates are in demand (K-17). Although oxygen has an even number of electrons, it is highly paramagnetic and can be detected by EPR induced transitions. Figure 6.1-8 shows six fine-structure lines and the energy levels involved in the transitions. Recombination rates can be examined by varying the drift distance between the discharge generating the free atoms, and the measuring cavity. Figure 6.1-9 shows the decrease in signal amplitude as this distance is increased and more atoms are lost through surface recombination. Measurements at several pressures from 1.0 to 2.1 mm Hg gave an exponential decay which increased with pressure. Similar decay curves for combustion products obtained with the sampler of Fig. 6.1-4 are shown in Fig. 6.1-10.

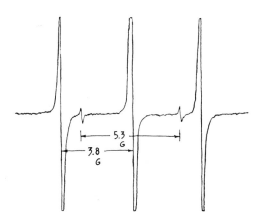

Fig. 6.1-7. EPR spectrum of atomic nitrogen: N_2 pressure, 11 mm Hg; flow, 125 cm^3/min; g, 2.002; spectrometer type RH1, X-band, 100 kc/sec modulation, TE_{102} rectangular cavity; 11 mm o.d. quartz sample tube. N_2 is dissociated with a 2450 Mc/sec discharge. (Courtesy U-2.)

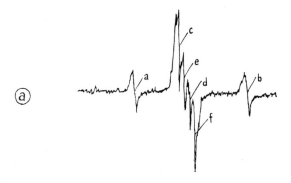

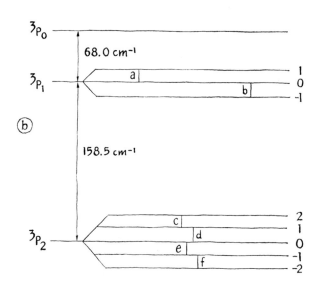

Fig. 6.1-8. (*a*) Atomic oxygen resonance showing a 6-line fine structure: spectrometer type RH3, *X*-band; cylindrical TE_{011} cavity; 6 kc modulation. The sample is 99.5% pure oxygen dissociated in an electrodeless discharge cavity at room temperature; pressure, 1 mm Hg (derivative spectra). (*b*) Energy levels and transitions associated with the absorption lines. (Courtesy K-17.)

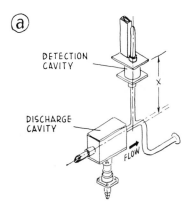

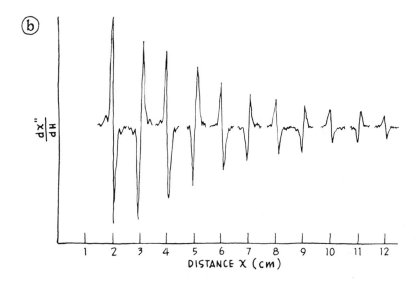

Fig. 6.1-9. (a) Detection and discharge cavities for the side-arm method of observing atomic oxygen produced by the dissociation of O_2 in an electrodeless discharge (b) Spectrometer signals $d\chi''/dH$ at various distances x along the side arm for 1 mm Hg pressure. For spectrometer data, see Fig. 6.1-8. (Courtesy K-17.)

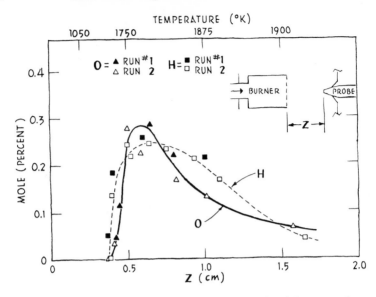

Fig. 6.1-10. Radical profiles in C_2H_6–O_2 flame: runs *1* and *2* were made on different days; gas flow is left to right; spectrometer type RH1, *X*-band, 100 kc modulation; 9 in. magnet; cavity, rectangular TE_{102}; 1 cm diameter sample tube; movable magnet and cavity; pressure, 0.1 mm Hg. (Courtesy W-16.)

6.2 SOLUTIONS

The traditional interest in studying dilute solutions of free radicals is tied to the abundant hfs and the possibility of translating this structure into a map of the unpaired electron density throughout the molecule. As is mentioned in Chapter II, much of this detail is lost in solids because of the line broadening caused by anisotropies in the *g* factor and hf coupling coefficients plus exchange and magnetic dipole–dipole interactions between spins of neighboring radicals. Rapid molecular tumbling averages out these anisotropies and dilution minimizes the exchange and dipole–dipole effects. A second reason for interest is the role played by radicals as reactive intermediates in chemical reactions. Here both identification and radical lifetimes are important and EPR permits the reaction to be followed without interfering in the process. In this section we will examine the techniques associated with radicals generated in a variety of ways:

1. Stable radicals dissolved in solution.

2. Negative and positive ions in solution.

3. Intermediate species in chemical reactions.

4. Radicals generated by photolysis and radiolysis of liquids.

In all cases the hfs is important for identification. Usually the g values are of secondary interest because they are normally very close to the free electron value, but precise measurements are finding small differences that become more significant as the theory reaches a similar level of accuracy. Measurements of the radical yield or G value* are vital to a quantitative understanding of chemical reactions, photolysis, and radiolysis. In pursuing the resolution and sensitivity necessary for these measurements the spectroscopist faces a number of choices, i.e., the type of spectrometer, method of radical production, solvent, temperature, and pressure. These parameters are considered further under the individual radical systems.

6.2.1 Spectrometer Considerations

Sections 3.4 and 5.5 contain the recommendations for high-resolution spectroscopy, namely, high sensitivity, homogeneity, and stability. In view of the homogeneity requirements on a magnetic field it is difficult to achieve the best resolution at high field strengths. Usually a sufficient sample is available to satisfy any filling factor; consequently, the sensitivity advantage of high frequencies is further reduced. For these reasons and also because of availability, the X band is the common frequency for measurements on radicals in liquids. As previously explained, a superheterodyne system is required to avoid broadening lines narrower than about 60 mG. A few lines impose this limitation but many do not; therefore, a homodyne system with 100 kc modulation is adequate for most of the measurements discussed here. A convenient arrangement is to have two spectrometers, i.e., a high-frequency modulated homodyne for exploratory measurements and a superheterodyne (with a 12 in. magnet) for the occasional narrow-line spectrum. In some laboratories there are two instruments (13); in others one spectrometer is arranged for both modes of operation. Both rectangular and cylindrical cavities are in use; however, when the liquid is dielectrically lossy, the rectangular cavity is slightly more efficient, as discussed in Section 7.7.

6.2.2 Sample Preparation

(a) Stable Radicals in Solution. When stable radicals such as DPPH are dissolved in an inert solvent, the spectrum changes from a single sharp line for the solid to a broad line for concentrated solutions; then as the dilution continues, the hf structure appears. Figure 6.2-1 illustrates this concentration dependence in DPPH dissolved in benzene where the first curve is narrow because of exchange narrowing in the solid. Under

---

* G value = number of free radicals generated per 100 eV of absorbed energy.

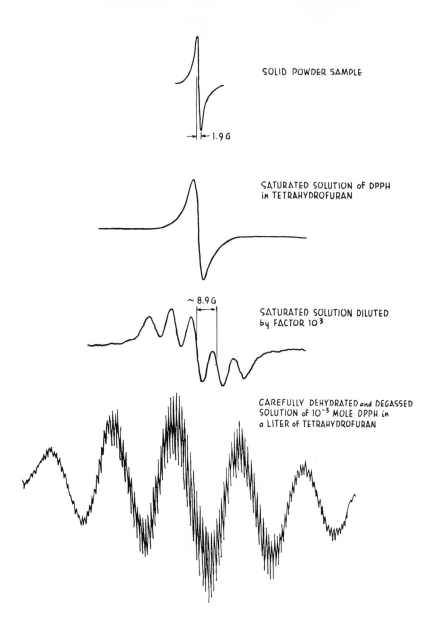

Fig. 6.2-1. Effect of dilution and solvent purity on the hfs of DPPH. (Solid sample, from B-9; solution samples, courtesy T-7.)

the conditions for the second curve the separation between spins is too great for exchange narrowing but spin–spin interactions are still sufficient for short relaxation times and the associated line broadening. In the dilute solution the radicals are sufficiently isolated so that the effects of the nuclear fields can be resolved, as in the two bottom curves. In the Section 5.5 discussion of requirements for resolving hf structure it was noted that in addition to being inert, the solvent should have a low viscosity to enhance tumbling of the molecules, and should be free of magnetic or electric dipoles both in the solvent molecules and in any resident impurities. The devastating effects of a strong paramagnetic impurity like dissolved oxygen are illustrated later in Fig. 6.2-12. Hausser (H-3) makes the specific point that this is a physical effect, i.e., the stable radicals are not reacting chemically with the oxygen. Most air saturated organic solvents contain on the order of 10^{-3} mole/liter or $\approx 10^{18}$ impurity spins/cm^3 (H-3). Frequently radical concentrations are limited to about 10^{-4} or 10^{-5} mole/liter for high-resolution EPR. Consequently, unless the solution is deaerated, the radicals may be severely outnumbered by the oxygens. In addition to the solvents listed in Table 5-6 methylcyclohexane, n-pentane, and propane are also suitable for high-resolution EPR.

(b) Negative Ions by Alkali Metal Reduction. In a traditional version of this process a dilute solution of the aromatic molecule in a polyether is mixed with an alkali metal under high-vacuum conditions to form a negative aromatic ion and a positive alkali metal ion. The main preparation problems are cleanliness and a suitable solvent. Henning (H-7) lists the following requirements for a suitable solvent.

1. It should be chemically inert to both the negative ion and the alkali metal.

2. It should have good solvating properties for both the positive and negative ions in order to suppress the formation of ion pairs.

3. It should not be proton active.

Several widely used polyethers are 1,2-dimethoxyethane (DME), tetrahydrofuran (THF), and dioxane.

Cooling DME and THF to -50 and $-80°C$, respectively, helps to reduce ion-pair formation and protonation. An excess of alkali metal will generate doubly charged negative ions which are not magnetic. One technique for suppressing this unwanted reaction involves reacting half the solution with the alkali metal (shaking) until conversion to the dinegative ion is complete; then the two halves of the solution are mixed in the absence of the metal to convert all the ions to the monovalent variety. Various purification rituals are available for cleaning the solvent of oxidizing agents such as water that would react with the negative ions.

Reference H-7 prescribes distilling the polyether three or four times from metallic sodium, followed by 24 hr of refluxing under a stream of dry nitrogen in a bulb containing sodium and a trace of anthracene indicator. When the solution is adequately clean, the anthracene negative ion will form and color the solution. Solution color is frequently the guide to adequate purity. Table 6.2-1 lists the colors exhibited by various hydrocarbon negative ions formed by reactions with sodium metal in clean solutions of THF.

Table 6.2-1

Colors of Hydrocarbon Negative Ions in THF (P-6)

Negative ion	Color
Naphthalene	Green
Anthracene	Brilliant blue
Phenanthrene	Olive green
Triphenylene	Lavender
Naphthacene	Blue green
Stilbene	Dark green in excess of stilbene, red in excess of sodium
Dibenz-[a,h]-anthracene	Dark green

A variety of arrangements are suitable for handling the sample, alkali metal, and solvent. Figure 6.2-2 shows one simple system and others are discussed in Section 6.3 in connection with alkali metal–ammonia solutions. The procedure prescribed with Fig. 6.2-2 is as follows (B-24):

(1) Wash a small clean piece of alkali metal in petroleum ether, place it in the side arm, add about 0.3 mg of hydrocarbon in the bulb, and evacuate the apparatus.

(2) If the hydrocarbon is at all volatile, cool the bulb in liquid nitrogen immediately after evacuation.

(3) Distil the alkali metal from the side arm by heating with a flame, being careful to form a mirror on the walls of the sample tube; then seal off the side arm.

(4) Distil about 1 ml of (previously cleaned) solvent into the sample tube and seal off the sample tube at the constriction.

(5) Tip some of the solution into the side arm for the EPR measurements.

Some of the rituals for handling and cleaning the alkali metal are described in Section 6.3 but a method used at Washington University (42)

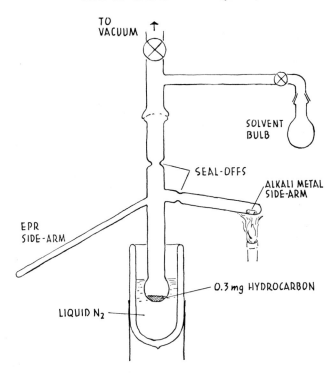

TO
VACUUM

SOLVENT
BULB

SEAL-OFFS

ALKALI METAL
SIDE-ARM

EPR
SIDE-ARM

0.3 mg HYDROCARBON

LIQUID N₂

Fig. 6.2-2. Arrangement for preparing anion radicals by reduction with an alkali metal (B-24).

appears to be particularly convenient for measuring out the small quantities required for these negative ion experiments. A bundle of fine glass tubes, cleaned and sealed at the top end, is inserted into the filling chamber of Fig. 6.2-3 along with chunks of sodium metal. After a good vacuum has been obtained, the metal is melted and an inert gas such as argon, dry nitrogen, or helium is admitted to force the metal into the tubes. Subsequently, the tubes are cut to provide the desired amount of alkali metal, dropped into the sample preparation apparatus, evacuated, and heated so that the metal will flow out of the tube ready for distillation.

(c) **Negative Ions by Electrolytic Reduction.** Electrolytic techniques are used quite widely and the reduction cells are commercially available. The electrical method offers several advantages over reduction with alkali metals, namely, convenience, stability, and simplicity: convenience because adequate concentrations of radicals can be generated without involving laborious high-vacuum techniques and simplicity because

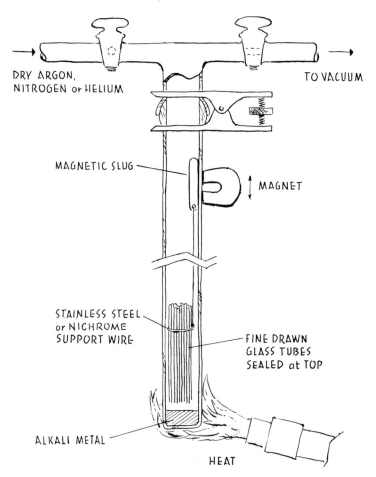

Fig. 6.2-3. Procedure for storing and handling alkali metals in fine glass tubes. Filling procedure: (*1*) assemble the tubes and alkali metal in the filling tube, then produce a good vacuum; (*2*) melt the alkali metal and degas; (*3*) lower the open ends of the fine tubes into the molten metal; (*4*) close off the vacuum and admit inert gas to force the metal into the tubes; (*5*) raise the tubes free of the metal and let it solidify. To use the metal, break the tube to the desired length of metal. Put it in the apparatus; heat under vacuum and the metal will run out of the tube (42).

interpretation of the spectra is not complicated by the presence of the metal (C-3); also the negative ions produced by electrical reduction appear to be more stable than the same species generated with the alkali metal (H-7). Figure 6.2-4 shows three electrolytic cells which illustrate the gamut of complexity normally encountered. In any case, the essential ingredients are the electrodes, an inert solvent appropriate for the sample, a supporting electrolyte to provide the charge transport, and the sample. The optimum operating voltage depends strongly on the concentration of the supporting electrolyte. Typical materials and operating parameters for the three cells are listed in Table 6.2-2. The important reaction in the cathode region is the transfer of an electron to the sample molecule to form the negative ion. Cell a is a single compartment type with electrodes at each end of a 4 mm diameter tube about 6 in. long. A melting point capillary tube provides electrical insulation over the center wire down to the reaction region that extends into the cavity. Cell b contains two compartments separated by a glass filter. Both compartments contain the same solvent and electrolyte but the sample is added only to the cathode room. Acetonitrile was selected for the solvent because (1) it is rather inert, (2) it is proton inactive, (3) it has a high dielectric constant ($\epsilon = 36$), and (4) it has a rather high solubility for heterocyclic molecules, as well as the supporting electrolyte. The solution was made more or less oxygen free by bubbling a stream of dry nitrogen through it for about $\frac{1}{2}$ hr.

Table 6.2-2

Materials and Operating Parameters for the 3 Electrolytic Cells
in Figure 6.2-4

Cell	a	b	c
Electrodes			
Cathode	Platinum, 0.3 mm	Tungsten	Mercury
Anode	Platinum, 0.3 mm	Mercury	Platinum
Solvent	Dimethyl sulfoxide	Acetonitrile	Dimethoxyetane
Electrolyte	Lithium perchlorate	n-Tetrabutyl-ammonium iodide	Tetra-n-butyl ammonium perchlorate
Typical sample		n-Hetrocyclic compounds	Anthracene
Voltage	~4 V	5–10 V	−2.3 V vs. Ag/AgClO$_4$
Current	63 μA	—	4 mA
Electrolyte concentration		0.03M	0.1M
Sample concentration		0.001M	0.002M
Reference	36	H-7	B-24

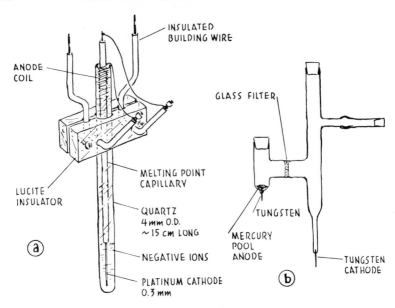

Fig. 6.2-4. Three styles of electrolytic cells. [(*a*) from 36; (*b*) after H-7; (*c*) courtesy B-24.]

During electrolysis anions originate at the cathode as a colored cloud and diffuse upward (H-7). For highly resolved spectra the reduction should be nearly complete because the presence of neutral sample molecules can seriously broaden the EPR line by transferring electrons from the negative ions. Optimum operating conditions are determined empirically but to achieve nearly complete reduction the current density should be as high as possible for a uniform cloud of ions. Cell *c* is designed to avoid contamination from absorbed gases and illustrates the complexity involved in going to a high-vacuum system. In return for this extra effort, the ions are found to be stable for several days or more (B-24). The apparatus consists of five compartments: a mixing chamber, reference compartment, mercury storage bulb, cathode chamber, and anode compartment. In addition, there is a provision for tapping off the colored radical-ion solution into a tube suitable for the EPR cavity.

Preparation procedure and construction details: The needle valves are 1 mm Teflon (Fisher and Porter). The reference electrode contains a fine asbestos fiber sealed into the glass tip of a 4 mm o.d. tube. The tip was ground on emery until the electrode resistance was about 5 MΩ. The reference electrode contains a 0.1*M* solution of silver perchlorate in contact with a silver wire which connects to the outside world through a nickel wire to glass seal. A small pinhole through the 4 mm

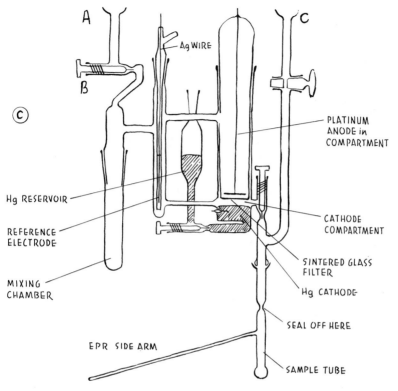

Figure 6.2-4c.

tube just below the taper joint permits evacuation, thus preventing leakage of the perchlorate into the rest of the system. When the black silver particles begin to precipitate, the silver perchlorate is replaced, which normally occurs after many runs. A 1 mm capillary tube connects the reference chamber to the cathode compartment which in turn is separated from the anode compartment by a 3 cm diameter "very fine" Corning sintered glass disk. The anode is a platinum disk and contact to the mercury cathode is by a tungsten wire sealed in the glass. To operate, weigh enough sample and electrolyte into the mixing chamber to make 15 ml of $0.002M$ hydrocarbon and $0.1M$ electrolyte; attach the apparatus to the vacuum line at A and evacuate to a pressure of about 1 µ Hg, distil about 15 ml of solvent into the mixing chamber from a storage reservoir on the vacuum line; seal off at valve B; and remove from the vacuum line. After melting and warming the solvent to provide thorough mixing with the sample and electrolyte, transfer the mixture into the anode, cathode, and reference chambers by judicious tipping. Next attach the system to the vacuum line at C, clamp a sample tube in place, and evacuate this section of the system. Add triply distilled mercury to the mercury reservoir, degas, and admit to the cathode compartment until the level is about 5 mm below the sintered-glass disk. When the solution has reached an equilibrium level, commence electrolysis with a power supply arranged so that the voltage between the cathode and the reference electrode can be controlled and measured, e.g., the potential is just above the first polarographic half-wave potential (-2.3 V vs. Ag/AgClO$_4$ for anthracene) and the current is initially about 4 mA. Essentially, complete reduction is obtained by continuing until the current drops to a very small value. Then about 2 ml of the colored solution is tapped off into the sample chamber and frozen in liquid nitrogen while the tube is sealed off at the constriction. After warming, the solution is tipped into the side arm for EPR measurements.

Operation in high vacuum introduces some new considerations in the selection of a solvent. Old standbys for cells a and b like dimethylformamide and dimethyl sulfoxide are inconvenient to transfer in vacuum because of their low volatility; however, solvents that would absorb water and oxygen in cells a and b are not necessarily excluded. The ethers tetrahydrofuran (THF) and 1,2-dimethoxyethane (DME) are in this second category but they are easily purified on the vacuum line; DME was used in cell c. Sample preparation is described in detail above (B-24).

(d) Positive Ions. Positive ion radicals have been produced by dissolving neutral aromatic hydrocarbons in concentrated sulfuric acid, e.g., pentacene, tetracene, perylene, and anthracene. Bolton and Fraenkel (B-24) prepared anthracene positive ions by dissolving the anthracene in 98% sulfuric acid. Below concentrations of $0.001M$ the EPR linewidth was independent of the concentration. Concentrations of up to $0.01M$ were used when resolution could be sacrificed for a larger signal. The anthracene positive ion had a half-life of about 1 hr at 20°C and 10 min at 50°C, respectively.

(e) Radicals by Radiolysis. Two general radiation techniques have been used successfully in EPR measurements of radiolysis products in liquids. In one the radicals are generated in a radiation source and pumped through the resonant cavity, as indicated in Fig. 6.2-5; in the other, radicals are formed in the cavity under direct bombardment by high energy electrons, as shown in Fig. 6.2-6. Both procedures are complicated by the high radiation levels which necessarily dictate some degree of remote control. In the flow system the maximum flow rate through the ^{60}Co source was 125 ml/sec requiring 4 sec to pass through the source and about 0.6 sec to go from the source to cavity. Flow rates were regulated with the calibrated throttling valve and a reservoir permitted control of the duty cycle before the solution was reirradiated (D-6). The source was capable of forming hydrogen at a rate of 2.3×10^{-7} moles liter^{-1} sec^{-1}. Assuming about 30 eV expended for each hydrogen atom released, this rate would require a 130 rad sec^{-1} exposure. One of the main problems with this arrangement is radical lifetime; in other words, the short-lived species

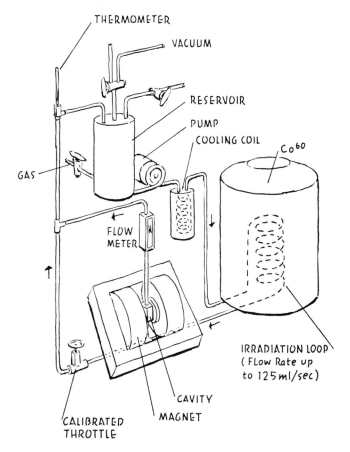

Fig. 6.2-5. Continuous-flow apparatus for measuring radicals produced in liquids by irradiation with ^{60}Co γ-rays. The flow system consists of a reservoir, pump, heat exchanger, irradiation coil, EPR cavity, flowmeter, and the necessary tubing and valves. (After D-6.)

do not reach the cavity. Also, in order to avoid unwanted modulation of the signal, it is important to maintain a uniform flow rate through the cavity. This system can also be used in stopped-flow type experiments where the spectrometer is locked on the peak of an absorption curve, the flow is abruptly stopped, and the spectrometer follows the decay in radical concentration.

The system of Fig. 6.2-6 eliminates the radical transport time problem but several factors limit the rate of production and thus the concentration of short-lived species available for detection. Usually the electron beam current was limited to less than 1 μA and frequently to 0.1 or 0.2 μA in

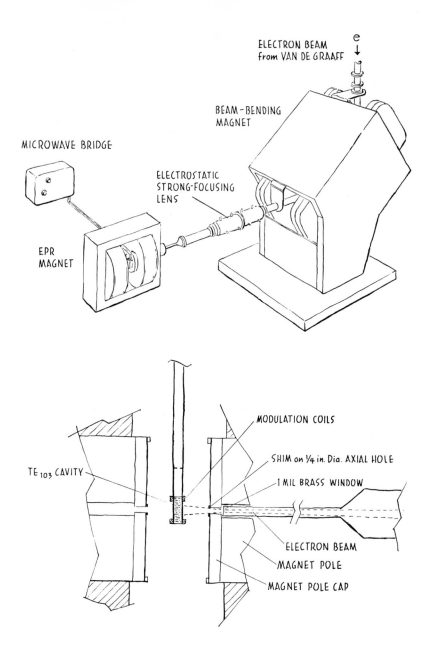

Fig. 6.2-6. Arrangement for measuring the EPR spectrum of radicals as they are formed by 2.8 MeV electron bombardment of a sample in the cavity. Electrons enter the bending magnet from above. Those of the correct energy pass through into the electrostatic focusing lens, then through an axial hole in the EPR magnet pole, and enter the cavity through a thin section in the wall, as indicated at the bottom of the figure. (After F-10.)

order to avoid (*1*) excessive heating of the sample, (*2*) excessive buildup of stable radiolysis products, and (*3*) instabilities in the electron beam (F-10). Sample heating is a problem because appreciable changes either in the sample volume or dielectric properties will alter the loaded cavity Q enough to detune the spectrometer. The concern with stable product buildup is a matter of sample purity. When these products become an appreciable fraction of the sample, products of the products will begin to appear and data analysis will be complicated further. Two types of instabilities were encountered. The first is of concern only with a Van de Graaff generator where the beam has to be bent 90° to enter the cavity. Slight changes in the terminal voltage alter the bending radius in the magnet, causing electrons to miss the sample. Since terminal voltage fluctuations increase with the electron beam current, small currents are required for stability. The second form of instability appears to be the result of excessive ionization in the vapor above the liquid sample.

Several advantages accrue from cooling the sample close to the freezing temperature: (*1*) Radical lifetime is increased, thus increasing the equilibrium concentration of these radicals and the chances of detection; (*2*) the Boltzmann factor is increased, thereby increasing the signal; and (*3*) the dielectric loss is sometimes reduced in materials that exhibit a small dipole moment, thereby improving the Q of the loaded cavity. Dielectric losses play a strong role in determining which materials can be observed and how they must be handled. Lossy dipoles were avoided in Ref. F-10 by starting with a good grade of hydrocarbon, Phillips Research Grade, which was then carefully outgassed and purified to avoid paramagnetic impurities. Vacuum-tight EPR cavities were loaded on a high-vacuum line to avoid oxygen. Outgassing by repeated freezing, pumping, and thawing was sufficient for most samples although trap-to-trap distillation was required for ethane. When necessary, i.e., when the sample did not give a detectable signal, further purification rituals involved passing the sample through a silica gel column to remove olifins or through a vapor-phase chromatograph. When the outgassing was not rigorously performed, a broad permanent EPR absorption peak developed during irradiation.

Three cavities of different lengths were used to cope with the dielectric properties of the samples: cavity I = 4.37 cm long, TE_{102}; cavity II = 3.61 cm long, TE_{102}; and cavity III = 4.93 cm long, TE_{103}. All were rectangular with 0.400 × 0.900 in. cross sections. Cavity I was used for lossy dielectrics where the sample was limited to a volume of 1 cm^3 or less in order to avoid lowering the cavity Q by a factor of more than 2. With cavity I vertical and the electron beam striking the sample as indicated in Fig. 6.2-7c, a considerable fraction of the electrons passes through

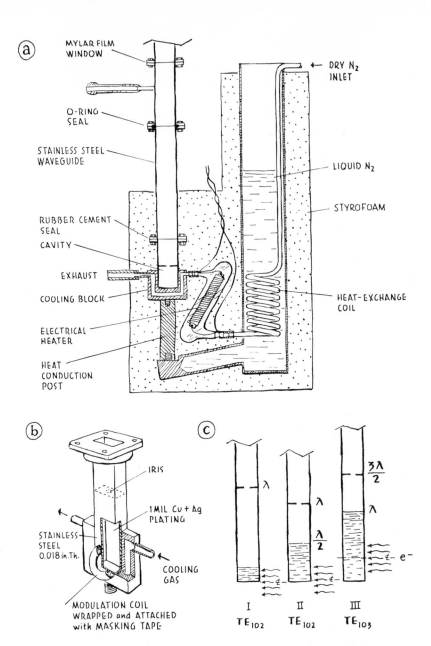

Fig. 6.2-7. (*a*) Arrangement for thermostating a cavity between 90 and 143°K. Dry nitrogen passes through the heat exchange coil in the liquid nitrogen bath, then over an electrical heater and through the cavity cooling block. The cavity is also cooled by conduction through the conduction post. (*b*) Details of the cavity, showing the cooling block and modulation coils attached. (*c*) Schematic representations of the three cavities involved in the electron irradiations, showing the liquid levels and areas bombarded by the electrons. (After F-10.)

the vapor above the sample, thus contributing to the instability. This vapor problem is nearly eliminated in cavities II and III where the larger samples keep the electrons mostly in the liquid. Cavity III gives the largest signal-to-noise ratio when the dielectric losses permit about 6 cm^3 of sample. It is important to fill cavity II to the $\lambda/2$ level and cavity III to the λ level, as indicated in Fig. 6.2-7, so that the liquid–vapor interface is at a node in the electric field where slight changes in the liquid level, due to either volume expansion or motion, will produce a minimum change in the rf field. Low temperatures are required to liquify the lighter hydrocarbons, and frequently measurements on other samples benefit by low temperatures. There are occasional exceptions such as propane which could not be used in cavities II and III at low temperatures because of dielectric losses; however, at temperatures above 203°K the losses are considerably less, presumably because more rapid molecular motion interferes with the loss processes. Figure 6.2-7 shows the temperature control system and the construction of the cavity which has to be compatible with the electron beam, 100 kc modulation, low temperatures, and a high vacuum. Over the range from 90 to 143°K this cooler maintained the temperature variation to within 0.5°K by means of a proportional controller which regulated the current in the heating coil. Higher temperatures were obtained with an external heat exchange coil. Heat conduction through the conduction post is important, particularly for reaching the lowest temperature, and a series of rods with different thermal conductivities were used to reach various temperatures.

The cavities were constructed of 18 mil, type 364, nonmagnetic stainless steel plated on the inside with copper topped by silver to form a thin conducting layer about 1 mil thick. Both the 2.8 MeV electrons and the 100 kc modulation penetrate this type of cavity wall satisfactorily. In the drift tube the electron beam is about 3 mm in diameter. After passing through the aluminum windows and cavity walls, the beam is about 1 cm in diameter. In operation, the cavity and cooler are surrounded by polystyrene foam.

Several precautions are in order with respect to the field modulation. Apparently the electron bombardment produces some heating effects which cause severe base-line drift when conventional 100 kc field modulation and phase-sensitive detection are employed. Double modulation at 100 kc and 200 cps plus an additional stage of phase sensitive detection at 200 cps eliminated the drift problem and provided an additional benefit, namely, discrimination against broad lines which are characteristic of the permanent signals produced in certain samples (F-10). Both modulation frequencies were applied to the same coils at about equal amplitudes. The modulation coils and their supports are exposed to extensive electron bombardment; consequently, many common insulators suitable for coil

Table 6.2-3

g Values of Semiquinones, Hydrocarbon Ions, and Hydrocarbon Radicals

Material	g Values[a]	
Semiquinones	B-21	
1,4-Benzosemiquinone	2.00468 ± 0.00002	
2-Methyl-1,4-benzosemiquinone	2.00462 ± 0.00002	
2-Chloro-1,4-benzosemiquinone	2.00486 ± 0.00003	
2-Bromo-1,4-benzosemiquinone	2.00512 ± 0.00004	
1,4-Naphthasemiquinone	2.00437 ± 0.00003	
9,10-Anthrosemiquinone	2.00413 ± 0.00002	
Hydrocarbon positive ions	B-21	S-6
Anthracene$^+$	2.00249 ± 0.00007	2.002565
Tetracene$^+$	2.00250 ± 0.00003	2.002598
Pentacene$^+$	2.00255 ± 0.00005	
Perylene$^+$	2.00250 ± 0.00002	2.002578
Hydrocarbon negative ions	B-31	S-6
Naphthalene$^-$	2.00263 ± 0.00010	2.002752
Anthracene$^-$	2.00266 ± 0.00003	2.002709
Tetracene$^-$	2.00262 ± 0.00002	2.002682
Pyrene$^-$	2.00266 ± 0.00002	2.002719
Perylene$^-$	2.00262 ± 0.00002	2.002667
Benzene$^-$		2.002850
Irradiated liquids	F-10	
CH_3	2.00255	
CD_3	2.00256	
C_2H_5	2.00260	
C_2D_5	2.00260	
C_2H_4D	2.00260	
C_2HD_4	2.00261	
C_2D_3	2.00220	
$CH_3{-}C{=}CH_2$	2.00222	

[a] *g* Values from Eq. 5-1 with slightly different values of K; in B-21, $K = 3.04197$; in S-6, $K = 3.04199771$; and in F-10, $K = 3.04194$.

forms are impractical. Plastic tapes are also short lived; therefore, the coils were made of Formvar-coated magnet wire taped together and supported with masking tape (2).

Experiments with high-energy electron accelerators usually involve remote operation so that some decisions are required about the location of the microwave gear and the associated spectrometer electronics, e.g., the cavity was located 70 ft from the control room in the Fessenden and Schuler arrangement (F-10). In the arrangement of Fig. 6.2-6 the Varian microwave bridge is located about 4 ft from the electron beam and all other controls are at the 70 ft point. Consequently, the bridge balance, rf attenuation, and coarse frequency adjustments are inaccessible during the period of bombardment. Another alternative was used with the apparatus illustrated in Fig. 7.5-21. All of the controls were located outside the target room and a long waveguide line connected the cavity to the microwave bridge. Both systems have worked satisfactorily with a wealth of samples.

6.2.3 Typical Results

"g Values" have been obtained with good precision for a variety of stable radicals, negative ions, and positive ions. Table 6.2-3 lists results from three investigations where the accuracy is adequate to detect small differences between radicals. All three determinations use Eq. 5-1 and measurements of ν_e/ν_p but slightly different values of K, as indicated in the footnote. All of the ions and stable radicals, and most of the reactive species have g values slightly in excess of the free electron value of 2.002319. The method of preparation, i.e., electrolysis or alkali metal reduction, has no effect on the g value and in most of the examples listed in Table 6.2-3 the g values are independent of temperature or solvent. However, a few temperature and solvent effects have been observed, as illustrated in Tables 6.2-4 and 6.2-5, respectively. In this particular case

Table 6.2-4

g Values of Nonhydrocarbon Radicals (S-6)

Radical	Method of preparation	Solvent[a]	Temp, °C	g Value[b]
p-Benzosemi-quinone	Air oxida-tion	Butanol with KOH	23	2.004679[c]
			−22	2.004651[c]
			−40	2.004631[c]
			−55	2.00460[c]
			−66	2.00450[c]
Durosemiquinone	Electrolytic reduction	DME	23	2.004915 ± 0.000005
			−71	2.004906 ± 0.000006
Tetrachlorosemi-quinone	Na reduction	DME	23	2.005819 ± 0.000008
			−71	2.005835 ± 0.000008
1,4-Dicyanoben-zene negative ion	Electrolytic reduction	DME	23	2.002713 ± 0.000006
			−47	2.002705 ± 0.000006

[a] DME is 1,2-dimethoxyethane.

[b] Correction for second-order shifts: p-benzosemiquinone, -1×10^{-6}; durosemiquinone, -2×10^{-6}; 1,4-dicyanobenzene, -1.2×10^{-6}.

[c] The linewidth increased from 0.09 G at 23°C to 1.1 G at −66°C, and the errors in g accordingly increased from ±0.000006 to ±0.000018.

Table 6.2-5

Effect of Solvent and Counterion on the g Value
of the Pyrene Negative Ion (S-6)

Solvent[a]	Cation	g Value[b]
THF	Na$^+$	2.002719
DME	Na$^+$	2.002722
TGL	Na$^+$	2.002720
THF	K$^+$	2.002714
DME	K$^+$	2.002726
THF	Li$^+$	2.002719
DME	Li$^+$	2.002724
DME	TNBA^{+c}	2.002726

[a] Prepared by Na reduction.
[b] All results are at room temperature, have been corrected for second-order shifts, and have errors of ±0.000006 or less.
[c] Electrolytic reduction.

lowering of the temperature increases the linewidth and complicates location of the center of the spectrum. The uncertainty in this step is too small to account for the observed g values; consequently, the shift appears to be real. Spin–Spin exchange interactions broaden the hf lines of most radical or ion spectra when the concentration of radicals is increased or the viscosity of the solvent is decreased. Edelstein et al. (E-2) have studied the variation of the linewidth with solvent viscosity when the viscosity was controlled by temperature and by pressure. Figure 6.2-8 shows the behavior of di-*tert*-butyl nitroxide (DTBN) radicals in liquid propane (top) and liquid *n*-pentane (bottom). At high viscosities, the linewidth is approximately linear with T/η as predicted by the theory of Pake and Tuttle, which relates the spin exchange frequency to temperature (T) and viscosity (η) (E-2). Linewidths range from a few gauss down to a minimum of about 17 mG (H-3), with a substantial population below 0.3 G, e.g., all but two of the values listed in Table 6.2-6 fall between 0.05 and 0.3 G and three-fourths of the materials in Tables 6.2-4 and 6.2-5 have lines in this range.

The number of hyperfine lines reported for liquid samples ranges from a minimum of two lines produced by transient hydrogen atoms (F-10) to over 400 components as in 1,3-bisdiphenyleneallyl (H-3). Corresponding splittings between lines, as indicated by the coupling coefficients, are

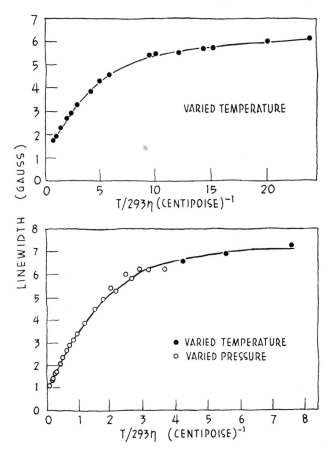

Fig. 6.2-8 (top). Line widths of DTBN in liquid propane, where $c \sim 0.01M$ at 20°C. The data were obtained in a sealed tube at variable temperatures. (Bottom) Linewidth of DTBN in liquid *n*-pentane. The open circles represent data at variable pressures with $T = 293°K$; the filled circles represent data at variable temperatures with $P = 1$ atm. Liquids are deoxygenated; $c = 0.012M$ for variable pressure data, and $c \sim 0.004M$ for variable temperature data. The linewidths were normalized for the concentration differences. (Courtesy E-2.)

506.6 G for the hydrogen atoms and $A_1 = 13.2$, $A_2 = 1.92$, $A_3 = 1.86$, $A_4 = 0.48$, and $A_5 = 0.36$ G for the 1,3-bisdiphenyleneallyl. Other hyperfine structures are listed in Tables 6.2-6 which shows the number of lines and the coupling coefficients for several series of materials. Figure 6.2-9 shows the spectra for the naphthalene and diphenyl anions, as well as the assignment of lines to the hydrogens responsible for the various coupling

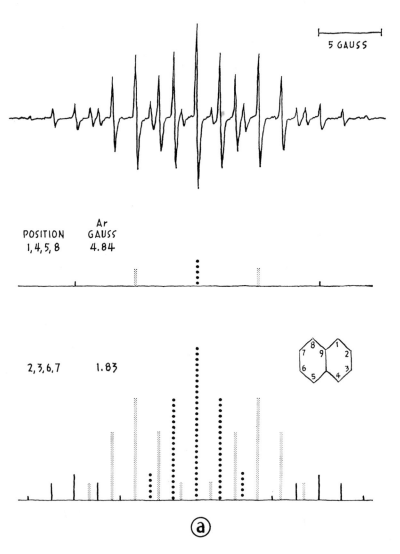

Fig. 6.2-9. EPR spectra of anions prepared by the reduction of hydrocarbons with potassium. (*a*) Naphthalene in DME: In unfolding the spectrum, four equivalent hydrogens, positions 1, 4, 5, and 8, produce a hf structure of 5 lines with intensity ratios of 1:4:6:4:1. Each of these lines is split into another quintet by interactions with the remaining four equivalent hydrogens, i.e., positions 2, 3, 6, and 7.

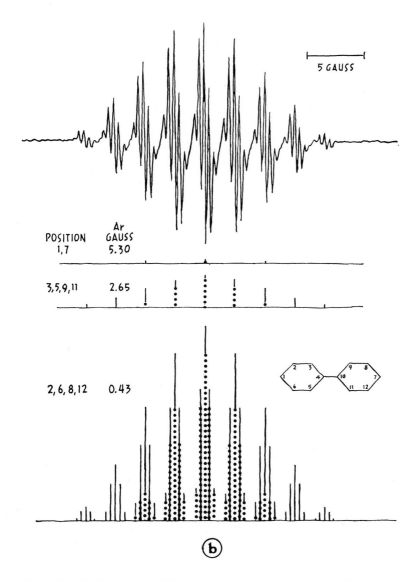

Fig. 6.2-9. (*b*) Diphenyl in THF: Two equivalent hydrogens, positions 1 and 7, produce a triplet with intensity ratios of 1:2:1. Equivalent positions 3, 5, 9, and 11 split these lines into superimposed quintets resulting in 9 lines which are further split into quintets by hydrogens in positions 2, 6, 8, and 12. (After H-7.)

Table 6.2-6. Hyperfine Characteristics of Typical Ions and Radicals in the Liquid Phase

Paramagnetic species	Method of production	Solvent	Number of lines	Linewidth, mG	Hf coupling coefficients, G			Ref.
					A_α	A_β	A_γ	
Benzene anion	Reduction with K	DME	7	700	3.715			H-7
Naphthalene anion	Reduction with K	DME	25	150	4.84	1.83		H-7
Diphenyl anion	Reduction with K	THF	45	150	5.30	0.43	2.65	H-7
Pyrazine anion	Electrochemical	Acetonitrile	25	200	7.18(N)[b]	2.63	1.54	H-7
Phenazine anion	Electrochemical	Acetonitrile	77	125	5.15(N)	1.80	1.86	H-7
1,3-bisdiphenylleneallyl	Electrochemical	CS_2	Over 400	30	13.2	1.92, 0.48, 0.36[c]		H-3
Wursters blue	Irradiation e^-		Over 240	150	7.02(N)		1.98	H-3
Methyl radical	Irradiation e^-	Liquid methane	4	290	23.04	6.74		F-10
Ethyl radical	Irradiation e^-	Liquid ethane	12	Between 130 and 310	22.38	26.87		F-10
Propyl radical	Irradiation e^-	Liquid propane	9	Between 130 and 310	22.1	33.2		F-10
Cyclopentyl radical	Irradiation e^-	Liquid cyclopentane	10	Between 130 and 310	21.48	35.16		F-10
Cyclohexyl radical	Irradiation e^-	Liquid cyclohexane	6	Between 130 and 310	21.0	46.0		F-10
Cycloheptyl radical	Irradiation e^-	Liquid cycloheptane	10	Between 130 and 310	21.79	24.69		F-10
Cyclooctyl radical	Irradiation e^-	Cyclooctane, 195°K	11	6000	21			F-10
	Irradiation e^-	Benzene,[a] 233°K	12		48	23–36		F-10

[a] Benzene irradiated at 193°K and annealed to 233°K to increase resolution.

[b] Splitting due to interaction with nitrogen nucleus.

[c] Five coupling coefficients were observed in this radical.

coefficients. In the naphthalene anion the hydrogens in positions 1, 4, 5, and 8 are equivalent; therefore, they produce five equally spaced lines. Similarly, positions 2, 3, 6, and 7 are equivalent and divide each line of the first quintet into five lines for a total of 25 resolved lines. In diphenyl there are three groups of equivalent hydrogens; Positions 1 and 7 make the strongest interaction and produce a triplet; positions 3, 5, 9, and 11 have the second strongest interaction so they generate a quintet; and positions 2, 6, 8, and 12 produce a second quintet, as indicated. When some hydrogens on the aromatic ring are replaced with nitrogens, the spectrum acquires more lines because $I_N = 1$ and because the nitrogen makes the neighboring hydrogens nonequivalent to their brethren. Figure 6.2-10 shows spectra for 1,4-diazanaphthalene and γ,γ-dipyridyl ions with the constructed spectra and the assignment of splitting factors.

The spectra of radicals generated by electron bombardment (F-10) often contain an additional complication for interpretation, namely, several radical species are produced and, as a result, the spectrum is a composite. This feature is most prominent in the larger molecules. Figure 6.2-11 shows a series of spectra for bombarded hydrocarbons which illustrates this complication. Simple molecules like methane and ethane exhibit lines corresponding to a single species but propane, butane, and larger molecules indicate the presence of several radical species. Figures 6.2-9 through 6.2-11 give only an inkling of the published spectra for liquid samples. Reference F-10 contains a good collection of spectra for radicals and Ref. H-7 shows a number of ions. Spectra for liquid samples are so plentiful that essentially every volume of *The Journal of Chemistry and Physics* contains a sprinkling of such curves. One last spectrum here will help to emphasize the importance of removing oxygen from solution samples. Figure 6.2-12 shows a portion of a Wurster's blue spectrum for a solution saturated with air (*a*) and after the oxygen has been excluded (*b*).

Several additional types of information pertinent to radiation damage studies were observed in the electron bombardment experiments (F-10). First, the elusive hydrogen atoms were observed in liquid methane, although they escaped in all the other samples of Table 6.2-6. Second, because of their high melting points some of the materials permitted enough diffusion when solid to keep the lines narrow and well resolved, e.g., the spectrum for neopentane in Fig. 6.2-13 is quite similar for both the solid and liquid. The diffusion rate is reduced in the solid so that the radicals cannot react and disappear as readily as in a liquid; consequently, for a given rate of bombardment the equilibrium radical concentration was 100 times larger than that for the liquid. In two cases, benzene and cyclooctane transient radicals were observed in the solid, although

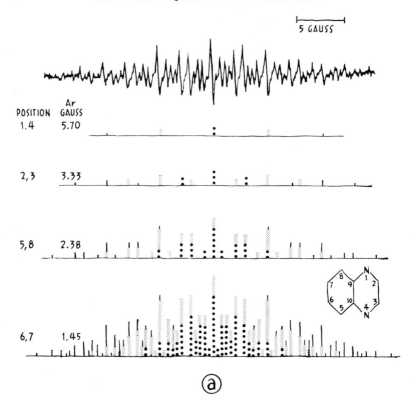

Fig. 6.2-10. Unfolding of the hf structure and the determination of coupling co-efficients. (a) 1,4-Diazanaphthalene: The nitrogens ($I = 1$) on positions 1 and 4 produce $(2nI + 1) = 5$ lines with the intensity ratios 1:2:3:2:1. Each of these lines is further split into triplets three times over by three equivalent pairs of hydrogens: positions 2 and 3 with 3.33 G splitting; positions 5 and 8 with 2.38 G splitting; and positions 6 and 7 with 1.45 G splitting. The lines are coded to assist in following the construction, particularly where lines are superimposed.

similar efforts on the liquids had been unsuccessful. Third, the presence of dissolved air causes the characteristic alkyl radical spectra to disappear, presumably because oxygen is a scavenger. No signals were observed in methane, ethane, and butane and the spectra for the higher hydrocarbons were reduced to a single broad line with a g value displaced about 20 G below the normal position (no hfs). Fourth, radical lifetimes and reaction rates can be determined from the equilibrium concentration of radicals

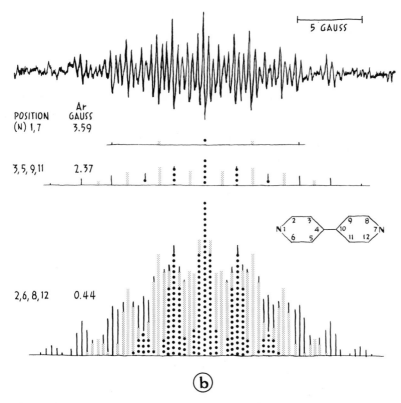

Fig. 6.2-10. (*b*) For γ,γ-dipyridyl: Again the nitrogens on positions 1 and 7 produce a quintet which is split twice over into quintets by groups of equivalent hydrogens; positions 3, 5, 9, and 11, 2.37 G splitting; positions 2, 6, 8, and 10, 0.44 G splitting. Intensities for 4 equivalent hydrogens are in the ratio of 1:4:6:4:1. (After H-7.)

at any rate of bombardment, particularly when only one species is involved. If the radicals disappear only by reacting with their brethren, then the radical concentration (R_i) is

$$R_i = (P_r/2K_{ii})^{1/2}$$

where P_r = the production rate and K_{ii} = reaction rate constant. Figure 6-2.14 shows the radical concentration as a function of exposure rate for irradiated ethyl, butenyl, and vinyl radicals.

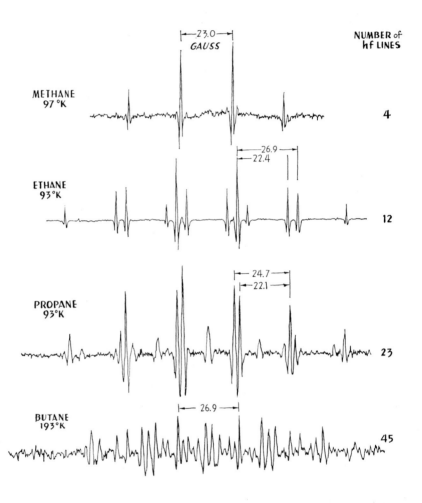

Fig. 6.2-11. EPR spectra of radicals in liquid hydrocarbons, measured while the sample undergoes irradiation with 2.8 MeV electrons: second-derivative presentation. The spectrometer and irradiation system are described in Figs. 6.2-6 and 6.2-7. (Courtesy F-10.)

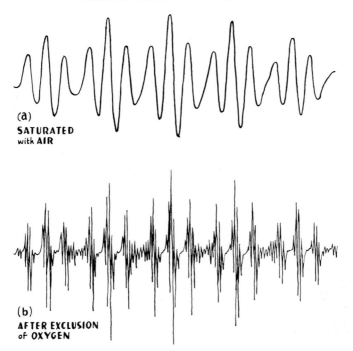

Fig. 6.2-12. Central part of the EPR spectrum of Wurster's blue, showing effect of dissolved oxygen: (*a*) saturated with air; (*b*) after exclusion of oxygen. (Courtesy H-3.)

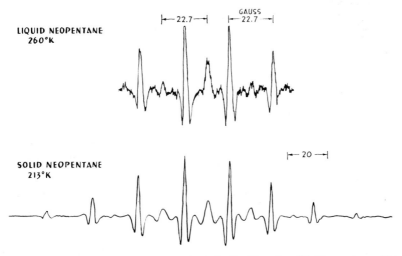

Fig. 6.2-13. Spectra of transient radicals in liquid and solid Neopentane. The signals are several orders of magnitude stronger in the solid than in the liquid samples. (Courtesy F-10.)

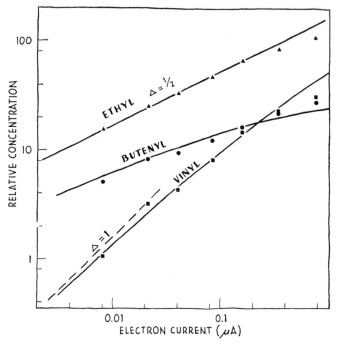

Fig. 6.2-14. Dose rate dependence of ethyl, vinyl, and butenyl radical signals at 113°K: normalized radical concentration $c \propto R^{\Delta}$, where R = dose rate and $\Delta = \frac{1}{2}$ for ethyl and 1 for vinyl; spectrometer type RH1–X; double modulation, 100 kc/sec and 200 cps. Liquid samples in cavities are shown in Fig. 6.2-7. (Courtesy F-10.)

6.3 ALKALI METAL–AMMONIA SOLUTIONS

Metal–ammonia solutions continue to be one of the most fascinating systems in chemistry despite their extensive history, which goes back 100 years to the work of Weyl (W-17). During this period over 1000 papers have appeared describing the important chemical and amazing physical properties of these solutions (J-7). Much of this intense interest developed because metal–ammonia systems apparently form true solutions of electrons. Few other systems permit a study of this fundamental particle of chemistry as the transition from nonmetallic to metallic bonding is produced by the simple expedient of changing the metal concentration (B-5,K-6). In recent years EPR has contributed substantially to the understanding of the "trapped electron" model for these solutions. In the following paragraphs we will first review some of the properties which are important both for conducting EPR measurements and for understanding metal-ammonia solutions and, second, describe typical EPR experiments and results.

6.3.1 Properties of Metal–Ammonia Solutions

(a) Solubilities (J-7). Under very clean experimental conditions all of the alkali metals dissolve readily in liquid ammonia to form true solutions. Initially there is no reaction and when the ammonia evaporates, the pure metal remains as a residue. However, these solutions are metastable and the metal ultimately reacts with the liquid to form the metal amide which is accompanied by the release of hydrogen. Elevated temperatures and foreign atom catalysts accelerate the reaction; therefore, general experimental practice includes low temperatures and very clean apparatus. Table 6.3-1 lists solubilities for a number of metals at various temperatures. The solubility depends slightly on the metal but shows no appreciable temperature dependence.

Table 6.3-1

Examples of Metals Soluble in Ammonia and Some of Their Solubilities
(J-7)

Metal	Solubilities at various temperatures in gram-atom metal/1000 g NH_3						
	168°K	173°K	209.5°K	223°K	239.5°K	273°K	295°K
Li			15.41		15.6	16.31	
Na	11.79			10.89	10.93	10.00	9.56
K		12.2		12.3	12.05	12.4	
Cs				25.1			

When models of these solutions are considered along with their properties, it is convenient to divide the concentrations into three ranges (J-7).

1. Extremely dilute (less than 0.005M) where the metal ions and electrons are essentially independent. It is generally accepted that the electrons are trapped in cavities surrounded by ammonia molecules centered with their protons nearest the cavity.

2. Moderately concentrated (about 0.005–1M) where ammoniated metal ions are bound together by electrons to form clusters.

3. extremely concentrated (greater than 1M) where the ammoniated metals are bound together by electrons much as in a molten metal.

Most EPR measurements have been made in the moderately concentrated range with a few observations extending to extremely dilute concentrations. At low temperatures fairly concentrated metal–ammonia solutions undergo an interesting separation into two liquid phases. For example, the phase diagram for sodium (Fig. 6.3-1) contains three phases: liquid, liquid + liquid, and liquid + solid. This phenomenon can be observed by isothermally diluting a solution which initially contains an excess of metal. If the temperature is held at 225°K, as indicated by the dashed line in Fig. 6.3-1, the process would commence in the liquid + solid phase at the extreme right. When the dilution reaches 10.8 M, all the metal is dissolved, the solution is saturated, and its color is bronze. Addition of more ammonia produces simple dilution down to a concentration of 3.95 M where the second liquid phase appears. This second phase is blue and has a higher specific gravity than the bronze phase. Throughout the liquid + liquid region the blue phase grows at the expense of the bronze phase until all the solution is converted at a concentration of 1.51 M. Below the 1.51 M concentration simple dilution again occurs. This liquid-phase separation has been observed with Li, Na, K, Ca, Sr, and Ba; Cs, however, apparently shows no miscibility gap (J-7). The shaded area in the liquid phase at the left of Fig. 6.3-1 covers the temperatures and concentrations generally encountered in past EPR measurements.

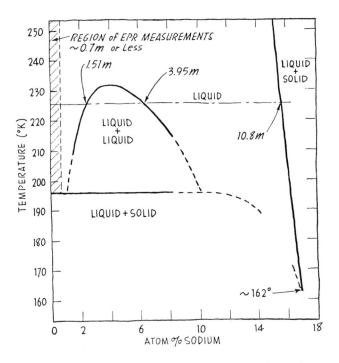

Fig. 6.3-1. Sodium–ammonia phase diagram. (After J-7.)

(b) Thermal Properties. Such properties as the melting point and vapor pressure require consideration when designing the apparatus and the experiment. Figure 6.3-1 shows that below the freezing point (195.3°K) the metal precipitates to form a liquid + solid phase. There the EPR spectrum is dominated by the conduction electrons in the metal. Pressure considerations normally establish the upper temperature limit. Pure

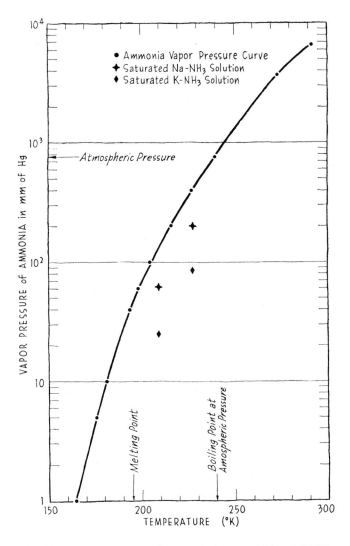

Fig. 6.3-2. Vapor pressure of ammonia between 165 and 290°K.

ammonia at atmospheric pressure boils at 239.6°K. The vapor pressure of ammonia at room temperature and therefore the pressure generally encountered in storage cylinders is about 100 psi. Figure 6.3-2 shows the vapor pressure in millimeters of mercury as a function of temperature. When an alkali metal is dissolved in the ammonia, the vapor pressure decreases slightly, as indicated by the points for saturated Sodium and potassium solutions. However, for the dilute concentrations used in EPR measurements the pressure reduction is negligible and the curve for pure ammonia is suitable for designing apparatus.

(c) Optical Properties. The blue color of the second liquid phase results from a strong infrared absorption band with a peak at about 15,000 Å and a short wavelength tail that extends into the visible part of the spectrum. Figure 6.3-3 shows the absorption spectra for a sodium–ammonia solution. Other alkali metals produce the same color, thereby lending support to the trapped electron model.

Metal–ammonia solutions are sensitive to ultra violet light and react to form the amide ion plus hydrogen. However, accidental ultraviolet irradiation is not a serious problem in the stability of stored solutions because the long wavelength threshold and the maximum effect occur at 2550 and 2300 Å, respectively (J-7).

(d) Electrical Properties. The electrical conductivity of metal ammonia solutions is an important factor in selecting the spectrometer frequency and the sample geometry for an EPR experiment. These solutions have conductivities ranging from that of a good electrolyte to a liquid metal.

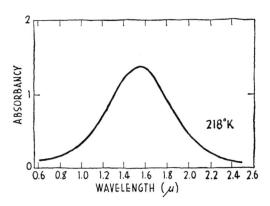

Fig. 6.3-3. Infrared absorption spectra of alkali metal–ammonia solution at 218°K.
(Courtesy G-8.)

Figure 6.3-4 shows the conductivity as a function of metal concentration for moderate and extremely dilute solutions. All three metals follow the same pattern, reaching a minimum equivalent conductance at about $0.05M$ (J-6). In the dilute region the equivalent conductivity approaches a value of about seven times that of salts in water. At the other extreme, saturated solutions are off the graph and approach the specific conductivity of mercury.

6.3.2 Objectives and Problems

Early EPR experiments were concerned with establishing the nature of the blue color centers; therefore, the linewidths, line shape, and the g value were measured in considerable detail as functions of metal concentration and temperature (G-2,H-26,L-4). After Kaplan and Kittel (K-4) put the "electron trapped in a cavity" model on a more quantitative basis, a number of experiments were designed to check this model and theory further (B-22,H-24,H-25,L-5). Table 6.3-2 summarizes the materials, parameters, and variables examined in some of these experiments. Sodium and potassium received the most attention; however, all the alkali metals were measured for at least one concentration in ammonia. Lithium

Table 6.3-2

Examples of Materials and Parameters Measured by EPR

Metal ammonia solution	Concentration, moles/liter	Temperature, °K	Spectrometer frequency, Mc	Parameters, determined	Ref.
Li–NH$_3$	0.2	201	300	ΔH	L-5
Na–NH$_3$	0.0001–0.1	195, 273, 294	49	ΔH, A	L-4
	0.1–0.5	195	19	ΔH	G-2
	0.049–0.98	240, 274, 298	7	ΔH, g, A, F, S	H-25
	0.1	198	300	ΔH	L-5
	0.02–0.65	297	17.4	T_1, T_2	B-22
K–NH$_3$	0.004–1.55	240, 274, 298	7	ΔH, g, A, F, S	H-25
	0.02–0.60	240, 274, 298	7	T_1, T_2	H-24
	0.08	203	300	ΔH	L-5
	0.7	296	23,700	ΔH, g	H-26
K–ND$_3$	0.020–0.800	240, 274, 298	7	T_1, T_2	H-24
Rb–NH$_3$	0.1	203	300	ΔH	L-5
Cs–NH$_3$	0.5	203	300	ΔH	L-5
Ca–NH$_3$	0.05	203	300	ΔH	L-5

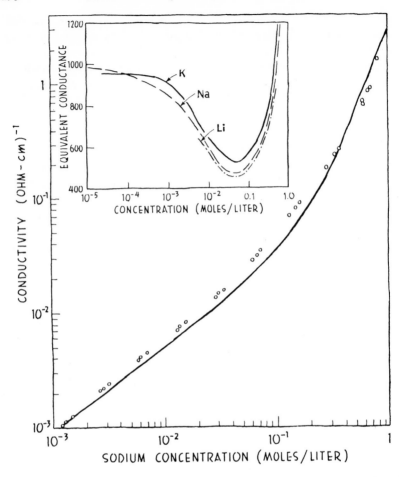

Fig. 6.3-4. Electrical conductivity in sodium–ammonia solutions at 239.5°K; the circles are experimental data and the solid line is theory. (After A-2 and J-7.)

has also been observed in methylamine and ethylenediamine although the higher rate of reactivity makes these solutions more difficult to use than ammonia. Concentrations range from 0.0001 to 1.55M, i.e., generally in the moderately concentrated region, and temperatures range from the melting point to room temperature.

Three characteristics of metal–ammonia systems require particular attention in planning an EPR experiment:

 1. Sample instability.
 2. High electrical conductivity.
 3. Extremely narrow EPR linewidth.

Reasonable sample stability can be purchased with very clean components and low temperatures. The electrical conductivity and linewidth are responsible for the predominance of megacycle frequency spectrometers in Table 6.3-2.

6.3.3 Sample Preparation

Sample holders and preparation systems are normally made of Pyrex glass. The design should withstand the anticipated pressure and permit easy cleaning. References B-22 and W-3 describe several satisfactory cleaning rituals which begin with a thorough cleaning of the stock, restrict contamination during fabrication, and conclude with a thorough washing.*

Preparatory procedures involving a wide range of fastidiousness will produce samples capable of exhibiting measurable spectra. These variations occur in the method of handling the alkali metal and in determining the metal concentration in the solution. No one system is universally superior and the degree of simplicity will depend on the equipment and procedures existing in a given laboratory. Figure 6.3-5 shows four satisfactory arrangements and lists typical procedures. In method *A* some purity of the metal is sacrificed for handling simplicity; however, the procedure will produce successful solutions of all the alkali metals and impurities are not troublesome with the relatively large samples of the size indicated. Various liquids are satisfactory for protecting the metal during the cutting and weighing operations, e.g., hexane (B-22), thiophene-free benzene (B-5), and liquid nitrogen (L-5). In the liquid nitrogen case purified alkali metal is encapsulated in thin-wall, glass capillary tubing so that the operation under the liquid consists of cutting a length of tubing, then crushing and removing the glass. Arrangement *B* provides a known amount of clean metal in the cell with a fairly simple arrangement; however, the technique is limited to sodium. Methods *C* and *D* employ several stages of distillation to purify the metal and thus cannot be used with lithium and calcium, which react with the glass at elevated temperatures.

* The procedure in Ref. B-22 is as follows:
 (1) Age glass stock in hydrochloric acid and water for 24 hr.
 (2) Wash with detergent and water.
 (3) Rinse repeatedly with distilled water.
 (4) Use Drierite and glass wool saliva traps in blow tubes during fabrication.
 (5) Wash finished system with detergent and water.
 (6) Immerse in hot chromic acid for 24 hr.
 (7) Rinse 10–15 times in distilled water.
 (8) Dry at 150°C.

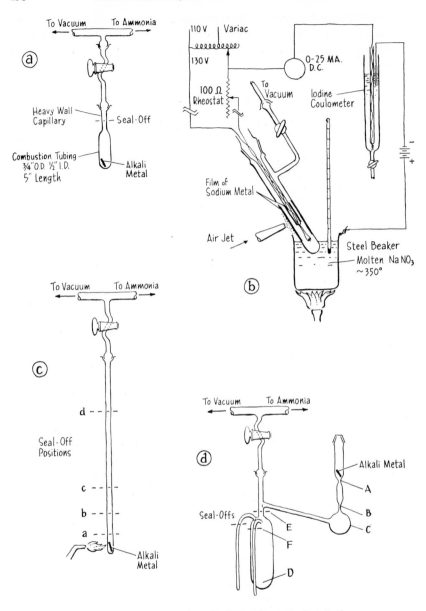

Fig. 6.3-5. Procedures for preparing alkali metal–ammonia solutions:

a. (1) Submerge the metal under hexane while cutting, weighing, and placing in the cell. (2) Evaporate the hexane under vacuum. (3) Flush the chamber and system with sodium-dried ammonia. (4) Repeatedly condense and melt the ammonia in the cell until the desired level is achieved, 2 in. (5) Seal off the cell while the solution is at 77°K. (6) Weigh the cell and detached glass to get the concentration by weight (B-22).

In all cases the 100 psi tank ammonia is dried and purified over sodium or potassium in a separate chamber until reactions cease and the metal dissolves to form a blue solution. In the absence of solid ammonia the blue color indicates the ammonia is adequately clean and dry (34). After removing the evolved gases in several freeze–pump–melt cycles, the desired amount of ammonia is distilled into the makeup chamber to form the metal–ammonia solution.

Several methods of determining the metal concentration are (1) direct measurement of weight or volume of constituents, (2) optical absorption, and (3) chemical analysis of the solution. Each method has some advantages and disadvantages. With direct measurements any reaction subsequent to the weighing will remove alkali metal and change the concentration. Since such reactions always occur, the EPR measurements should be made while the solutions are fresh. Impurities in or on the metal also reduce the accuracy of the direct determination. The optical method can be used at any time, and the solution concentration can be measured as a function of time. However, the accuracy depends on existing data relating optical absorption to concentration (G-8). Several methods of chemical analysis are in use and all measure the composition some time after the EPR measurements have been completed. Reactions occurring in the intervening time produce an error; consequently, this time should be minimized.

(1) Gold and Jolly (G-8) described a determination based on the hydrogen liberated by the addition of ammonium chloride, i.e.

$$NH_4^+ + Na \rightarrow NH_3 + Na^+ + \tfrac{1}{2}H_2$$

---

b. Arrangement for preparing sodium free of hydrogen and carbohydrates by electrolysis through soda glass; (1) Evacuate the bulb and heat the filament. (2) The electrons emitted from the filament go to the glass walls, thereby completing the electrolysis circuit through the walls, the $NaNO_3$ bath, and the steel beaker to the positive terminal of the battery. During this phase the current is a few milliamperes. (3) When sufficient sodium has entered the bulb to form a sodium discharge, the current can increase to a few hundred milliamperes. (4) The sodium discharge is controlled by the air blast which cools the bulb and causes the sodium metal to deposit on the wall. (5) Faraday's law applies. Therefore, the amount of purified metal can be measured with the iodine coulometer. (Courtesy 34.)

c. (1) Cut the metal under oil, wash it in benzene, quickly transfer to the bottom of a long tube, and evacuate the tube. (2) Distil the metal up the tube 3 or 4 times and seal off the lower section after each distillation, i.e., at a, b, and c. (3) Condense the purified ammonia into a cell and seal off at d (34).

d. (1) The opened capsule of purified metal is inserted at A. (2) Melt the metal under vacuum and allow it to flow through the constrictions into C. (3) Seal off at B; heat and degas the system for 6 hr to a vacuum of 10^{-5} mm Hg. (4) Distil the metal into the makeup cell. (5) Condense the purified ammonia into the makeup cell D and seal off at E. (6) Rinse the absorption cells several times with the solution; then seal off the sample tubes at F.

This is a sensitive method suitable for small samples.

(2) In Hutchison's titration procedure, water is added to take up the metal, the ammonia is evaporated off by heating the solution, and the remaining solution is titrated with a standard acid (H-20).

(3) In Ref. D-7 ammonia is evaporated off, leaving the metal residue which is taken up with water. Then the metal concentration is determined with a flame photometer by comparison with standard solutions of the chlorides.

For increased stability, metal ammonia solutions are kept cold, particularly when in storage. Below 233°K reaction rates can usually be kept below 0.5% per hour. Dry Ice temperature (about 195°K) is convenient for storage and Douthit and Dye (D-7) report no evidence of decomposition for 1 week storage at 196°K. Levy (L-5) stored samples of all the alkali metal–ammonia solutions at 77°K for several months without detecting a change in the EPR signal amplitude.

6.3.4 EPR Equipment and Techniques

All but one of the measurements reported in Table 6.3-2 were obtained with low-frequency spectrometers. Two factors dictated this selection: (1) the narrow width of the absorption line and (2) the high electrical conductivity of the solutions. The narrowest lines have a ΔH of 20–30 mG; therefore, to avoid distortions the magnetic field should be uniform over the sample and stable with time to a few milligauss. With the 2 G field required for a 5.5 Mc spectrometer the required homogeneity is about 1 part in 10^3, which is much easier to achieve than the corresponding uniformity of 1 part in 10^6 required at X-band frequencies. Modern magnets can achieve the stability required at X-band frequencies; consequently, measurements of the narrow lines are not restricted to low-frequency spectrometers. At the low fields the earth's magnetic field is an appreciable factor requiring either a correction or alignment of the solenoid field.

Although most of the early measurements were made at low frequencies, the current prevalence of X-band instruments will shift much of the future work to higher frequencies, particularly for samples with broader lines where 100 kc modulation is already in use (34). With moderately dilute metal concentrations, e.g., less than about 0.3–0.5 mole/liter in Fig. 6.3-6, the linewidth becomes comparable with the modulation side-band positions which occur at about ± 34 mG. The minimum line width, 20 mG, corresponds to about 60 kc/sec (B-22); therefore, low-frequency modulation or superheterodyne spectrometers are desirable to avoid line broadening and distortion with the narrowest lines. Figure 6.3-7 shows sample cavity arrangements typical of low-frequency operation. Pyrex is generally

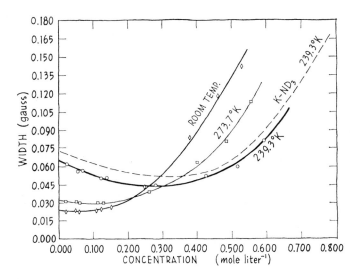

Fig. 6.3-6. Width of resonance at maximum slope versus concentration. Solid lines
are for K–NH₃. (Courtesy H-24.)

satisfactory for the sample container because the narrow lines are not
appreciably distorted by the broad impurity lines normally present in
Pyrex. Temperatures can be conveniently controlled by cooling baths:
for example, Levy (L-5) used 200°K Dry Ice and acetone, 230°K Dry
Ice and watered ethanol, and 273°K ice bath.

A sealed Faraday tube arrangement (L-4) provides a method of varying
the concentration at will; however, this variability complicates concentration measurements. In Ref. L-4 concentrations are estimated by visual
color observations.

6.3.5 Examples of Experimental Results

(a) *g* **Values.** Hutchison and Pastor (H-25) measured the spectroscopic
splitting factor of potassium by the comparison method using DPPH
($g = 2.0037$) and tris-*p*-nitrophenylmethyl as standards. They found that
$g_K = 2.0012 \pm 0.0002$ and was independent of the metal concentration
for solutions ranging from 0.0036 to 0.276 mole/liter. Also, measurements
at both 23,500 and 7 Mc gave the same *g* values (H-25). Levy (L-5)
compared sodium and calcium solutions by placing samples in adjacent
positions in the cavity. No difference in the *g* value was observed within
the limit of detection, namely, 0.005.

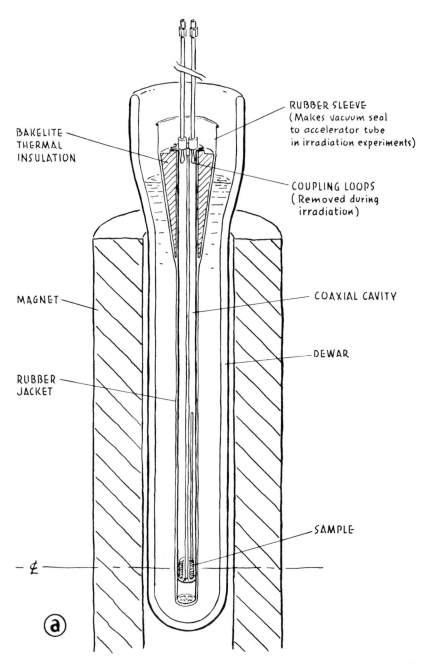

RUBBER SLEEVE
(Makes vacuum seal
to accelerator tube
in irradiation experiments)

BAKELITE
THERMAL
INSULATION

COUPLING LOOPS
(Removed during
irradiation)

MAGNET

COAXIAL CAVITY

DEWAR

RUBBER
JACKET

SAMPLE

₵

ⓐ

Fig. 6.3-7. (a) Coaxial cavity for 300 Mc spectrometer located in the solenoid magnet and dewar. The alkali–ammonia solution is sealed in an annular Pyrex vial that fits around the center conductor. A Neoprene rubber jacket keeps the cooling liquid out of the cavity (L-5).

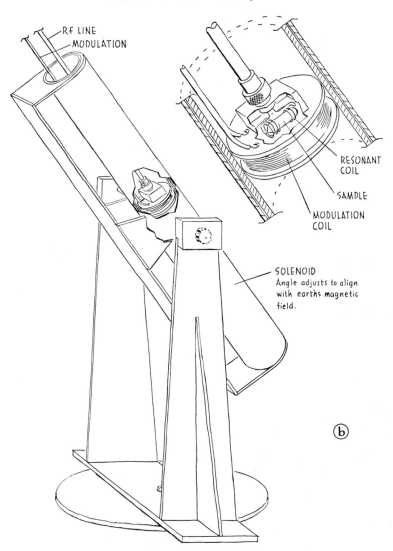

RF LINE
MODULATION

RESONANT
COIL

SAMPLE

MODULATION
COIL

SOLENOID
Angle adjusts to align
with earths magnetic
field.

(b)

Fig. 6.3-7. Reference to irradiation applies to the use of this cavity for radical production in solids (Section 7.5). (*b*) Sample in a resonant coil megacycle spectrometer located in a solenoid magnet tipped to avoid disturbances in the field H_0 due to the contribution from the earth's magnetic field. (Courtesy H-25.)

(b) Line Shape. Hutchison (H-20) obtained resonance curves that were very close to a Lorentzian shape. In Fig. 6.3-8 a resonance curve for potassium is compared with normalized Lorentzian and gaussian curves. Throughout the central absorption region the Lorentzian curve fits very

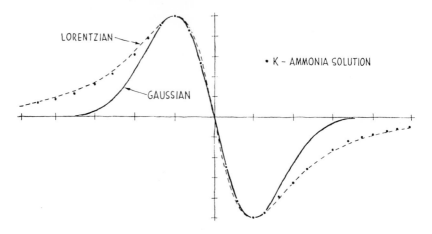

Fig. 6.3-8. Comparison of line shape for potassium–ammonium solution with Lorentzian and gaussian derivative curves. The concentration is 0.201 mole/liter. (After H-20.)

closely and departure occurs only in the wings. Changes in temperature and metal concentration within the region examined had no effect on the shape, i.e., 240–300°K and 0.0111–0.185 mole/liter, respectively (H-20).

(c) **Linewidths,** ΔH. Most of the work on linewidths involved air core solenoids; therefore, field values were calculated from coil dimensions and the measured magnetizing current. ΔH varies with both the metal concentration and the temperature. Figure 6.3-6 shows a family of curves of ΔH versus concentration for three different temperatures. Below a concentration of about $0.200M$, ΔH is nearly constant; however, there is always an observable minimum. The narrowest line is 23 mG wide at a concentration of $0.02M$ and a temperature of $\sim 300°K$. Hutchison and Pastor (H-25) remark that the rapid increase in ΔH at the larger concentrations may be associated with the increased electrical conductivity, noting that the rise coincides with the concentration where the skin depth corresponds to the sample dimensions, namely, about 1 cm. The dependence of linewidth on the alkali metal is not well known but the effect appears to be minor on the basis of the evidence in Table 6.3-3, which lists observed linewidths for all of the alkali metals in ammonia at concentrations below the level where a small concentration effect was found in potassium.

(d) **Relaxation Times,** T_1 **and** T_2. Relaxation time measurements have been made by both CW and pulse techniques (B-22,H-24,H-25) with results that agree on the equality of T_1 and T_2 but show some dispersion in

Table 6.3-3

Width of EPR Absorption Line for Alkali Metal–Ammonia
Solutions (L-5)

Solution	ΔH Peak-to-peak of derivative curve, Oe	Temperature, K°	Concentration, M
Li–NH$_3$	0.1	201	0.2
Na–NH$_3$	0.13	198	0.1
K–NH$_3$	0.1	203	0.08
Rb–NH$_3$	0.16	203	< 0.1
Cs–NH$_3$	0.4	203	0.5
Ca–NH$_3$	0.14	203	0.05

the absolute values. Using continuous wave techniques Hutchison and
O'Reilly observed T_1 and T_2 in K–NH$_3$ and K–ND$_3$ as a function of
potassium concentration and solution temperature. Since the line shape
was Lorentzian and inhomogeneous broadening of the line was negligible,
T_2 is given by

$$T_2 = 2/\sqrt{3}\ \gamma\Delta H$$

where $\gamma = 2\pi\nu\ 2.8$ Mc/sec G and ΔH is the width measured between points
of maximum slope when H_1 is extrapolated to zero. T_1 follows from

$$T_1 = (D_{ex}^{-2/3} - 1)/\gamma^2 H_1^2 T_2$$

where D_{ex} = maximum derivative signal/maximum derivative signal at
zero H_1.

Figure 6.3-9 shows the results at room temperature where the relaxation
times cover the widest range, namely, from about 0.5 to 4.0 μsec. Above
concentrations of 0.15M, $T_1 = T_2$; however, at lower concentration T_1
is slightly longer than T_2. Figure 6.3-10 shows the relaxation time dependence on temperature for various potassium concentrations. At low
temperatures both T_1 and T_2 are relatively insensitive to the concentration.
Blume (B-22) obtained T_2 for a series of Na–NH$_3$ solutions by measuring
the decay time of the free-induction signal, following the method of Hahn.
His values of T_2 are also given in Fig. 6.3-9. The T_1 obtained by the Carr-
Purcell method gave values of $T_1 = T_2$ with an error of about $\pm 10\%$.

6.3.6 Other Alkali Metal Solutions

A few other liquids have been used as solvents for lithium and sodium
but the stabilities achieved were usually inadequate for convenient EPR

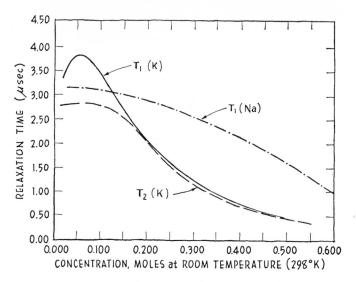

Fig. 6.3-9. Relaxation times (T_1 and T_2) versus concentration for K–NH$_3$ and Na–NH$_3$ solutions at room temperature. [T_1(Na), B-22; T_1(K) and T_2(K), courtesy H-24.]

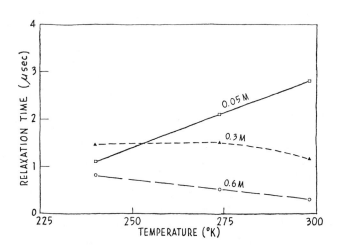

Fig. 6.3-10. Relaxation time T_2 versus temperature for various concentrations of K in NH$_3$ (H-24).

experimentation. For example, Levinthal et al. (L-4) observed EPR resonances for lithium dissolved in both methylamine (CH_3NH_2) and ethylenediamine. Levy (L-5) used lithium in methylamine and found the following ratio for a concentration of about $0.1M$ at $203°K$.*

$$\Delta H_{CH_3NH_2}/\Delta H_{NH_3} \approx 0.6/0.1 \approx 6$$

---

* In the theory of Kaplan and Kittel (K-9)

$$\Delta H \sim 1/\omega_c \approx 3\eta V/kT$$

where ω_c = the frequency for rotational dipolar relaxation, η = the viscosity, V = the molecular volume, k = the Boltzmann factor, and T = the temperature. When methylamine and ammonia are compared on this basis

$$\frac{\Delta H_{CH_3NH_2}}{\Delta H_{NH_3}} = \frac{(\eta V)_{CH_3NH_2}}{(\eta V)_{NH_3}} = \frac{(0.7)(67)}{(0.5)(34)} \approx 3$$

and the temperature dependence of ΔH is comparable for both NH_3 and CH_3NH_2.

CHAPTER VII

EPR in Solids

7.1 FREE ELECTRONS

7.1.1 Metals

Only modest vigor has been applied to spin resonance of the conduction electrons in metals, partly because few materials yield detectable spectra, but largely because of the success of cyclotron resonance. Both techniques are of interest because they supply information about the electronic states in metals; however, cyclotron resonance with its information about effective mass and multiple orbits is the most informative.

From the standpoint of prevalence EPR has been reported in Na, Li, Be, K, and W while cyclotron resonance includes also Al, Cu, Bi, Sn, and Zn. The traditional excuse offered for the dirth of EPR observations is the short relaxation time which results in an undetectably broad signal. With reference to a mechanism proposed by Elliott (E-8), Wertz (W-11) mentions that one will perhaps not find EPR absorption with heavy metals which have large spin–orbit coupling. In discussing unsuccessful attempts to observe EPR in Mg, Al, Pd, and W, Feher and Kip (F-7) also refer to the attractive features of Elliott's mechanism and point out that these metals have larger spin–orbit couplings than Na, Li, and Be where resonance was observed. Impurities with strong spin-orbit coupling would also interfere with resonance detection. This resort to relaxation time limitations is not completely satisfying for materials that give a measurable cyclotron resonance signal but no EPR. Cyclotron resonance requires that $\omega_c \tau \geq 1$ in order to obtain a distinctive resonance, where $\omega_c =$ angular rotational cyclotron frequency and $\tau =$ the collision relaxation time (D-9). Another factor favoring cyclotron resonance detection is the transition probability which is a factor on the order of 10^{12} larger for cyclotron resonance than for EPR. Although other considerations reduce this factor somewhat, the advantage remains with cyclotron resonance (D-9). A brief look at the other side of the coin reminds us that perhaps the EPR of conduction electrons should remain hard to find. Otherwise the spectroscopist could become overwhelmed

308

with spectra from the metal cavities, i.e., the same features: pure materials, perfect crystal lattice, and low dislocation concentration contributing to a high Q cavity also favor EPR.

The information of concern in the EPR spectrum of conduction electrons involves the spectroscopic splitting factor and the relaxation time. In metals the EPR line shape is a function of the sample size; therefore,

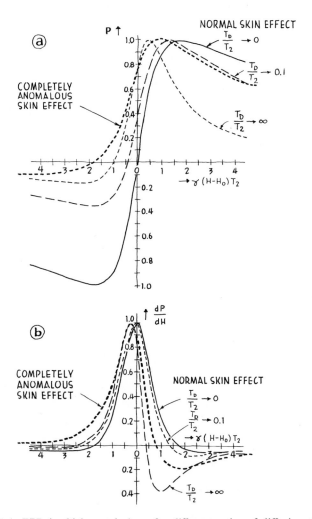

Fig. 7.1-1. EPR in thick metal plates for different ratios of diffusion time T_D to relaxation time T_2: (a) power absorption; (b) derivative of power absorption: solid and dash, normal skin effect; dotted, anomalous skin effect. (Courtesy F-7.)

some theory is required to extract g, and T_2 from the unsymmetrical spectra frequently encountered. Here we follow Dyson's theory (D-12) as modified by Feher and Kip (F-7).

Briefly, three general experimental situations arise:

1. Thin case $[\theta < 4\delta; T_T \ll T_D]$: in small particles or thin films where the thickness is small compared to the skin depth the diffusion time (T_D) is unimportant and the line has an ordinary symmetrical Lorentz shape.

2. Intermediate case: where the metal is not thick compared with the skin depth, e.g., 10^{-4} to 10^{-5} cm. This case is difficult to treat but easy to avoid experimentally.

3. Thick case $[T_T \gg T_D; T_T \gg T_2$, e.g., $\theta > 40\delta]$: Feher and Kip (F-7) have worked out expressions for three limiting thick sample cases

a. $T_D/T_2 \to 0$, symmetrical Lorentzian line

b. $T_D/T_2 \ll 1$

c. $T_D/T_2 \gg 1$, e.g., slowly diffusing magnetic dipoles as from paramagnetic impurities.

Here δ = classical skin depth, T_D = time for an electron to diffuse through the skin depth; T_T = time for an electron to traverse the sample; T_1 = electron spin relaxation time, in metals $T_1 = T_2$ (F-7); and θ is the sample thickness. The skin effect is normal when $\delta > \Lambda$ and anomalous when $\Lambda > \delta$, where Λ = mean free path where an electron loses its memory.

Figure 7.1-1 shows line shapes of the absorption and derivative curves for the three limiting cases of thick samples in the normal skin effect region. The importance of the T_D/T_2 ratio is apparent and as the diffusion time becomes small compared with the relaxation time, the absorption curves begin to look like normal derivative curves and vice versa. Therefore, guidance is needed in locating the proper values of frequency or magnetic field to use in determining g and T_2. Figures 7.1-2, 7.1-3, 7.1-4, and 7.1-5 show asymmetry relations in absorption and dispersion curves for the normal skin depths case. The point on the curve corresponding to the resonance condition used in evaluating g is given by Figs. 7.1-2 and 7.1-3, while Figs. 7.1-4 and 7.1-5 provide a convenient evaluation of $(T_D/T_2)^{1/2}$.* Feher and Kip (F-7) also show how the A/B ratio can be used

---

* One ritual involves the following:

(1) Measure A/B; find $(T_D/T_2)^{1/2}$ from Fig. 7.1-4 or 7.1-5.

(2) Use the $(T_D/T_2)^{1/2}$ ratio to find value of $\gamma(\Delta H)T_2$ from Fig. 7.1-2 or 7.1-3.

(3) Measure ΔH at the half-power point and use to solve for T_2 from $T_2 = [\gamma(\Delta H)T_2]_{graph}/\gamma(\Delta H)_{measured}$.

(4) Also from the $(T_D/T_2)^{1/2}$ ratio find the value of $\gamma(\delta H)T_2$ and solve for δH, which leads to the magnetic field strength required to evaluate g.

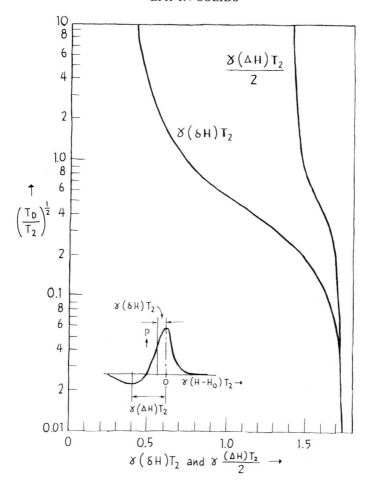

Fig. 7.1-2. $\gamma(\delta H)T_2$ and $\gamma(\Delta H)T_2/2$ vs. $(T_D/T_2)^{1/2}$ for the power absorption due to EPR in thick metal plates: T_D = diffusion time; T_2 = electron spin relaxation time. (Courtesy F-7.)

to determine that the resonance in thick samples arises from conduction electrons, i.e., for derivatives curves:

1. Paramagnetic impurities on the surface give $A/B = 1$.

2. Paramagnetic impurities in the volume give $A/B = 2.7$ for a Lorentzian line and 2.0 for a gaussian line.

Figure 7.1-5 shows that A/B can never be less than 2.7 for conduction electrons and even the value of 2.7 has not been observed in practice. This

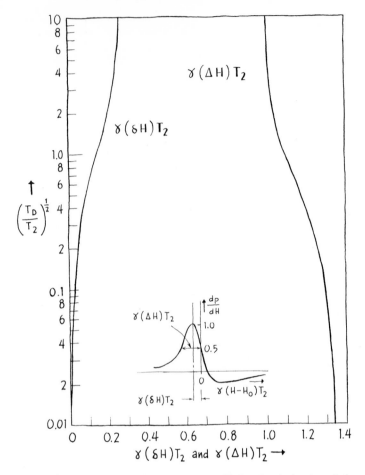

Fig. 7.1-3. $\gamma(\Delta H)T_2$ and $\gamma(\delta H)T_2$ vs. $(T_D/T_2)^{1/2}$ for the derivative of the power absorption due to EPR in thick metal plates: T_D = diffusion time; T_2 = electron spin relaxation time. (Courtesy F-7.)

identification possibility is a definite advantage provided by thick samples in contrast to "thin case" samples where the Lorentzian line with $A/B = 1$ cannot be readily differentiated from impurities.

In the region of anomalous skin effect the resonance curves are distorted to the shapes shown as dotted curves in Fig. 7.1-1. These curves apply only to diffusion times that are short compared with the relaxation time; however, this is the situation encountered experimentally at low temperatures where the anomalous skin effect becomes important.

(a) **Sample Preparation.** *Thin Samples.* In this category we find two general geometries, i.e., fine particles and thin layers. Because the alkali metals were studied most extensively, protective coatings were required for both the particles and films. Feher and Kip (F-7) produced small particles of the alkali metals by ultrasonically dispersing the bulk metal in mineral oil at a frequency of 700 kc/sec. The small particles were separated out by

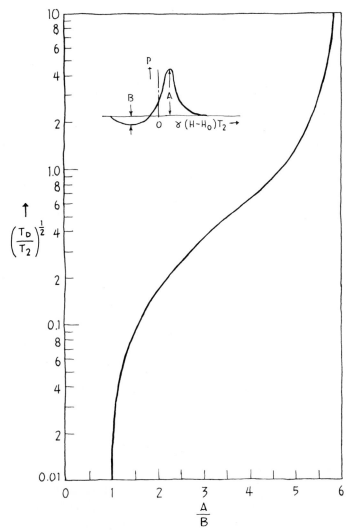

Fig. 7.1-4. A/B vs. $(T_D/T_2)^{1/2}$ for the power absorption due to electron paramagnetic resonance in thick metal plates. (Courtesy F-7.)

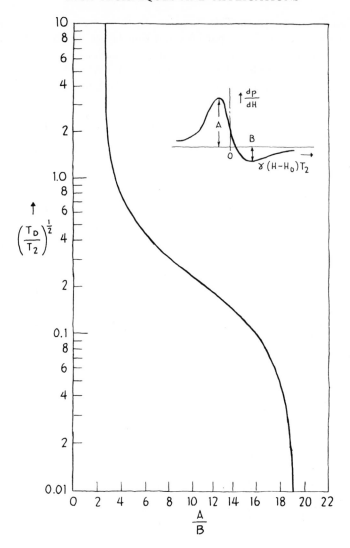

Fig. 7.1-5. A/B vs. $(T_D/T_2)^{1/2}$ for the derivative of the power absorption due to EPR in thick metal plates. (Courtesy F-7.)

centrifuging at 200g for several hours and mounted in paraffin for measurements. Levy (L-5) prepared fine dispersions of Na, K, and Li by freezing metal–ammonia solutions. Table 7.1-1 lists the metal concentrations and temperatures involved in several metal–ammonia experiments. Techniques for preparing these solutions are described in Section 6.3. In

Table 7.1-1

Metal–Ammonia Samples for Conduction Electron EPR

Metal	Concentrations, moles	Temp, °K	Sample size	Ref.
Na	0.1 and 0.01	4–220	1–50 mg	L-5
K	0.08 and 0.4	4–180	1–50 mg	L-5
Li	0.2 and 0.35	4–140	1–50 mg	L-5
Na		14–77	3 mm diameter, 2 mm long	V-9

a variation of the metal–ammonia ritual, Pressley and Berk prepared Li samples for g-factor measurements by evaporating the ammonia (P-17). The metal particles left behind ranged in size from 5 to 50 μ and were subsequently dispersed ultrasonically in purified mineral oil, which also supplied the protons for the NMR measurement used to determine g.

Another method of generating colloidal sodium or potassium is the decomposition of sodium or potassium azide, respectively (K-7,M-7). In Ref. K-7, polycrystalline NaN_3 was sealed in evacuated quartz tubes and irradiated at 573°K with a mercury lamp,* until the sample turned to a deep purple. In Ref. M-7 KN_3 similarly sealed in quartz was irradiated at 303°K with x-rays† for 15 hr which turned the sample a light brown color. Two min of heat at 573°K changed the color to a dark green, which was the color of the specimen studied by EPR. While the decomposition of metal azides appears to be a convenient way to produce collodial metal particles, King, et al. (K-7) note that many of the metal azides are highly explosive and poisonous; therefore, due precautions should be observed.

Metal coatings can be evaporated onto a dielectric substrate to provide another form of thin sample. For example, Feher and Kip (F-7) evaporated alkali metal films up to 0.15 mm thick onto thin mica sheets. Before these coatings were removed from the vacuum, a thin protective coating of paraffin was evaporated onto the suface to exclude air. An added advantage of this technique is that some purification of the metal occurs during the evaporation.

Thick Samples. In Ref. F-7 thick samples of sodium and lithium were prepared by rolling the bulk material under a protective medium such as molten paraffin or between sheets of Parafilm.‡ Other thick specimens

---

* Hanovia type SH 616A.

† 40 MA of 40 kV electrons on a tungsten target.

‡ A thin strengthened film of paraffin available from Central Scientific Company.

used in the coaxial cavity system of Fig. 6.3-7*a* were vacuum cast into glass molds whose concentric walls fit the cylindrical cavity.

Pure samples from single metal crystals should offer the best opportunities for detecting the EPR signal. In this case, samples can be prepared by the techniques developed for cyclotron resonance. The problem involves obtaining a flat polished face in the desired crystalographic orientation without too much damage to the crystal at the surface. Some crystals can be grown with a satisfactory surface; others must be cut. Three procedures that have been successful in preparing samples for cyclotron resonance are:

1. Copper single crystal (K-10); resistivity ratio $\rho_{300°K}/\rho_{4°K} \approx 5000$–10,000; cut with concentrated nitric acid on a continuous string saw; smoothed with acid saturated felt, and finally electropolished in a 60–40 phosphoric acid–distilled water solution. With the sample horizontal and facing up, a current density of about 50 mA/cm^2 gave the best mirror surface.

2. Aluminum single crystal (S-20), residual resistivity ratio $\rho_{300°K}/\rho_{4°K}$ = 10,000. Two cutting techniques were used successfully: the string saw and the electrical discharge machine. In the string saw cuts, the string is wet with a saturated solution of cupric chloride at room temperature. During cutting, the copper that plates out on the bottom of the cut is periodically removed with HNO_3. An electrical discharge machine (e.g., Elox process*) produces a smoother surface so that less material has to be removed in the lapping step. The lap is a piece of garment interfacing material dampened with an approximately 50% saturated solution of $CuCl_2$. If the cloth is too wet, rapid etching pits the surface. In all cases of chemical lapping the sample is kept in continual motion to avoid irregularities in the chemical activity. Mechanical force is limited to avoid damage to the surface. The aluminum is electropolished in 10–20 min with a 50% ethanol–40% H_2PO_4–10% glycerine solution at a temperature of 60–80°C, using 20 V and 0.25–0.3 A/cm^2. Figure 7.1-6 shows the bath and sample arrangement. The plastic sample support keeps the specimen a few mils above the Teflon cloth which separates the specimen from the stainless steel anode. Again the sample is continually moved during the polishing process.

3. Tin single crystals (K-12). Tin crystals were grown by the Bridgman process in a mold with optically flat quartz sides so that no subsequent surface treatment was required.

(b) EPR Considerations. Many of the early measurements (F-7,L-5) were made at 300 and 600 Mc/sec, using the coaxial cavity shown in Fig.

---

* Electric discharge machining.

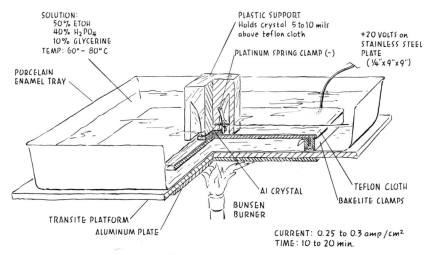

Fig. 7.1-6. Arrangement for electropolishing aluminum crystals (34).

6.3-7*a*. For "thin case" samples the usual high-frequency advantage applies; however, for "thick case" specimens the effective volume of the sample decreases with frequency. Considering the factors in Eq. 3.1, Feher and Kip (F-7) conclude that a spectrometer at 9 kMc would be about six times more sensitive than one at 300 Mc; however, the noise value in the respective detectors nearly nullifies this advantage.

In several more recent studies of finely divided sodium and potassium samples, the measurements were made with types RH1 and RS3 *X*-band spectrometers (V-9,K-7,M-7). Above about 30°K, at least for sodium, the spectrometer requirements are considerably relaxed and the simple homodyne systems are adequate because the relaxation time is short enough to eliminate rf saturation problems (V-9). At temperatures below 20°K Vescial et al. (V-9) observed line broadening due to the Overhauser effect*; therefore, it was necessary to operate with weak rf fields, e.g., in a RS3-type spectrometer with a klystron operating at 50 mW, saturation was observed with 20 db attenuation but the linewidths were power independent with 40 db attenuation.

A variety of cavities are satisfactory for "thin case" samples, e.g., coaxial 300 Mc arrangements (F-7,L-5), the *X*-band cylindrical TE_{011} cavity (V-9) and the *X*-band rectangular cavity (K-7,M-7). Also the

---

* When the rf field is strong enough to partially saturate the EPR resonance, the Overhauser polarization of the sodium nuclei adds another component to the magnetic field seen with the electron and the resonance may shift by as much as 5 G (V-9).

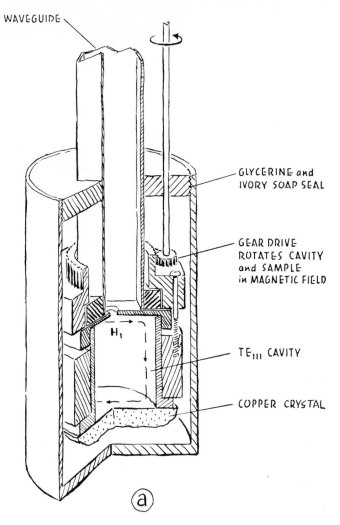

WAVEGUIDE

GLYCERINE and
IVORY SOAP SEAL

GEAR DRIVE
ROTATES CAVITY
and SAMPLE
in MAGNETIC FIELD

H_1

TE_{111} CAVITY

COPPER CRYSTAL

(a)

Fig. 7.1-7. Two cyclotron resonance cavities arranged for EPR measurements. Both arrangements permit rotation of the sample with respect to H_1 and/or H_0. [(a) After K-10; (b) after S-20.]

low-temperature dewar systems of Fig. 7.6-4 are satisfactory for this type of sample. Thick multicrystal samples were used in the coaxial cavity. However, if single crystals are to be studied, an adaptation of one of the cyclotron resonance cavities would probably prove to be the best choice. For example, in the cavities shown in Fig. 7.1-7, the carefully flattened and polished sample forms part of the cavity wall. In cyclotron resonance the rf

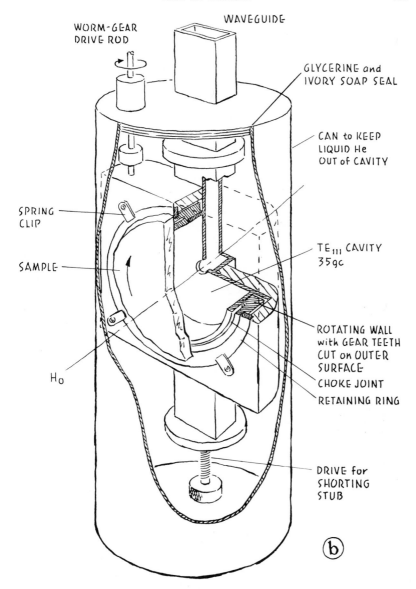

WORM-GEAR
DRIVE ROD

WAVEGUIDE

GLYCERINE and
IVORY SOAP SEAL

CAN to KEEP
LIQUID He
OUT of CAVITY

SPRING
CLIP

SAMPLE

H_0

TE_{111} CAVITY
35 gc

ROTATING WALL
with GEAR TEETH
CUT on OUTER
SURFACE

CHOKE JOINT

RETAINING RING

DRIVE for
SHORTING
STUB

ⓑ

Figure 7.1-7*b*.

electric field is arranged parallel to the external magnetic field; consequently, for EPR the coupling and mode splitting pin would be oriented to make the magnetic field H_1 perpendicular to H_0. Cavity *a* only provides for rotation of the sample in one plane of the H_0 field while arrangement *b*, coupled with a rotating magnet, permits orientation along any crystalline axis. When samples are too small to cover the entire end of the cavity or only the most parallel H_1 field lines are used, the sample can be mounted over a small hole in the end of the cavity. Various materials have been used for these cavities: electrodeposited copper (K-10); silver-plated brass (S-20); and for higher frequency cavities, coin silver G-1. However, the more recent cavities are silver-plated brass. Due to the high friction of silver on silver, the silver is polished off at the rotating joint. It is necessary to take into consideration several opposing factors in mounting the samples: They must be securely attached to avoid vibration due to interactions between the field H and the eddy currents induced in the sample by the field modulation, yet the sample strain should be minimized. Grimes and Kip (G-19) found that sodium and potassium could not be clamped tight enough at room temperature to eliminate the vibration problem without extruding the sample into the cavity with disastrous consequences. The solution was to clamp the sample lightly at room temperature then cool the assembly to 77°K where the hardened metals could support the necessary clamping force without excessive distortion. In another experiment (K-10) a copper crystal was successfully attached with indium solder which remains pliable at 4°K. The choke joint in cavity *b* helps to minimize microwave losses when the contact is not ideal. Liquid helium is excluded from the cavity by a threaded copper can sealed to the lid with the Ivory Soap and glycerine mixture. Helium exchange gas in the cavity increases the rate of heat transfer from the sample.

(c) Typical Results. *g* Values have been measured both by comparison to the free radical DPPH and by simultaneous measurements of the rf frequency and H_0, as indicated in Table 7.1-2. In Refs. K-7 and M-7, H_0 was measured with external proton-resonance probes but in Ref. P-17 the oil suspending the metal particles provided the protons so that field inhomogeneities were avoided. The observed *g* shifts listed in Table 7.1-2 are small and in various states of agreement with theory.

As indicated earlier, the shape of the resonance line depends on the sample dimensions. In the small particle case a symmetrical Lorentzian curve is obtained, as shown in Fig. 7.1-8, where the sodium particles are less than 5 μ in diameter. When the sample contains a range of particle sizes extending from thin to thick, the spectrum will be an unsymmetrical composite curve (Fig. 7.1-9) that does not fit any of the A/B ratios. Thick samples exhibit the T_D/T_2 dependent shapes as calculated in Fig. 7.1-2 and measured in Fig. 7.1-10. The qualitative agreement is apparent.

Linewidths and relaxation times vary with the temperature and are sensitive to impurities. Figure 7.1-11 shows the temperature dependence of linewidth in frozen lithium, potassium, and sodium–ammonia solutions.

Table 7.1-2

Shift in g Factors for Conduction Electrons in Metals

Metal	Sample case	Preparation technique	Method[a]	$\Delta g \times 10^{-4}$, experimental	$\Delta g \times 10^{-4}$, calculated (B-14)	Fre-quency, kMc	Ref.
Li	Thin	Evaporated Li–NH$_3$ and dispersed, Li in mineral oil	ν and H	0.02 ± 0.02 0.02 ± 0.02	—	9.5	P-17
Na	Thick	Bulk metal	DPPH	-8 ± 2	-7	9.5	F-7
Na	Thin	Decomposed sodium azide	ν and H	-6 ± 2	-7	9.1	K-7
K	Thin	Irradiated KN$_3$	ν and H	-41 ± 5	14–25	9.1	M-7
Cs	Thin	Cs–NH$_3$	DPPH	~ 700	100–300	0.3	L-5
Be	—	—	DPPH	$+9 \pm 1$	—	9.5	F-7

[a] ν and H = independent measurements of ν and H; DPPH = by comparison to DPPH.

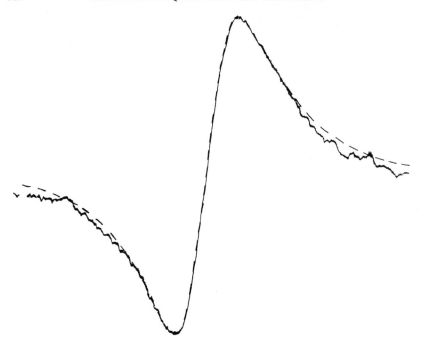

Fig. 7.1-8. EPR in small sodium particles of diameter smaller than $5\,\mu$: $T = 296°K$; $\nu = 320$ Mc. The dashed line is a theoretical curve for the case of thickness, small compared to the skin depth, i.e., a Lorentzian curve. (Courtesy F-7.)

Peak-to-peak values for the derivative curve range from 0.5 to 5 G for sodium and lithium, and from 5 to 25 G for potassium, (L-5). Higher-temperature regions are discussed in Refs. L-5 and M-7. Figure 7.1-12 shows the effect of impurities on the relaxation time of lithium samples. In this temperature region the observed value of $T_2 = 2.7 \times 10^{-7}$ sec for the purest material. Beryllium also had a temperature-independent relaxation rate and $T_2 = 2.0 \times 10^{-8}$ sec (F-7). In keeping with the observed wider linewidth for potassium the relaxation time was short, i.e., $T_2 = 5 \times 10^{-9}$ sec at 4°K. For sodium between 4°K and room temperature, the relaxation time is $T_2 \sim 1/T$ and ranges from about 6×10^{-6} to 10^{-8} sec.

7.1.2   Semiconductors

Historically, the EPR of conduction electrons in semiconductors was first reported in 1953 (P-15) about a year after the first report on such electrons in metals. A few other notes or papers were published about this time (W-19,F-13,F-12) but generally this resonance has been studiously

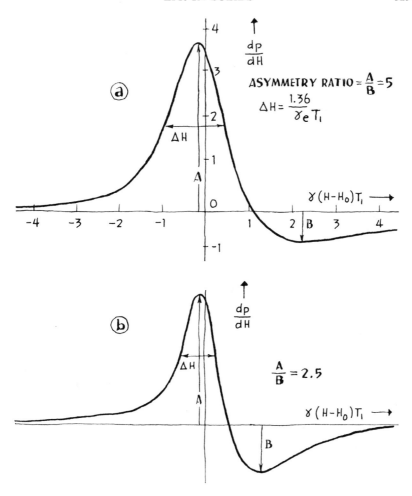

Fig. 7.1-9. (*a*) Derivative of ideal Dyson absorption line in the region of the anomalous skin effect. (*b*) Typical absorption derivative observed in sample of frozen sodium–ammonia solutions. (Courtesy V-9.)

avoided rather than studied. Primary interest centered on the status of donors and acceptors in the lattice and, as we will see in Section 7.2, experiments designed to observe the hfs of these centers require experimental conditions that eliminate the conduction electrons, i.e., moderate concentrations of donors or acceptors and low temperatures. Experimentally there is an area where the conduction electrons in silicon have been useful in EPR, that is, as stable *g* markers and yardsticks. Thin

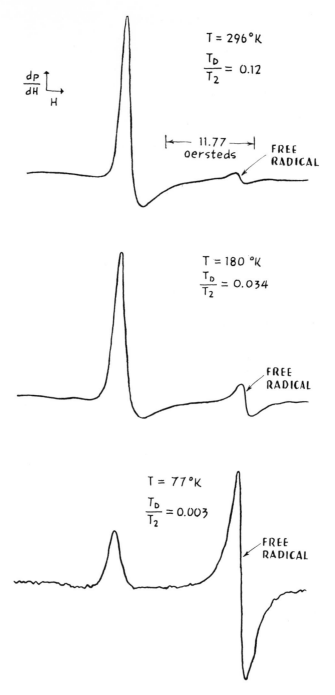

Fig. 7.1-10. EPR in thick plates of lithium for different ratios of T_D/T_2. Compare the shapes with the theoretical curves of Fig. 7.1-1. (Courtesy F-7.)

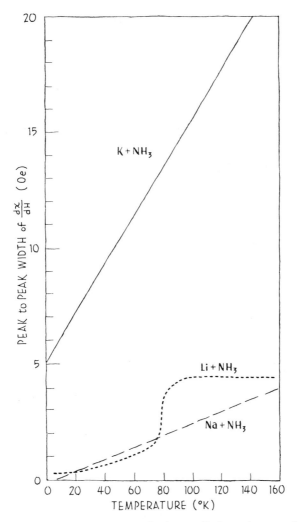

Fig. 7.1-11. Linewidth versus temperature for frozen alkali metal–ammonia solutions. (After L-5.)

wafers of n-type silicon doped with about 3×10^{18} phosphorus atoms per cubic centimeter and calibrated for spin concentration by electrical measurements have been supplied as yardsticks (L-12).

(a) Sample Preparation. The main requirements are high carrier concentrations, particularly for observations at low temperatures, and thin sections appropriate for the skin depth. In the original work (P-15) n-type

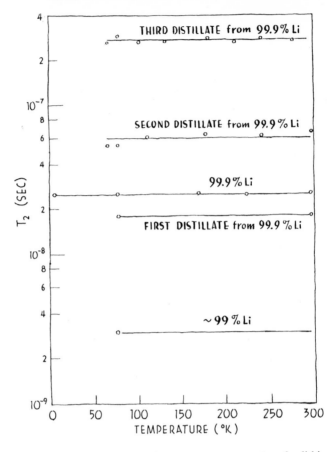

Fig. 7.1-12. Electron spin relaxation time T_2 versus temperature for lithium samples of different purity. (Courtesy F-7.)

silicon crystals containing 1×10^{18}–2×10^{18} phosphorus atoms per cubic centimeter (i.e., between 0.01 and 0.02 Ω cm) were crushed in a steel die, sieved through a 325 mesh screen, washed overnight in hydrofluoric acid, and suspended in paraffin wax. Each sample contained about 0.2 cm³ of silicon and almost all of the particles were under 10 μ diameter. The calculated skin depth for this material is about 100 μ at 300°K. Willenbrock and Bloembergen (W-19) observed EPR for both electrons and holes in silicon crystals containing 5×10^{17}–5×10^{18} donors or acceptors per cubic centimeter. Fletcher et al. (F-12) and Feher (F-2) used thin, n-type silicon wafers, 0.76 and 0.25 mm thick, respectively, and containing from 2×10^{18} to 6×10^{18} donors per cubic centimeter.

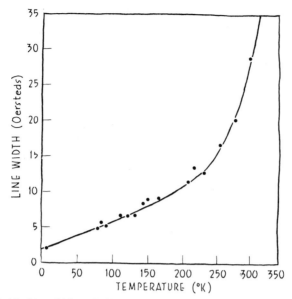

Fig. 7.1-13. Linewidth at half-maximum absorption versus temperature. (Courtesy P-15.)

(b) Spectrometer Considerations and Results. Spectrometer requirements are not a particular problem. Various X-band and 24 kMc systems have been used mostly with rectangular cavities (F-12,F-4,W-19,P-15). Apparently rf saturation is not a problem in the temperature range from 4 to 300°K, where measurements were made by Portis et al. (P-15).

The results are very similar to the thin sample case for the alkali metals. For example, Portis et al. (P-15) found that the splitting factor was independent of temperature over the range from 4 to 300°K in n-type silicon and $g = 2.001 \pm 0.001$. Willenbrock and Bloembergen (W-19) found the same g value for both electrons and holes in silicon, namely, 2.00. The line shape is Lorentzian in the fine particle case and varies with temperature, as shown in Fig. 7.1-13. Willenbrock and Bloembergen (W-19) reported widths at half maximum for n- and p-type silicon of 4–5 G at 78°K in agreement with Fig. 7.1-13. The relaxation time at 4°K appears to be less than 10^{-3} sec (P-15).

7.2   IMPURITY OR DEFECT CENTERS IN SEMICONDUCTORS

We had a brief brush with semiconductors in connection with the conduction electrons of the previous section, now it is time to examine these materials in more detail. Semiconductors are attractive for both scientific and commercial reasons; consequently, a substantial EPR effort and a sizable literature have evolved since Fletcher et al. reported the spin resonance of donors in silicon (F-12, 1954). Two good reviews, Refs. L-15 and F-1, cover the literature in much greater detail than is appropriate here. Reference L-15 gives an indication of the published work by listing 219 references prior to 1961. Semiconductors provide an ideal system for resonance studies for the following reasons (F-1):

1. They are probably the best understood solids.

2. They are commercially available with a high degree of purity and perfection.

3. Impurities can be introduced and controlled in various electronic states.

4. Interpretation and theoretical treatment is facilitated by the simple crystal structure.

5. Beyond providing an ideal host for the study of introduced impurities, EPR is an important tool for determining the band structure of these solids.

For example, the high purity and crystal perfection in silicon leads to long spin relaxation times; therefore, this substance is ideal for detailed studies of relaxation mechanisms.

7.2.1   Materials and Defects

Table 7.2-1 indicates the principal semiconductors studied to date; however, silicon has received more attention that all the other materials combined. The compounds are difficult to obtain with adequate purity, and resonance in germanium escaped detection during the early searches, apparently because of line broadening. Ludwig and Woodbury (L-15) divided the paramagnetic centers in semiconductors into three types, i.e.,

Case 1: electrons localized at isolated defects such as impurity ions.

Case 2: electrons in a partially filled band.

Case 3: electrons at broken bonds, analogous to free radical electrons.

For example, when Group V elements such as P, As, Sb, or Bi are introduced into silicon, four of the valence electrons form bonds to neighboring silicons but the fifth electron remains unpaired and available for EPR detection. At sufficiently low temperatures in dilute concentrations, this electron remains bound to the impurity as in Case 1. If the sample temperature is raised, the electron escapes from the donor and moves through the lattice as a conduction electron (Case 2), yielding the EPR spectrum of the preceding section. For this reason, the bound electrons are studied at low temperatures, usually at liquid helium temperature or below. Other examples of localized electrons are encountered in

Table 7.2-1

Some Semiconductors Studied by EPR Techniques

Group IV elements and compounds	Group III–V compounds	Group II–IV compounds
Si	InSb	ZnS
Gr		
C (graphite)		
C (diamond)		
SiC		

acceptor impurities, transition metal ions, and impurity pairs. Case 3 centers are believed to result from atoms that were displaced to form interstitials and vacant lattice sites. Some of these defects either singly or in consort now have pedigree names such as *A*, *E*, *J*, *C*, and *B* centers, somewhat analogous to the nomenclature of defects in the alkali halides.

All EPR parameters are of interest and have been measured on some of the numerous variations of materials and defects. Table 7.2-2 lists representative examples of measured materials and parameters along with their literature references.

7.2.2 Sample Preparation

In common with other spin systems involving a host crystal containing paramagnetic impurities, sample preparation involves incorporating enough of the desired impurities for a detectable signal without generating unwanted species or interactions. An additional restraint is the solubility of the impurity in the host. In the semiconductors studied to date, these limitations lead to spin concentrations ranging from about 10^{15} to 10^{17} centers per cubic centimeter. At higher concentrations, new lines begin to appear in the hfs due to clusters of spin centers; at lower concentrations, the relaxation times can become extremely long with the accompanying complications from rf saturation and weak signals. Recipies for sample preparation can be cataloged either according to the host crystal or according to the defect. Because the emphasis in this section is on defects, we will follow the nomenclature in Refs. F-1 and L-15 where localized defects are further subdivided into (*1*) shallow donors and acceptors and (*2*) deep impurities which include the transition elements.

(a) Shallow Donors: P, As, Sb, Bi. *Silicon Host. n-*Type doped with phosphorus or arsenic is readily available from commercial sources. For an

Table 7.2-2

Examples of Spin Centers and EPR Parameters Studied in Semiconductors

Donor or acceptor			Spin center or impurity						
Host crystal	Element	Concentration	Treatment	Studied	Concentration per cm³	Temp, °K	Observed parameters	Mode	Ref.
Silicon	P	10^{15}–10^{16}	Strained, irradiated (e)	Si-A center	$\sim 10^{18}$	20 and 77	g, hfs, τ	Dispersion	W-7
Silicon	Sb, P, As	10^{16}	Strained	Donors		1.25	Δg, T_s	Dispersion	W-22
Silicon	P	10^{15}–10^{16}	Strained, irradiated (e)	Si-E center		4.2–155	hfs, g, τ	Dispersion and ENDOR	W-5
Silicon	B, Al, Ga, I		Strained, irradiated (e)	Si-G6 Si-G7		40–110	hfs, g, τ	Dispersion	W-4
Silicon	B, P	$\sim 2 \times 10^{16}$ (B) $\sim 2 \times 10^{15}$ to 5×10^{16} (P)	Irradiated (e)	Si-G6 formerly Si-A	$\sim 10^{15}$	20.4	hfs, g	Dispersion	C-22
Silicon	B, P	$\sim 10^{16}$	Transition metals diffused in at 1250°C	V^{2+} Cr^+ Mn^- Mn^{2+} Fe^0	10^{15}–10^{16}	1.3 and 20.4	hfs, g	ENDOR	W-28
Silicon			Metals diffused in at 1300°C	Pd and Pt	1–4×10^{16}	Up to 20	hfs, g	ENDOR	W-26

Material	Impurity	Concentration	Species	Condition	Temperature	Measured	Method	Reference
Silicon	P, As, Sb	5×10^{16}– 6×10^{18}		Strained	4.2	hfs, g	Dispersion	J-4 F-12, F-13
Silicon	P	3×10^{6}– 10^{17}			12 to 4	hfs, τ		F-2, F-4, F-5
Silicon	^{121}Sb, ^{123}Sb	5×10^{6}			1.2	hfs, g	ENDOR	E-6
Silicon	B, As	10^{15} As, residual B	N(II, III) IX, (I, I′), (V, VI), (VII, VIII)	Neutron irradiated, 10^{18}–10^{19} NVT^a	300, 77, 4.2	hfs, g	Absorption	J-9
Silicon	P	6×10^{16} and 8×10^{16}			1.3	hfs	ENDOR	J-4
Germanium	P, As	8×10^{14}– 5×10^{15}			1.3	hfs, ΔH, g		F-8
SiC		5×10^{17}–10^{18} 5×10^{17}	S, N, B, Ni B		78	g, ΔH, hfs		W-19 L-15
SiC		3×10^{16}	N		14 and 20.4	hfs, g	ENDOR	W-27

^{a}NVT = neutrons per cm^2.

undistorted hf structure of $(2I + 1)$ lines the donor concentrations should be limited to $6 \times 10^{16}/cm^3$ for phosphorus or arsenic (J-4) and $\sim 10^{17}/cm^3$ for antimony according to Ref. E-6. Figure 7.2-1 illustrates the growth of additional lines from clustering centers which become detectable in phosphorus-doped silicon at concentrations of about 7×10^{16} P/cm^3. At the 3×10^{18} P/cm^3 concentration, the overlap between donor centers

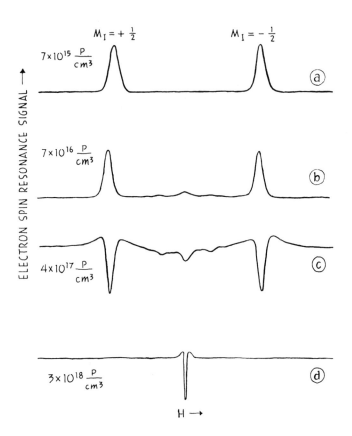

Fig. 7.2-1. Electron spin resonance signal from silicon doped with varying amounts of phosphorus. The range covers the transition from localized centers (*a*) to free carriers (*d*). Between these extremes the signal is due to clusters of phosphorus atoms (*b*, *c*) and marks the beginning of the impurity band conduction process. The different line shapes are a result of the change in relaxation times which cause the transition from "adiabatic fast" to "slow" passage conditions. Spectrometer, Type RS1 X-band; superheterodyne with balanced mixer, AFC; cavity, reflection, rectangular TE$_{101}$, $Q \sim 5000$, silvered Pyrex, Fig. 7.2-4a; temperature $= 1.25°$K, modulation, 100 cps; mounted on pole faces (rotating magnet); magnet, 12 in. Varian; sample size, $9 \times 15 \times 1$ mm. (Courtesy F-2.)

becomes so extensive that the electrons are no longer localized; therefore, a conduction electron spectrum is obtained. Fletcher et al. (F-13) examined this transition to a conduction electron spectrum for donors of phosphorus, arsenic, and antimony and in all cases the hfs had disappeared at 6×10^{18} donors per cubic centimeter, as indicated in Fig. 7.2-2.

When silicon crystals are cut, sandblasted, polished, or broken, resonance centers associated with the surface develop. For example, in both n-type ($\sim 2 \times 10^{14}$ P/cm^3) and p-type ($\sim 5 \times 10^{14}$ B/cm^3) silicon, sandblasting with about 600 mesh SiC generated about 3×10^{14} centers/cm^2 of surface. These centers can be removed by etching away about 10^{-4} cm of silicon with an acid etch consisting of 3 parts by volume of nitric acid to 1 part of hydrofluoric acid (W-22). Such precautions are of concern only when

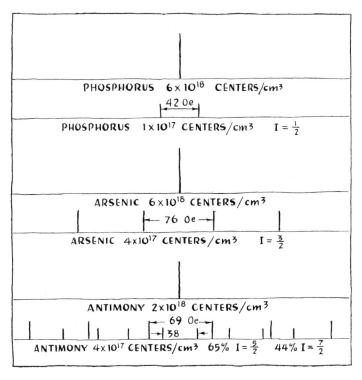

MAGNETIC FIELD

Fig. 7.2-2. Hyperfine splittings for group V donors in silicon. At 4×10^{17} centers/cm^3 the hfs is resolved but at concentrations of 2×10^{18} to 6×10^{18} centers/cm^3 only a single line is observed, i.e., the conduction electron spectrum: cavity—reflection, rectangular; temperature = 4.2°K. (Courtesy F-13.)

working with very dilute donor concentrations or when it is desirable to increase the effectiveness of photoexcitation.

Some typical sample sizes are $1 \times 9 \times 15$ mm for TE_{101} rectangular cavities at (X-band frequencies) and $3 \times 3 \times 10$ mm for a TE_{011} cylindrical (14 kMc) cavity.

Germanium Host. Although germanium in the form of high-purity single crystals was available before silicon, germanium has not shared silicon's popularity as a host for EPR studies because spectra were hard to find. References L-15 and F-1 suggest several factors hindering detection: (*1*) a large spin–orbit interaction with an accompanying relatively short relaxation time; (*2*) a broad anisotropic width of the resonance line related to local strains in the sample, and (*3*) a low solubility for certain impurities. Spectra of phosphorus, arsenic, and antimony donors have been detected, particularly when the magnetic field H_0 points along the (100) crystallographic direction (L-15,F-1). Donors are limited to concentrations comparable to those in silicon for satisfactory hf measurements.

(b) Shallow Acceptors: B, Al, Ga, Id. Feher (F-1) reports that the electron spin resonance of shallow acceptors was even more difficult to find than the resonance for donors in germanium. Again the problem was excessive line broadening, but this time orientation in the external magnetic field proved ineffective and it was necessary to apply uniaxial stresses to remove the degeneracy of the valence band responsible for this situation. Figure 7.2-3 illustrates the development of a detectable signal as a uniaxial stress is applied parallel to the [100] plane and perpendicular to H_0 in boron-doped silicon. The concentration of 1.5×10^{17} B/cm³ is close to the concentrations encountered in other experiments. Apparently no shallow acceptors have been observed by EPR techniques in germanium and Feher (F-1) points out that they will be even more difficult to find than in silicon.

The hfs of boron acceptors have been measured in SiC doped to a level of 5×10^{17} B/cm³ (W-27). Apparently most of the boron disappeared during heating in the furnace because the original doping level was about 3×10^{19} B/cm³ in the change. At still higher boron concentrations the hyperfine structures are no longer resolved and a single resonance line is observed (W-27).

(c) Deep Traps. The most frequently studied deep traps involve transition metal ions such as V, Cr, Mn, Fe, Ni, Pd, and Pt, which usually are incorporated in a silicon host crystal. Other elements such as lithium, sulfur, and nitrogen have been used but not as extensively. These ions are difficult to study (L-15) because their solubilities limit concentrations to modest values from about 10^{14}–10^{17}/cm³ and, furthermore, the ions tend

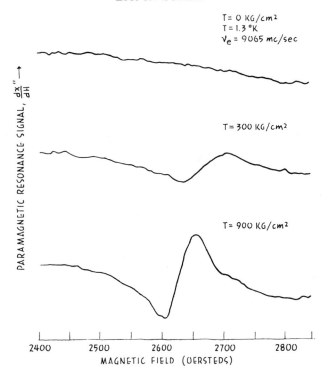

Fig. 7.2-3. EPR from holes in boron-doped silicon (1.5×10^{17} B/cm^3) subject to uniaxial stress T parallel to (100); $T \perp H$, note the broadening and disappearance of the line as the strain is reduced. (Courtesy L-12.)

to precipitate instead of remaining supersaturated. In contrast to these limitations, silicon was the first host in which the charge on the ion was controlled. When the host is undoped, the impurities remain neutral but doping with donors or acceptors leads to negative or positive metal ions respectively, e.g., in manganese, four charge states Mn^{2+}, Mn^+, Mn^0, and Mn^- have been so produced. In some cases such as chromium and sulfur, the neutral and doubly charged atoms show no EPR; therefore, when these impurities are diffused into crystals doped with an acceptor, a EPR signal develops which increases in amplitude until the acceptor concentration equals the chromium or sulfur population. An increase in the acceptor concentration beyond this point causes the signal to decrease apparently because Cr^{2+} and S^{2+} ions form, i.e., the signal drops to zero when there are two acceptors for every ion.

The procedure followed by Woodbury and Ludwig (W-28) in preparing V^{2+}, Cr^+, Mn^-, and Fe^0 illustrates the general practice. Silicon samples about 3 × 3 × 10 mm cut from crystals containing appropriate acceptor or donor concentrations are alloyed to a small amount of the transition metal which is then allowed to diffuse at about 1250°C. This is a convenient diffusion temperature because the solubilities of transition elements apparently reach a maximum close to 1250°C. Generally, the samples are encapsulated in quartz tubes during the diffusion step; however, two procedures are followed, depending on the rate of quenching required to keep the impurities from coagulating or precipitating. When a comparatively slow quench is adequate, the samples are sealed in evacuated quartz tubes. After the diffusion step the tubes are quenched in water. For faster quenching, samples treated in an open tube under an argon atmosphere are blown directly from the furnace into a cooling bath of ethylene glycol.

Chromium, manganese, and iron diffuse at room temperature at rates detectable over time periods of several weeks or months (W-28). Table 7.2-3 summarizes the preparation of various samples reported in the literature.

(d) Irradiation Induced Centers. As previously indicated, irradiation induced atomic displacements in a perfect crystal generate two basic defects: interstitial atoms and vacant lattice sites. In practice, these basic defects interact to generate a variety of compound defects (L-12). For example, Watkins and Corbett (W-7) indicate that approximately 20 different centers have been observed in electron irradiated silicon. Several factors are important in controlling the centers produced during irradiation (J-9).

1. Sample temperature: affects the defect configuration by controlling the mobilities of the basic imperfections.

2. Particle energy: control of the bombarding particle energy can give information about the threshold energies required for various defects.

3. The Fermi level: controlled by the donors and acceptors present is important in determining the charge state of the center and its magnetic characteristics.

Various radiation sources are appropriate: x-rays, electrons, and neutrons. However, substantial energies are required for basic defect production by the light particles, e.g., in silicon, the threshold energy of 12.9 eV to create an interstitial atom, and a vacant lattice site requires a 145 keV electron. Sample thicknesses are usually less than several millimeters, particularly when electrons are the bombarding particles. Irradiation from both sides improves the uniformity of defect concentration. Rituals, radiations, and materials for several of the named centers are collected in Table 7.2-4.

Table 7.2-3 Conditions for Preparing Deep Traps in Semiconductor Host Crystals

Ion	Host crystal	Diffusing temp, °C	Approximate solubility limit, transition ions per cm³	Required shallow impurity type	Rate of quenching	Ref.
V^{2+}	Si	1250	$< 10^5$	Low resistivity, p-type acceptor		W-28
Cr^+	Si	1250	$\sim 8 \times 10^{15}$	Low resistivity, p-type acceptor		W-28
Mn^+	Si	1250	$\sim 2 \times 10^{15}$	Donor (phosphorus)	Rapid	W-28
4 Mn atom cluster	Si	1250	$\sim 2 \times 10^{15}$	Donor (phosphorus)	Slow	W-28
Mn acceptor pair	Si	1250	$\sim 2 \times 10^{15}$	B, Al, Au, Pt acceptor	Slow	W-28
Fe^0	Si	1250	1.5×10^{16}	n-type		W-28
Fe^+	Si	1250	1.5×10^{16}	p-type B, Ga, Al, In	Rapid	W-28
Pairs, Fe acceptor	Si	1250	1.5×10^{16}	p-type, B, Ga, Al, In	Slow	W-28
Li	Si	1250	3×10^{16}	Probably oxygen[a]		F-2
Pd^-	Si	~ 1250	$1–4 \times 10^{16}$	Donor p-type		W-26
Pt^-	Si	~ 1250	$\sim 1–4 \times 10^{16}$	Donor p-type		W-26
S^+	Si	~ 1300	$\sim 3 \times 10^{16}$	Acceptor B	Rapid[c]	L-14
Ni^-	Ge	850	7×10^{15}	n-type, As[b]		L-16

[a] A pulled crystal has about 10^{18} oxygens /cm³. When a zone refined crystal was used, no resonance developed.

[b] No resonance was observed for Ni^0 or Ni^{2-}. Signal grows with concentration of Ni^- until 7×10^{15} spins; then signal decreases as Ni^{2-} concentration builds up.

[c] After heating overnight, the samples were removed from the quartz ampoules, reheated to $\sim 1300°C$ for a few minutes, then rapidly quenched by being blown from furnace directly into a beaker of ethylene glycol.

Table 7.2-4

Production of Defect Centers by Irradiation

Center[a] and model	Host	Doping	Particle type	Energy	Dose rate	Total dose	IRR temp	Ref.
Si-E	Grown in vacuum by floating zone technique	n-type; $\approx 10^{15}$–10^{16} P/cm^3	Electrons	1.5 MeV	≈ 2.5 μA/cm^2	Not given	Room temperature, maximum temperature rise 25°C	W-5
Si-A; Si-B1	Pulled silicon in argon	n-type; $\approx 10^{15}$–10^{16} P/cm^3	Electrons	1.5 Mev	≈ 2.5 μA/cm^2		Room temperature, maximum temperature rise 25°C	W-7
Si-N			Fast neutron	Pile spectrum		7×10^{17} to 10^{19} NVT	~50°C	N-1
Si-J; Si-G5	Pulled silicon	p-type; B, Al, Ga, In; low resistance	Electrons	1.5 MeV	≈ 2.5 μA/cm^2		Room temperature, maximum rise 25°C, also at 20.4°K	W-4
Si-C; Si-G7	n-type Si; P doped; high resistivity	n-type; P doped; high resistivity	Electrons	1.5 MeV	≈ 2.5 μA/cm^2		Room temperature, maximum rise 25°C, also at 20.4°K	W-4

[a] At least two nomenclatures are used in the literature of irradiation induced defect centers, thereby accounting for the dual labeling in the "center" column.

Table 7.2-5

Typical Spectrometers and Features Encountered in the Literature of Semiconductor EPR Measurements

Spectrometer type	Frequency	Detector	Absorption or dispersion	Temperature down to °K	Modulation frequency	Cavity mode and material	Ref.
RH3	14 kMc	Bolometer	χ'' and χ'	1.3	80–100	Cylindrical TE_{011} brass, Ag coated quartz	L-15, W-27, L-16, W-26, L-14, W-28
RS1	X band	ENDOR	χ'	1.25	100	Rectangular TE_{101}, Ag coated Pyrex	F-2, F-5, E-6, W-22
RS1	K band, X band	Balanced mixer	χ''	4.2	500	Rectangular TE_{102}	J-9
RS1	K band	Bolometer	χ'	20 and 77	94	Cylindrical TE_{011}	W-7, W-5
RH1	X band	Single crystal	χ'' and χ'	4.2 and	500	Rectangular TE_{102}	N-1
	K band	bolometer	χ'' and χ'	300°K	500	Rectangular TE_{102}	N-1

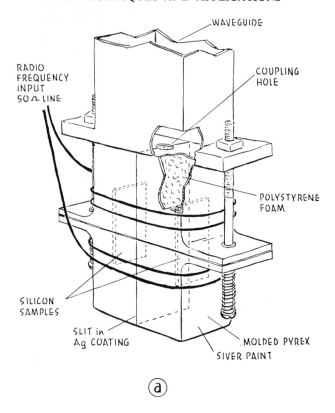

Fig. 7.2-4. Three coil and cavity arrangements used with EPR or ENDOR measurements on silicon crystals. (*a*) Rectangular TE$_{101}$ split cavity molded out of pyrex and coated on the inside with silver (after F-2).

7.2.3   Spectrometer Requirements and Techniques

All of the measurements and techniques described here involved home-made spectrometers, frequently of elegant design. Both homodyne and superheterodyne circuits and X-band to K-band frequencies have been used; X-band superheterodyne systems predominate; however, rf saturation is a serious problem with the pure semiconductors; consequently, the spectrometers are frequently operated in the dispersion mode and a separate cavity is required for frequency control. This ease of saturation coupled with the inhomogeneous broadening of the lines fulfill the requirements for the ENDOR technique which has been used extensively to resolve hfs. Both the spectroscopic splitting factor and the hyperfine interactions are commonly measured as a function of the sample orientation

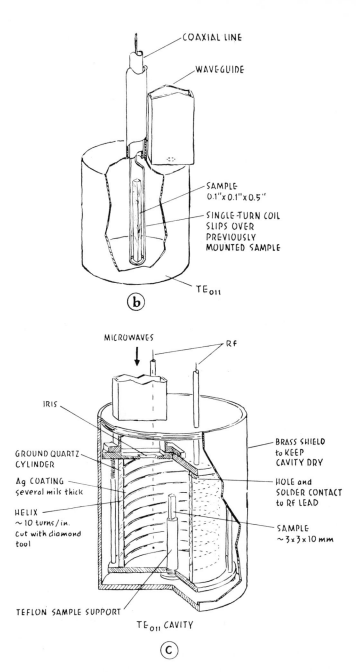

Fig. 7.2-4. (*b*) Cylindrical TE_{011} microwave cavity with internal coil assembly for ENDOR studies (after W-5). (*c*) Quartz cylindrical TE_{011} cavity with combination rf coil and cavity wall (W-28).

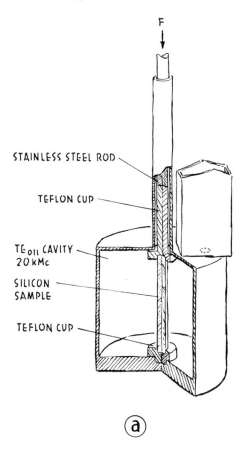

Fig. 7.2-5. Methods of stressing samples in cavities at cryogenic temperatures. (*a*) Silicon sample (2–4 mm thick) supported and compressed between teflon cups which become sufficiently hard at low temperatures to serve as compression blocks. Max stress 880 kg/cm^2 at 120 and 77°K. Silicon samples 3.5 × 3.5 × 15 mm glued between two phosphor-bronze compression blocks were stressed in an arrangement similar to (*a*). A jig held the rods and crystals coaxial during the gluing (after W-7).

in the magnetic field; therefore, the spectrometers are generally equipped with magnets that rotate about the cavity and the modulation coils are mounted on the pole faces. Modulation frequencies are low, usually below 500 cps. Table 7.2-5 lists the type of circuit and particular spectrometer features encountered in a substantial portion of the EPR studies on semiconductors. The preference for superheterodyne systems is apparent along with a general use of balanced mixer detectors. In addition to

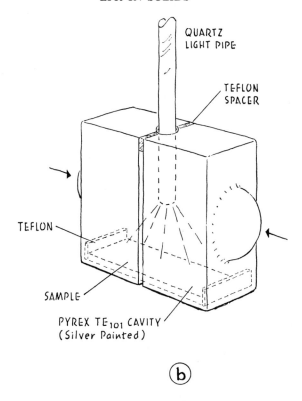

QUARTZ
LIGHT PIPE

TEFLON
SPACER

TEFLON

SAMPLE

PYREX TE$_{101}$ CAVITY
(Silver Painted)

(b)

Fig. 7.2-5. (b) Rectangular TE$_{101}$ squeeze cavity. The load applied to the hemispheres (see Fig. 7.2-6) is shared by the sample which is slightly longer than the inside length of the cavity and the Teflon strip. A quartz light pipe provides illumination which reduces the relaxation time for the spins. (Courtesy W-22.)

provisions for (1) ENDOR, some cavities have been designed to permit stressing the samples (2) electrically or (3) mechanically during the EPR measurement in order to develop detectable lines, as indicated in Fig. 7.2-3. From a chronicler's point of view, it is noteworthy that these three techniques were first tried on semiconductors (F-1).

Figure 7.2-4 shows three cavity arrangements used for ENDOR measurements on silicon. The Feher cavity (a) consists of molded Pyrex with a coating of Dupont No. 4545 silver paint fired on the inside at a temperature of 550°C. Eddy currents induced by the radio frequency coil are reduced by the indicated slot through the coating. Since the two halves of the cavity are $\lambda/4$ long, their junction does not disturb the currents in the cavity walls. Two samples $9 \times 15 \times 1$ mm were held in position with Styrofoam which filled the entire cavity, thereby reducing the amount of liquid helium bubbling in the cavity. This arrangement had an unloaded Q

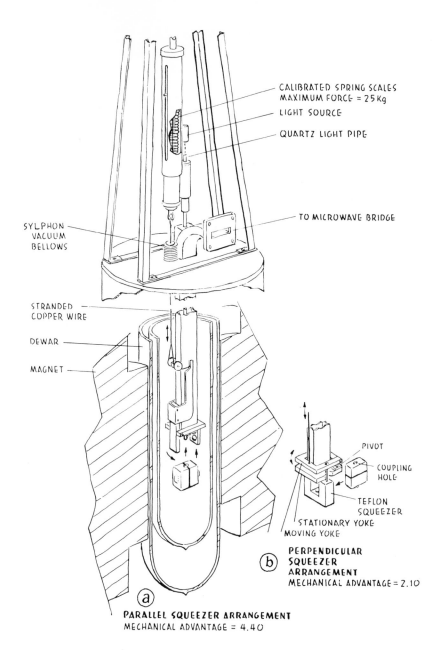

CALIBRATED SPRING SCALES
MAXIMUM FORCE = 25 Kg

LIGHT SOURCE

QUARTZ LIGHT PIPE

TO MICROWAVE BRIDGE

SYLPHON
VACUUM
BELLOWS

STRANDED
COPPER WIRE

DEWAR

MAGNET

PIVOT

COUPLING
HOLE

TEFLON
SQUEEZER

STATIONARY YOKE
MOVING YOKE

(b) PERPENDICULAR
SQUEEZER
ARRANGEMENT
MECHANICAL ADVANTAGE = 2.10

(a)

PARALLEL SQUEEZER ARRANGEMENT
MECHANICAL ADVANTAGE = 4.40

Fig. 7.2-6. Mechanical assemblies for applying stress to the samples in Fig. 7.2-5. (a) The spring loaded parallel squeezer used to compress sample in squeeze cavity in the direction of the magnetic field (courtesy W-22). (b) The spring loaded perpendicular squeezer for stressing samples at right angles to the magnetic field (courtesy W-22).

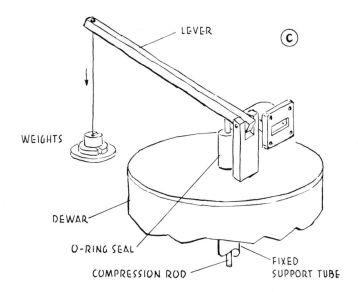

Fig. 7.2-6. (c) Simple weight and lever for loading cavity a in Fig. 7.2-5.

of about 5000 at 4°K. The cylindrical TE_{011} cavity (b) contains a single turn coil to supply the rf field for the nuclear transitions (W-5). No details of the cavity construction are included in Ref. W-5; however, any of the low-temperature metal cavity constructions of Chapter IV would be suitable. Cavity c is similar to the example in Fig. 4-26; however, here the helix serves both to control the mode of the microwave field and to supply the radio-frequency field for the nuclear transitions. A diamond tool is used to cut through the coating. Holes drilled through the quartz cylinder permit a solder contact between the lead-in wires and the coating. A brass shield around the cavity excludes the refrigerant (W-28).

Uniaxial stress effects have been measured in both cylindrical and rectangular cavities with the arrangements indicated in Figs. 7.2-5 and 7.2-6. In the cylindrical TE_{011} example, samples are maintained in compression by a simple lever and weight system which forces a stainless steel rod against the crystal supports. In one adaptation of cavity 7.2-5a the supports were phosphorus–bronze glued to the specimen in an alignment jig (W-5). The sketch shows a crystal supported by a pair of Teflon cups. At low temperatures, the Teflon becomes hard enough to withstand the forces involved, i.e., about 880 kg/cm². An O-ring seal between the stainless steel pressure rod and the supporting tube isolates the cavity from the atmosphere. The rectangular TE_{101} cavity, system b, permits illumination of the sample while it is under stress. As in Fig. 7.2-4a the cavity consists of two molded Pyrex quarter-wavelength sections coated with silver paint. Hemispheres ground on the ends align the cavity and distribute the applied force to the sample through cardboard or Teflon strips which deform plastically to further distribute stress uniformly over the sample surface. Under pressure the gap between halves of the cavity is about 0.5 mm and the Q is not adversely affected. Light for photoexcitation comes into the cavity in a quartz light pipe through the coupling iris. Figure 7.2-6 shows the mechanisms for compressing the rectangular cavities. The "parallel squeezer" and "perpendicular squeezer" labels refer to the alignment of the force with respect to the magnetic field H_0 (W-22). In both cases a calibrated spring applies a tensile force up to 25 kg to a flexible copper wire which couples through a flexible bellows seal to a pivoting lever, which in turn squeezes the cavity. Hemispherical holes in the parallel squeezer jaws engage the cavity hemispheres to align the cavity and assure a uniaxial force on the sample. In the perpendicular squeezer the wire pulls up on the movable yoke which lifts the Teflon C-clamp and squeezes the cavity up against the fixed flange. Here the iris position is not the most convenient for illuminating samples directly; however, light should reflect to the samples. Assembly c suggests a simple lever and weight arrangement suitable for loading the cylindrical cavities.

7.2.4 Typical EPR Characteristics

(a) Shallow Donors and Acceptors. The original work of Fletcher et al. (F-13) and others indicated that the spectroscopic splitting factor for all the donors measured was essentially the same as those for the conduction electrons. Table 7.2-6 illustrates this uniformity. However, more recent measurements with the improved precision of the sandwiched technique

Table 7.2-6

Electron Spin Resonance Spectra of Donors in Silicon (L-13)

Nucleus	Nuclear spin	g Factor	Hyperfine structure constant, G	Line-width, G
^{7}Li	3/2	1.998	0.3	3.0
^{31}P	1/2	2.000	44	2.9
^{75}As	3/2	2.0004	76	3.6
^{121}Sb	5/2	2.000	69	2.7
^{123}Sb	7/2	2.000	38	2.7

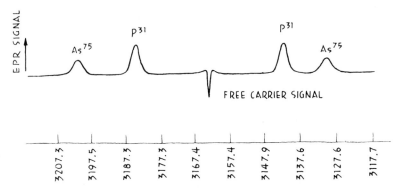

Fig. 7.2-7. EPR dispersion signals from a two silicon-crystal sandwich consisting of a heavily doped marker sample responsible for the free carrier signal and a lightly double-doped wafer with localized electrons which produce the hf structure. Field measurements are by proton resonance. Again the change in line shape indicates "slow" passage conditions for the dilute sample and "fast" passage for the free carrier signal. Spectrometer data are the same as those for Fig. 7.2-1. (Courtesy F-2.)

reveal definite differences in the fourth decimal place. Figure 7.2-7 illustrates these results with spectra for ^{75}As, ^{31}P, and free carrier electrons on one trace. In this technique the silicon sample consists of a thin (0.25 mm thick) heavily doped (3×10^{18} P/cm^3) wafer sandwiched to a double-doped wafer containing $\approx 5 \times 10^{15}$ As/cm^3 and $\approx 5 \times 10^{15}$ P/cm^3 (F-2). When all the donor g values (g_D) were referred to the conduction electron g values (g_{ce}), the values for the conduction electrons were consistently slightly larger. Table 7.2-7 lists values of $g_D - g_{ce}$ for the three commonest donors. Feher (F-2) notes that a silicon sample containing 3×10^{18} donors per cubic centimeter possesses a number of ideal characteristics as a g marker:

1. It exhibits a narrow symmetrical resonance line.

Table 7.2-7

Difference between the g Value of Donor Electrons (g_D)
and the Unbound Conduction Electrons (g_{ce})[a] (F-2)

Donor	E_i,[b] Mv	$g_D - g_{ce}$
Sb	39	$-(1.7 \pm 0.1) \times 10^{-4}$
P	44	$-(2.5 \pm 0.1) \times 10^{-4}$
As	49	$-(3.8 \pm 0.1) \times 10^{-4}$

[a] $g_{ce} = 1.99875 \pm 0.00010$.
[b] E_i = ionization energy at donor.

2. The line is isotropic; no variation with the angle of the magnetic field (H_0) has been found.

3. The samples are stable for an indefinite period.

4. Its magnetization even at 1°K is low enough so that corrections due to demagnetization fields are negligible.

About 3×10^{18} donors per cubic centimeter appears to be the optimum doping level because higher concentrations lead to broadening due to collisions and lower concentrations fail to generate enough nonlocalized electrons. Two other factors influencing the g values are crystalline strain and the orientation of the stress axis to the magnetic field. Wilson and Feher (W-22) suggest two mechanisms for the g shift under strain: (*a*) the "repopulation effect" and (*b*) the strain dependence of $g_{\parallel}$ and $g_{\perp}$. If the lattice is deformed by uniaxial compressive or tensile stresses, the crystal

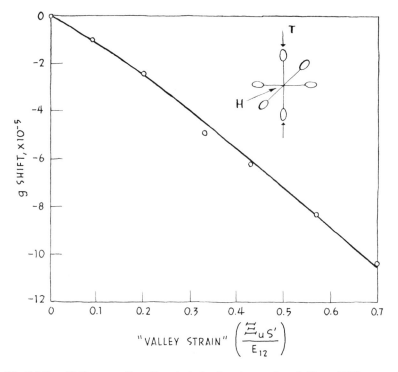

Fig. 7.2-8. g Shift versus the valley strain in phosphorus-doped silicon (10^{16} centers/cm³); $T = 1.25$°K. Uniaxial compression applied in the perpendicular squeezer along the (100) direction. Points are average shift of magnetic field in the (010), (001), and (011) crystallographic directions, normal to applied stress. The solid line is a calculated curve; $g_{\parallel} - g_{\perp} = 1.1 \times 10^{-3}$ (spectrometer data, see Fig. 7.2-1). (Courtesy W-22.)

symmetry is altered so that the valleys in the conduction band are no longer equivalent and the population of electrons in the various energy states is altered. The degree of this admixture of states depends on the ratio $\Xi_u S'/E_{12}$, where Ξ_u is the deformation potential; $S' = T/C'$, where T is the stress, $C' =$ appropriate elastic constant, and E_{12} is the splitting between the single and the doublet states. Figure 7.2-8 shows how the g shift ($g - g_0$) increases as a function of this valley strain for a phosphorus-doped crystal. Some of these shifts are an order of magnitude smaller than

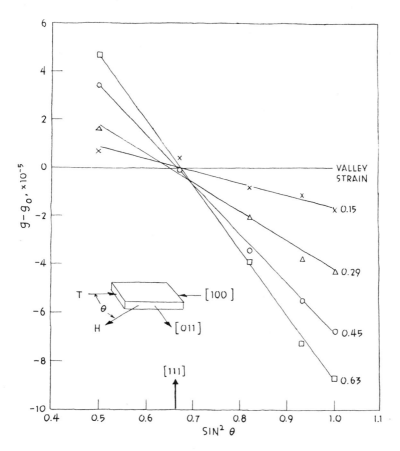

Fig. 7.2-9. g Shift vs. $\sin^2 \theta$, where θ is the angle between the stress axis; T and the magnetic field for a uniaxial compression in the (100) direction for arsenic-doped silicon; $T = 1.25°K$; $\nu = 9$ kMc/sec. The measurements were made in the "parallel squeezer" (Fig. 7.2-6a). Since the microwave field coincides with the stress axis, the EPR signal decreases rapidly at small values of θ. Hence observations at angles less than 45° were not possible. Note that the g shift vanishes in the (111) direction. (Spectrometer data same as Fig. 7.2-1.) (Courtesy W-22.)

the values in Table 7.2-7; consequently, high accuracy is required for the measurement. The value of g also varies with the orientation of the strained crystal in the magnetic field. Figure 7.2-9 shows the increase in this orientation dependence as the valley strain is increased for an arsenic-doped silicon crystal. The g shifts were the same for the three donors studied, which were phosphorus, arsenic, and antimony. In Ref. F-8 Fehr et al. report on phosphorus and arsenic donors in germanium for a magnetic field parallel to the (100) direction and temperatures between 1.3 and 4°K. Their results for both germanium and silicon show that the g shift in germanium is about two orders of magnitude larger than that in silicon (see Table 7.2-8). This shift coupled with the previously mentioned low solubility for these donors and the line broadening for other field orientations made the resonance difficult to find. As indicated in Fig. 7.2-3,

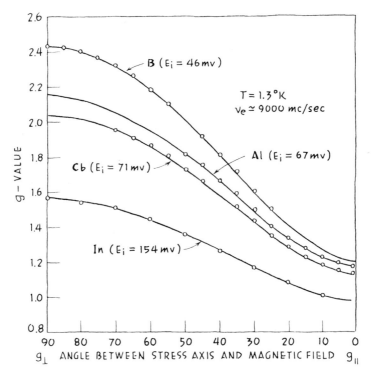

Fig. 7.2-10. g Value versus crystal orientation in the magnetic field: Acceptor concentration, $\sim 10^{17}$ acceptors/cm^3; stress 700–900 kg/cm^2 applied in the (100) direction; H_0 rotated in the [110] plane of the sample. The solid line represents the theoretical fit $g^2 = g_\perp{}^2 \sin^2 \theta + g_{||}{}^2 \cos^2 \theta$ (note the strong dependence of the g value on the binding energy E_i of the hole); spectrometer data, see Fig. 7.2-1. (Courtesy F-6.)

Table 7.2-8

Summary of Electron Spin Resonance Data on Phosphorus- and Arsenic-Doped Germanium and Silicon[a]

Donor	Donor concentration, cm^{-3}	g Value	Linewidth ΔH, Oe	Total hf splitting, Oe
		Germanium		
Phosphorus	8×10^{14}	1.5631 ± 0.0003	10	21
Arsenic	5×10^{15}	1.5701 ± 0.0003	11	107
		Silicon		
Phosphorus	1.5×10^{16}	1.99850	2.8	42
Arsenic	1.8×10^{16}	1.99837	3.2	212

[a] Because of different passage conditions the linewidth in silicon has to be multiplied by 0.85 before comparing it to that in germanium (F-8).

acceptors require some strain in the crystal to develop a detectable line. Figure 7.2-10 (F-13) shows the dependence of the spectroscopic splitting factor for four acceptors on the magnetic field orientation.

When the donor concentration is below about $10^{17}/cm^3$, interactions between spin centers are negligible and the hf structure follows the $(2I + 1)$ pattern controlled by the nuclear spin. Table 7.2-6 lists the nuclear spins for the common donors along with the splittings between hyperfine lines. In silicon, ^{31}P produces a doublet with about a 42 G splitting as indicated in Figs. 7.2-1 and 7.2-2; arsenic generates four lines with a 76 G separation; and the two isotopes of antimony, ^{121}Sb and ^{123}Sb, give six- and eight-line spectra with 69 and 38 G splittings. Similar spectra were observed in germanium, as illustrated by Fig. 7.2-11, which shows the quartet for ^{72}As and the doublet for ^{31}P. The experimental derivative curve for the arsenic-doped sample has a line shape that is nearly gaussian. Values of the linewidth between inflection points are listed in Tables 7.2-6 and 7.2-8, i.e., about 3 G in silicon and 10 G in germanium. Table 7.2-8 also shows that the interaction between the unpaired electron and the donor nucleus is weaker in germanium than in silicon, i.e., the hyperfine splitting is about half. Reference E-6 contains very precise ENDOR measurements of the hf splitting for the two isotopes of antimony in silicon.*

* High precision was required because the numbers were used to determine the hfs anomaly. As mentioned above, the interaction between the unpaired electron and the nuclear magnetic moment is given by the hyperfine interaction constant a. For two isotopes 1 and 2 in the same electronic state the ratio is found to be $a_1/a_2 = (g_1/g_2)(1 + \Delta)$ where Δ is called the hyperfine structure anomaly and is on the order of a fraction of a per cent (E-6).

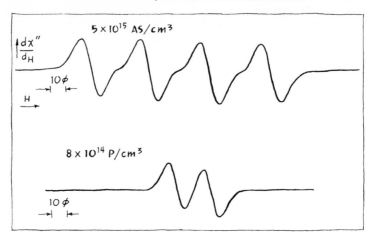

Fig. 7.2-11. EPR signal from arsenic and phosphorus donors in germanium with H parallel to the (100) direction: $T = 1.3°K$, $\nu_e = 9000$ Mc/sec (spectrometer data, see Fig. 7.2-1). (Courtesy F-8.)

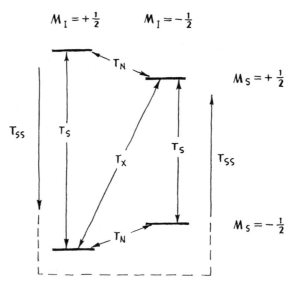

Fig. 7.2-12. Transitions between energy levels corresponding to four different relaxation processes in a system corresponding to phosphorus-doped silicon where $I = \frac{1}{2}$ and $S = \frac{1}{2}$. The $(+\frac{1}{2}, +\frac{1}{2}) \leftrightarrow (-\frac{1}{2}, -\frac{1}{2})$ transition is not indicated because it is forbidden. (Courtesy F-5.)

In contrast to donors, spectra for acceptors are relatively scarce. Figure 7.2-3 shows one of the few examples; however, boron has no nuclear magnetic moment and, as a result, the spectrum is a singlet.

In Ref. F-1 Feher points out that many relaxation processes can be operative in silicon. Four processes studied in phosphorus-doped silicon are indicated on the energy level diagram of Fig. 7.2-12.

T_s = electron spin flip, $\Delta M_s = \pm 1$, $\Delta M_I = 0$

T_n = nuclear spin flip,* $\Delta M_I = \pm 1$, $\Delta M_s = 0$

T_{ss} = double electron spin flip $\Delta M_{s1} = \pm 1$, $\Delta M_{s2} = \mp 1$

T_x = simultaneous electron nuclear spin flip $\Delta M_s = \pm 1$, $\Delta M_I = \mp 1$

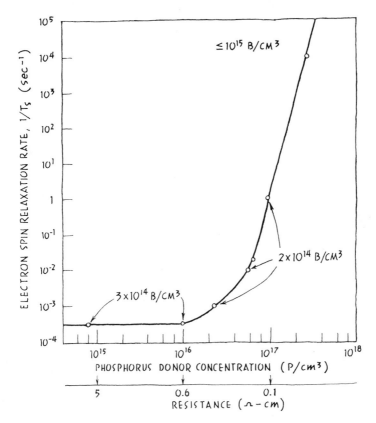

Fig. 7.2-13. Effect of donor concentration on the electron spin relaxation rate in phosphorus-doped silicon: $T = 1.25°K$ (spectrometer data, see Fig. 7.2-1; cavity, see Fig. 7.2-4a). (Courtesy F-5.)

* This process can either involve the flip of a nuclear spin or the transfer of an electron from one donor to another of different M_I state.

Because of the variety of relaxation processes, it was necessary to distribute the equilibrium population of spins in different ways in order to separate the different processes; T_s predominated in most cases. The adiabatic fast passage inversion technique was employed for relaxation times longer than 1 sec. Light and room-temperature radiation were carefully excluded from the samples during the relaxation measurements by wrapping the glass cavities in several alternate layers of aluminum foil and carbon paper. In addition, the inside of the waveguide leading to the cavity was filled with Styrofoam and a glass window 1 mm thick absorbed the room temperature radiation (F-5).

Various internal and external parameters influence the relaxation times and the predominant mechanism. For example, Fig. 7.2-13 shows the dependence of the electron spin flip relaxation (T_s) on phosphorus donor

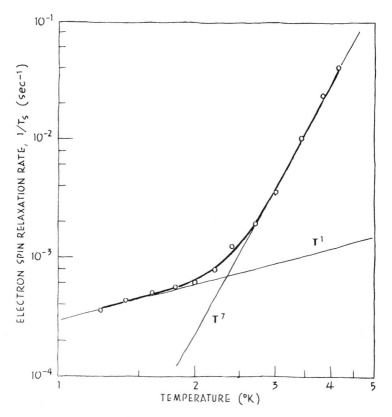

Fig. 7.2-14. Effect of temperature on the electron spin relaxation rate in silicon-doped with 7×10^{15} P/cm³ (spectrometer data, see Fig. 7.2-1; cavity, see Fig. 7.2-4a). (Courtesy F-5.)

concentration for crystal samples containing a nearly constant number of acceptors. At low concentrations the relaxation time is constant and T_s approaches 1 hr; however, above 10^{16} donors per cubic centimeter, T_s decreases rapidly. Similarly, Fig. 7.2-14 shows the T_s relaxation rate temperature dependence in the concentration-independent region of Fig. 7.2-13. At low temperatures over the limited temperature range observed T_s exhibits a $1/T$ dependence consistent with the direct phonon process discussed in Chapter II. Above about 3°K the curve follows the T^7 behavior characteristic of Raman processes. The influence of illumination on T_s is illustrated in Fig. 7.2-15, which shows the reduction in relaxation rate as a function of the light wavelength. At long wavelengths, the relaxation rate increases by a decade but for illumination with energies equal to the band gap, the rate increases over a hundredfold. Reference F-5 should be consulted for further detail on these results and the studies of the other relaxation mechanisms, i.e., T_{ss}, T_x, and T_n. Also Ref. W-22 discusses some effects of strain on T_x processes. Studies of the changes in EPR spectra for crystals under strain have been helpful in understanding the interacting fields which cause the electrons to relax. Figure 7.2-16 gives one example of the relaxation behavior of boron acceptors in silicon. At the higher temperature T_s becomes very short as the stress is reduced and the resultant line broadening prevents detection at zero stress (L-15).

(b) Deep Impurities—Mostly Transition Metal Ions. Various transition elements have been studied in semiconducting host crystals by both EPR and ENDOR techniques. As a result, considerable detailed information is available for the various types of spin resonance centers mentioned in Section 7.2.2, i.e., isolated single atoms or ions, clusters of like defects, and pairs with acceptor atoms. In addition to these groupings, isotopes such as ^{29}Si can interact to generate further alterations or additions to the spectrum. The examples given here are concerned principally with the isolated ion or atom and spectra that can be resolved with EPR techniques. The higher resolution of ENDOR has generally been required to resolve interactions with host isotopes as in the problem of interstitial versus substitutional location of the spin system. Table 7.2-9 contains a modest sampling of deep impurities, their hosts, their spectroscopic splitting factors, and their hfs characteristics. Spectroscopic splitting factors were obtained from measurements of the resonance frequency and the magnetic field strength and the values generally are close to the free-electron value, i.e., 2.0023. In the silicon host crystal, both the g factor and the hf interactions with the V, Cr, Mn, and Fe nuclei are isotropic; however, anisotropic centers are indicated by the interaction coefficients for some of the other defect–host combinations. Table 7.2-9 also lists the nuclear magnetic moments and the number of hf

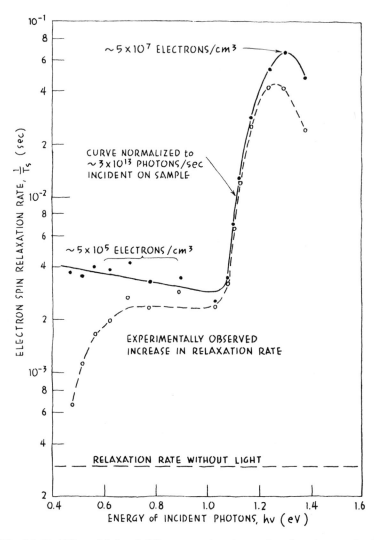

Fig. 7.2-15. Effect of light of different wavelengths on the relaxation rate in phosphorus-doped silicon (7×10^{15} P/cm^3): $T = 1.25°$K; $H \approx 3200$ Oe. The sharp increase in relaxation rate occurs at the band gap where electron-hole pairs are produced. The number of free carriers produced by the light was obtained from the Hall coefficient (spectrometer data, see Fig. 7.2-1; cavity, see Fig. 7.2-4a). (Courtesy F-5.)

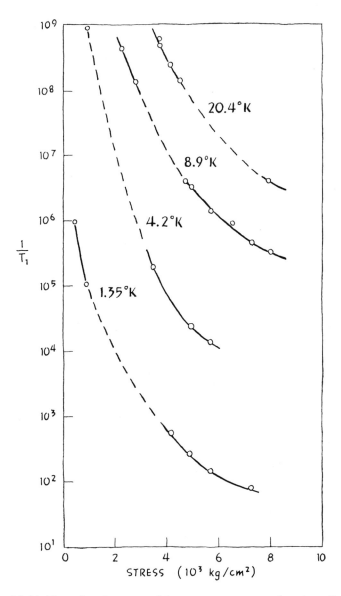

Fig. 7.2-16. The relaxation rate of boron acceptors as a function of uniaxial stress: spectrometer, Type RH3-K reflection homodyne with balanced mixer bolometer detector magic T bridge; cavity, cylindrical TE_{011}; modulation, 80 cps coils on magnet poles; magnet, Varian, rotates in horizontal plane. (Courtesy L-15.)

Table 7.2-9

Deep Impurity Centers in Semiconductor Host Crystals

Host	Impurity	Nuclear moment	Hf lines reported	A, 10^{-4} cm^{-1}	g	Splitting, G	Temp, °K	$H_0 \parallel$ to	Ref.
Si	$^{51}V^{2+}$	$\frac{7}{2}$	8	-42.10	1.9892	45.3	1.3		W-28
Si	$^{53}Cr^{+}$	$\frac{3}{2}$	4	$+10.67$	1.9978	11.4	20.4		W-28
Si	$^{55}Mn^{-}$	$\frac{5}{2}$	6	-71.28	2.0104	76	20.4		W-28
Si	$^{55}Mn^{2+}$	$\frac{5}{2}$		-53.47	2.0066				W-28
Si	$^{55}Mn^{0}$	$\frac{5}{2}$		12.8	2.0063				W-28
Si	$^{57}Fe^{0}$	$\frac{1}{2}$	1		2.0699				W-28
Si	$^{32}S^{+}$	$\frac{1}{2}$	1	6.98					
Si	$^{33}S^{+}$	$\frac{3}{2}$	4	104.2 ± 0.2	2.0054 ± 0.0002	114			L-14
Si	$^{105}Pd^{-}$	$\frac{5}{2}$		12.2	1.9190		<20	[$\bar{1}$10]	W-26
				6.0	2.0544			[001]	
				~ 36	1.9715			[110]	
Si	$^{195}Pt^{-}$	$\frac{1}{2}$		184.2	1.4266		<12	[$\bar{1}$10] or [110]	W-26
				127.0	2.0789			[001]	
				147.0	1.3867			[110] or [$\bar{1}$10]	
Si	^{195}Pt	$\frac{1}{2}$		156	2.021		<20	$\parallel$ to [111]	W-26
				62	2.126			$\perp$ to [111]	

Material	Nucleus	S		A	g			Site	Ref.
Ge	^{61}Ni	$\frac{3}{2}$	4	$A_1 = 10.3$ $A_2 \leq 1.6$ $A_3 = 12.2$	$g_1 = 2.1128$ $g_2 = 2.0294$ $g_3 = 2.0176$				L-16
SiC	^{11}B	$\frac{3}{2}$	4	$A_1 = 1.7$ $A_2 = 1.3$	$g_\| = 2.0020$ $g_\perp = 2.0068$		21	Site I	W-27
SiC	^{11}B	$\frac{3}{2}$	4	2.1	$g_\| = 2.0056$ $g_\perp = 2.003$		21	Site II	W-27
SiC	^{11}B	$\frac{3}{2}$	4	1.7	$g_\| = 2.0062$ $g_\perp = 2.005$	~ 1.8	21	Site III	W-27
SiC	^{14}N	1	3	11.08 11.20	$g_\| = 2.0036$ $g_\perp = 2.0030$ $g_\| = 2.0040$ $g_\perp = 2.0026$	12	20.4		W-27
C(dia-mond)	^{14}N	1	3		2.0024 $\pm$ 0.0005		33.6		S-17

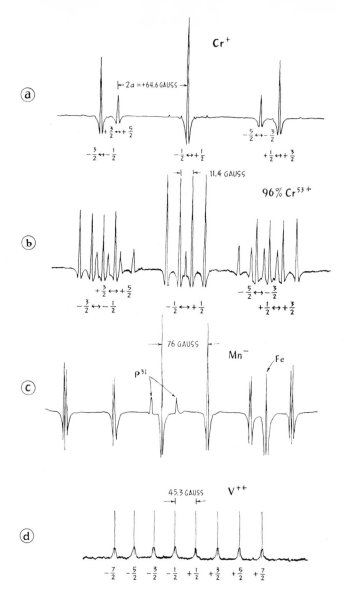

Fig. 7.2-17. EPR spectra for transition metals in silicon: (a) (Cr)$^+$ five fine structure lines for the magnetic field in the (001) direction: $T = 20.4°$K. (b) Cr$^+$ enriched
to 96% ^{53}Cr. Each fine structure line is split into four by the hyperfine interaction;
$T = 20.4°$K. (c) Mn$^-$: six manganese hyperfine lines with a splitting of 76 G, each
split into two fine structure lines. Lines for iron and phosphorus are also present.
(d) V^{2+}: eight vanadium hyperfine lines with 45.3 G splitting, each split into three
fine structure lines that are not resolved in this trace; temperature 1.3°K (spectrometer data, see Fig. 7.2-16; cavity, see Fig. 7.2-4c). (Courtesy W-28.)

lines observed. Figure 7.2-17 shows the hyperfine spectra for Cr^+, V^{2+}, and Mn^- in a silicon host; Cr^+ has a fine structure of five lines with intensity ratios of $8:5:9:5:8$, as indicated. These lines are further split by the four-line hf structure appropriate for $I = \frac{3}{2}$. Mn^- and V^{2+} exhibit hf structures of six and eight lines separated by 76 and 45.3 G, respectively. In addition, a single line for neutral iron was observed on the high-field side of the Mn^- spectrum in agreement with the g value of Table 7.2-9. Figure 7.2-18 contains spectra for some of the other donors in Table 7.2-9. Curve a contains the single line of nonmagnetic ^{32}S and four lines for the ^{33}S isotope with $I = \frac{3}{2}$. Curve b for nickel enriched to 83% ^{61}Ni contains the four hf lines for $I = \frac{3}{2}$ plus a small signal in the middle for zero spin nickel nuclei. According to Ref. L-16 this was the first experimental determination of the spin of ^{61}Ni. Spectra c and d are for nitrogen and boron, respectively, in SiC. Such three-line nitrogen spectra have been observed both in undoped SiC and diamond crystals as resident impurities (W-27, S-17). Boron-11 with an 80% abundance and a spin of $\frac{3}{2}$ dominates the spectrum for boron in SiC, which has been resolved into three sets of four hyperfine lines, as indicated. The sets are believed to result from boron nuclei substituting for carbon in three nonequivalent sites.

Information on line structure and relaxation times is meager for most of the deep trap impurities. For V^{2+}, Cr^+, Mn^-, or Mn^{2+}, the relaxation times are reported to be relatively long at liquid hydrogen temperatures (W-28). At $1.3°K$, they are on the order of seconds or longer. At $10°K$ the lines are on the order of 1 G wide. Reference L-15 should be consulted for g values and interaction coefficients for additional deep donors, as well as groups and pairs of impurity centers.

(c) **Radiation Damage Centers.** Most of the radiation effects studies have been made on variously treated silicon crystals and the centers are listed in Table 7.2-4. Proposed models for these centers are listed in Table 7.2-10. Apparently most of the centers are compounds of the primary radiation products interacting with each other or with foreign atoms in the lattice. The spectroscopic splitting factors are close to the free electron value and similar for all the centers listed in Table 7.2-10. The g factors are anisotropic. All of the examples of spectra to follow exhibit hfs due to interactions with ^{29}Si ($I = \frac{1}{2}$ and 4.7% abundant) and in some cases with magnetic impurity nuclei.

Si-E Center. Presumably vacancies generated at random locations by the ionizing radiation can migrate through the crystal until trapped by substitutional phosphorus atoms. Figure 7.2-19 shows a schematic diagram of the center along with the EPR spectrum for crystals oriented with H_0 parallel to the [011] axis. The unpaired electrons and the spectral lines

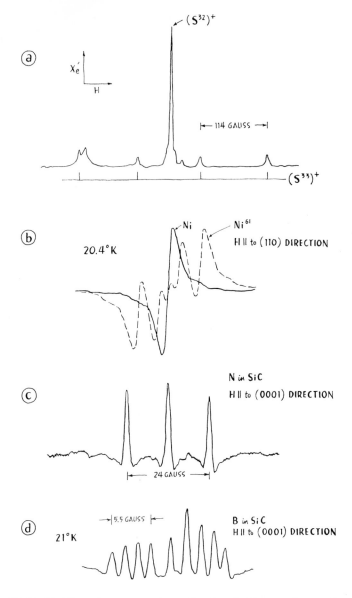

Fig. 7.2-18. (*a*) Dispersion spectra for sulfur-doped silicon under rapid passage conditions, sulfur enriched to contain 20% ^{33}S (courtesy L-14). (*b*) Absorption derivative for nickel-doped germanium at 20.4°K. Nickel enriched to contain 83% ^{61}Ni, which produces the four hyperfine lines; brass TE_{011} cylindrical cavity (courtesy L-16). (*c*) Derivatives of the dispersion spectrum for nitrogen in SiC at 20.4°K showing 3 hyperfine lines with 12 G splitting between lines (courtesy W-27). (*d*) Derivative of the dispersion spectrum for boron-doped SiC, with boron enriched 92% ^{10}B and H_0 parallel to the hexagonal axis (spectrometer data, see Fig. 7.2-16). (Courtesy W-27.)

Table 7.2-10

Proposed Models for Radiation Damage Centers

Center	Model	Ref.
Si-E	A lattice vacancy adjacent to a substitutional phosphorus atom.	W-5
$\begin{bmatrix} \text{Si-}A \\ \text{Si-}B1 \end{bmatrix}$	A lattice vacancy trapped at an interstitial oxygen vacancy.	W-7
$\begin{bmatrix} \text{Si-}J \\ \text{Si-}G6 \end{bmatrix}$	A divacancy in a single positive charge state.	W-4
$\begin{bmatrix} \text{Si-}C \\ \text{Si-}G7 \end{bmatrix}$	A divacancy in a single negative charge state.	W-4
Si-B	Presumably a defect structure involving one or more vacancies in which the resulting atom rearrangements have one dangling bond. Found in both p- and n-type electron irradiated silicon.	W-6
$\begin{bmatrix} \text{Si-}N \\ \text{Si-}P1 \end{bmatrix}$	Similar to a B center but definitely not the same imperfection—produced by neutron irradiation.	N-1
Si-II, III	Believed to involve two unpaired electrons localized in dangling tetrahedral orbitals centered on nuclei which are separated by about 5 Å.	J-9

associated with the several orientations of the defect center are indicated. Each center contains a phosphorus nucleus with $I = \frac{1}{2}$ which produces the doublet structures marked in Fig. 7.2-19. In the few E centers containing a ^{29}Si nucleus the hyperfine interaction is much stronger leading to satellites with about 16 times the separation of the phosphorus doublet; however, the intensity is too low for clear resolution on the scale of this figure. Measurements as a function of temperature or compressional stress reveal rather drastic changes in the line shapes and size (see the amplitude shifts in Fig. 7.2-19 when an axial compression stress of 12,500 lb/in² is applied along a [110] axis). Watkins and Corbett (W-5) explain this behavior in terms of "bond switching" motion in which the phosphorus-vacancy direction remains fixed but the bonds switch between the indicated multiplets to seek out the lowest energy orientation. The total area under the curve remains unchanged during this switching process.

Si-Bi Center. These centers develop only in crystals containing substantial concentrations of oxygen impurities and the model consists of an interstitial oxygen atom which has captured a lattice vacancy with bonds as indicated in Fig. 7.2-20, i.e., two of the four silicon atoms adjacent to the

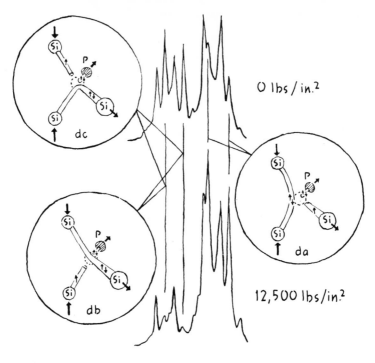

Fig. 7.2-19. Dispersion spectrum of Si-*E* center in silicon irradiated with 1.5 MeV electrons: temperature, 20.4°K; H_0 parallel to [011]; top, zero stress; bottom 12,500 lb/in² uniaxial compression stress along a [110] axis. Typical defect orientations responsible for the lines are shown in insets; spectrometer type, RS1 − K with balanced mixer and bolometer detectors; cavity, cylindrical TE_{011}, internal coil for ENDOR (see Fig. 7-2.4*b*); temperature, 20°K and 77°K; modulation, 94 cps; uniaxial stress arrangement (see Fig. 7-2.5*b*). (Courtesy W-5.)

vacancy bond together while the other two bond to the oxygen with paired electrons. In the neutral state the center is not paramagnetic; therefore, donors must be present in the crystal to provide the electrons which make the centers paramagnetic. A *Bi* center can have six possible orientations and six possible resonance lines corresponding to the ways the oxygen atom can be located between two of the four silicon atoms (W-7). The splitting factor is anisotropic; consequently, the lines will normally be separated and since all orientations are equally probable, the amplitudes should be the same. Some of the lines in Fig. 7.2-20 are superimposed for this orientation in the field; however, it is apparent from the amplitudes how they can be resolved into six equal lines. The figure also shows the change in population of the various orientations resulting from a 12,500 lb/in² axial

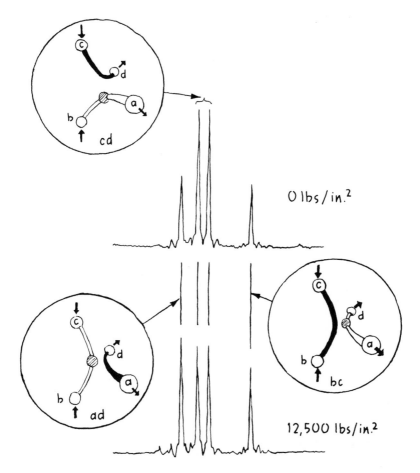

Fig. 7.2-20. Dispersion spectrum of Si-*A* center in silicon irradiated with 1.5 MeV electrons. Spectrum changes from *A*-center reorientation under stress along [110] axis. Stress applied at 125°K and frozen in by quenching to 77°K. Defect orientations corresponding to various lines are shown in the insets (spectrometer data, see Fig. 7.2-19). (Courtesy W-7.)

stress which makes all orientations no longer equally probable. Hyperfine structure due to interactions with ^{29}Si are not resolved in this figure because of the low amplitude and wide splitting involved.

Si-G6 (Si-J)(Si-G7)(Si-C). Reference W-4 explains the formation of *G*6 and *G*7 centers in terms of the diagram in Fig. 7.2-21, which shows the six broken bonds of the divacancy rearranged to form two "bent" pair

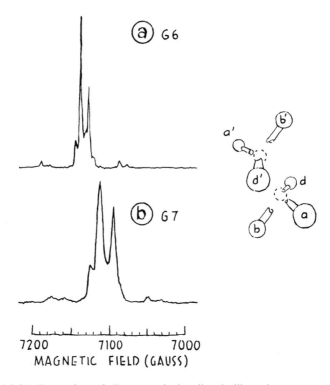

Fig. 7.2-21. Formation of divacancy in irradiated silicon by rearrangement of bonds and the spectra for silcon *G*6 and *G*7 centers at 20.4°K, with H_0 parallel to the [100] axis (spectrometer data, see Fig. 7.2-19). (Courtesy W-4.)

bonds *a–d* and *a'–d'* plus an extended orbital *b–b'* containing the unpaired electrons responsible for the EPR. In low-resistivity *p*-type material *G*6 centers are formed by the loss of an electron from the center (to an acceptor) leaving one electron in the *b–b'* bond. Conversely, *G*7 centers form in high-resistivity *n*-type silicon when an electron is added to make a total of three in the *b–b'* orbital. Figure 7.2-21 also shows spectra for both centers with the crystal oriented so that the [100] axis is parallel with the magnetic field. These centers are sensitive to motional effects generated either thermally or by compressional stresses. Figure 7.2-22 shows the effect of a 875 kg/cm² compression load applied along the [011] axis and the postulated centers responsible for the various lines. Under strain all possible divacancy orientations are no longer equally probable and alignment prefers the lowest energy position. Stressed samples containing *G*7 centers exhibited spectral changes similar to the results for the *G*6 centers.

The small hyperfine satellites well out on the tails of the main absorption

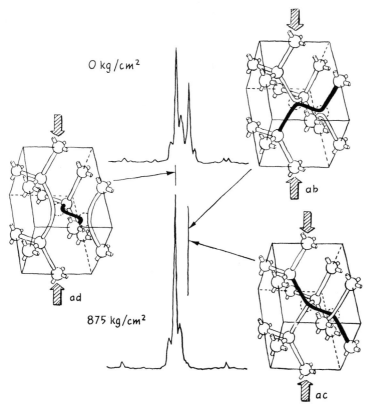

Fig. 7.2-22. Change in the G6 spectrum under [011] compressional stress at 30°K; H_0 is parallel to [011] axis. The defect orientations responsible for the various lines are shown in the insets (spectrometer data, see Fig. 7.2-19). (Courtesy W-4.)

peaks in both Fig. 7.2-21 and Fig. 7.2-22 result from interactions with ^{29}Si nuclei.

Si-N (II, III), etc. Neutron irradiation generates a complex EPR spectrum in silicon which has been interpreted in terms of at least five centers. Jung and Newell (J-9) explain the Roman numeral nomenclature as follows: $S = \frac{1}{2}$ centers in silicon are designated Si-IX, the two transitions of $S = 1$ centers are designated separately and given compound names such as Si-II, III; Si-V, and Si-VII, VIII. As indicated in Table 7.2-10, the centers have not been identified; however, their properties and behavior as a function of magnetic field orientation, temperature, defect concentration, and oxygen dependence have been thoroughly examined (N-1,J-9). Again the g values are near the free electron value and fall within the range

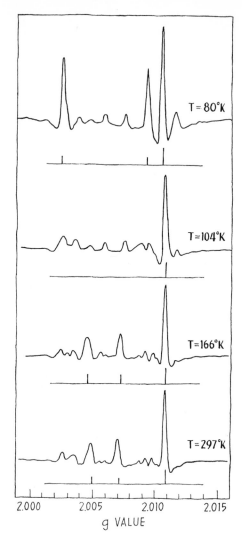

Fig. 7.2-23. Dispersion spectra for neutron irradiated silicon, with H_0 parallel to the [111] axis. Line drawings indicate the position and relative intensities of lines attributed to Si-$P1$ (formerly Si-N) centers. Spectrometer type, RS1 K-band with bolometer detector; temperature 80–297°K; modulation, 500 cps). (Courtesy N-1.)

covered by the other defects. Figures 7.2-23 and 7.2-24 illustrate the spectra associated with $P1$, IX, and II, III centers. Feeble hf structures due to ^{29}Si nuclei are labeled in Fig. 7.2-24. The relative amplitudes and spacing of the $P1$-center lines vary with temperature (Fig. 7.2-23). Because of the

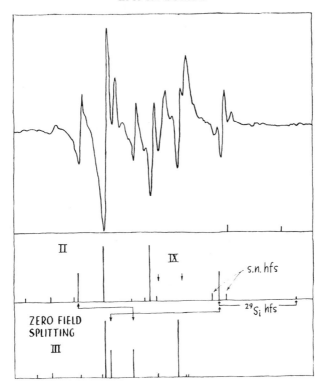

Fig. 7.2-24. Absorption spectrum for (II, III) centers in silicon irradiated with 1.8 × 10^18 NVT and annealed 30 min at 100°C. Principal lines belonging to set II or set III are so labeled along with hfs satellites due to the ^29Si nearest and next nearest neighbors: Crystalline axis [110]. Spectrometer type, RS1 K-band reflection superheterodyne with balanced mixer detector; cavity, rectangular TE_{102}; temperature, 300°K; modulation, 500 cps; sample size quarter wavelength slab; magnet, Varian 12 in. rotated through 90°. (Courtesy J-9.)

long relaxation times at low temperatures, these signals were observed in dispersion. Measurements of the absorption spectrum at room temperature gave a gaussian line shape with a width at half maximum of 4 G.

7.3 COLOR CENTERS, PRINCIPALLY IN ALKALI HALIDES

7.3.1 Interest in *F* Centers

Wood and Joy have expressed the interests in *F* centers nicely, "This defect is one of the simplest which can occur in ionic crystals, and in the physics and chemistry of lattice defects in these crystals it occupies a position of importance roughly comparable to that of the hydrogen atom in ordinary chemistry" (W-25). This interest extends back at least 50 years to the pioneering work of Pohl and his students and shows no signs of abating. The present F-center model, namely, an electron trapped in a negative ion vacancy, was proposed by deBoer in 1937. Subsequent investigations have amassed a tremendous quantity of evidence supporting this model and the interaction of the electron with its surroundings is well described. EPR and particularly ENDOR have contributed substantially to the understanding of the detailed interactions with neighboring ions. Hutchison was the first to report the detection of F centers by EPR techniques (A-9).

The main problems in observing the EPR of F centers are:

1. Generating a detectable quantity of F centers by themselves. Careful preparation and handling of samples are required to avoid the host of other possible centers.

2. In most of the alkali halides only a broad gaussian line is observed because the hfs is not resolved by EPR. LiF and NaF are exceptions. ENDOR techniques have been quite successful in resolving the hfs of most of the alkali halides.

3. Since the lines are broad, large concentrations of F centers are required for good signal-to-noise ratios.

7.3.2 Sample Preparation

Four general coloring techniques capable of producing adequate concentrations of F centers are chemical, electrical, radiation, and conversion. In the chemical process a stoichiometric excess of the alkali metal is diffused into the crystal, thereby generating negative ion vacancies which trap electrons to form F centers. Electrical refers to injecting electrons into heated crystals under the influence of a strong electric field. Radiation involves bombarding the sample with ionizing radiation to generate free electrons that can be trapped to form F centers. Finally conversion applies to the (U center + $h\nu \rightarrow F$ center) reaction where U centers (H-ions) are converted by illumination in the U absorption band.

The F centers are the same irrespective of their origin so a choice is usually based on the ease of preparation for a particular alkali halide and the risk of forming other centers. Table 7.3-1 summarizes the techniques selected for a variety of EPR investigations. The lithium and sodium salts are difficult to color by the chemical and electrical methods without generating clusters of defects; therefore, radiation has been used exclusively on these salts. The potassium salts color readily by all four techniques.

(a) **Chemical Method.** Figure 7.3-1 illustrates the chemical method for generating F and U centers. The literature abounds in rituals for this

Table 7.3-1. Production of F Centers for EPR Observation

Crystal	Coloring technique	Centers/cm^3	Measuring method	Sample size, mm	Ref.
LiF	50 kV x-rays, $\frac{1}{2}$–15 hr, 300°K	10^{17}–10^{18}	Optical		H-14
	Neutrons, flux = 10^{12} n/cm^2-sec, 1–24 hr				H-17
	360 MeV protons				J-3
	^{60}Co γ-rays, $\frac{1}{2}$–180 hr, 225,000 rep/hr	to 3.4 $\times$ 10^{18}	Optical	2 $\times$ 2 $\times$ 6	H-27
	180 kV x-rays	5 $\times$ 10^{16}– 15 $\times$ 10^{16}			S-3
LiCl	50 kV x-rays, 20 hr, 300°K	10^{18}	Optical		H-14
NaF	50 kV x-rays, 15 hr	10^{18}			H-14
	x-rays				L-11
KCl	Chemically, heat crystal 10 hr at 600°C, while K at 150–400°C, quench in paraffin oil	5 $\times$ 10^{16} to 10^{18}			H-14
	Neutrons, flux = 10^{12} n/cm^2 1–24 hr				
	40 kV x-rays, Cu target, 20 mA, 300°K	10^{16}–10^{17}	Optical	7 $\times$ 7 $\times$ 1	B-33
	γ-rays, 0.667 MeV, ^{137}Cs, several hours at 77 or 300°K	10^{16}		2 $\times$ 2 $\times$ 2	F-9
	Electrical, Alkadag electrodes, 500 V, 600°C, 1 mA in dry N$_2$				F-9
	Chemically, heat crystals 8 hr at 560°C	8 $\times$ 10^{16} to 10^{18}			O-6
	U $\rightarrow$ F conversion with x-rays, 150 kV, 12 mA, for 10 min	3 $\times$ 10^{17}	Optical	10 $\times$ 10 $\times$ 1	M-14
KBr	Chemically, quench in mineral oil	10^{18}	Optical		H-14
	Electrical	$\sim10^{19}$	Optical		T-3
	Radiation, 18 MeV electrons	10^{19}–10^{20}	Optical		T-3
	50 kV x-rays, 40 mA, up to 24 hr				D-8
NaCl	50 kV x-rays, 4–10 hr	10^{18}	Optical		H-14
	50 kV x-rays, 40 mA, up to 24 hr				D-8
NaBr	50 kV x-rays, 20 hr, 300°K	5 $\times$ 10^{17}	Optical		H-14
CsCl	Radiation, 2 MeV electrons, 3 $\times$ 10^6 to 6 $\times$ 10^8 R, 80 and 230°K				H-18
NaH	X-rays, 30 min				W-20
	50 kV, x-rays, 40 mA, to 24 hr				D-8
^{7}LiH	Neutrons, flux = 4 $\times$ 10^9 n/cm^2-sec, dose = 10^{12} n/cm^3 at 78°K	$>10^{17}$		2	L-9
^{6}LiH	Neutrons, flux = 4 $\times$ 10^9 n/cm^2-sec, dose = 10^{12} n/cm^3 at 78°K	10^{17}		2	L-9
^{7}LiD	Neutrons, flux = 4 $\times$ 10^9 n/cm^2-sec, dose = 10^{12} n/cm^3 at 78°K	10^{17}		1	L-9
^{6}LiD	Neutrons, flux = 4 $\times$ 10^9 n/cm^2-sec, dose = 10^{12} n/cm^3 at 78°K	10^{17}		1	L-9
MgO	Neutrons 1 to 3 $\times$ 10^{19} n/cm^2				A-14
	Heat in Mg vapors at 1500°C, quench and irradiate with x-rays				A-14

operation, running the gamut from samples sealed in Pyrex tubes which collapse during heating in a simple muffle furnace to elaborate arrangements to grow the crystals with the centers in place. The two temperature zone arrangement of Fig. 7.3-1 allows the crystals temperature to be maintained at 50–75°C below its melting point for a maximum diffusion rate while the color-center concentration is independently controlled by the alkali metal vapor pressure, i.e., the temperature (T_2) of the vapor generator. Since the heating cycle is controlled by the time for alkali metal atoms to diffuse to the center of the crystal, the sample thickness should be limited to roughly the finished size. A thin layer is usually split off each surface to remove contamination. Potassium bromide and potassium chloride samples with a $\frac{1}{2}$ in. minimum dimension were successfully colored at 50–75°C below their respective melting temperatures in about 3 hr. Simple stainless steel wire supports with negligible contact areas support the crystals away from the container surface and from each other for free access to the vapor and a minimum contamination of the surface. Rapid cooling of the samples is important if extraneous defects are to be avoided, particularly in NaCl. Quenching the entire chamber in motor oil is one satisfactory method; however, all the red hot metal should be submerged to avoid igniting the oil. When U centers are desired, the chamber is filled with hydrogen at a pressure of about 400–450 psi. The outlet tube permits the air to be purged from the chamber before the heating cycle and can be used to assist in cooling the crystals rapidly by circulating hydrogen during the quenching period. Quenching is not essential in the U-center process, particularly if the alkali metal vaporizer is cooled first so that the hydrogen

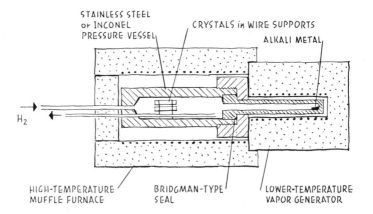

Fig. 7.3-1. Two-zone furnace and chamber for chemical method of generating F centers or U centers in alkali halide crystals.

has a few additional minutes to convert any remaining F centers to U centers. Then the chamber can be removed from the furnace and cooled in air while hydrogen continues to circulate around the crystals.

(b) Electrolytic Coloring. Figure 7.3-2 illustrates the essential features of the electron injection method. Here KCl is heated to a temperature of about 600°C where the ions can migrate to prevent space charge buildup when electrons are injected from the pointed platinum cathode. The voltage and temperature are adjusted until the crystal colors in a few minutes without electrical breakdown. Feldman et al. (F-9) used about 500 V and 1 mA, with Alkadag electrodes covering both ends of the crystal. Platinum or carbon electrodes are used to avoid contaminating the crystal with foreign metal ions, e.g., Cu, Au, or Ag anodes will inject the corresponding ions into the crystal where upon the electrons combine with the ions to form visible imperfections. Prolonged electrolysis can ultimately generate metal dendrites. A shell $\sim \frac{1}{2}$ mm thick next to the surface remains free of F centers; consequently, samples must be slightly larger than required for the EPR measurement. As in the chemical method, the crystal must be quenched to avoid forming other types of defects.

(c) Radiation Methods. According to Table 7.3-1, F centers have been generated by irradiation with neutrons, protons, electrons, γ-rays, and x-rays. Neutrons, γ-rays, and x-rays require long exposure times, frequently

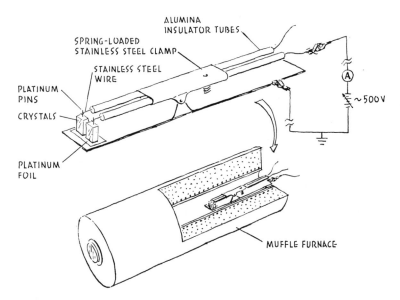

Fig. 7.3-2. Furnace and electrodes for electrolytic production of F centers.

hours, while the charged particles permit short exposures limited usually by the heating of the sample. The yield of F centers depends on the sample temperature, as shown in Fig. 7.3-3 where the highest efficiency occurs somewhat below room temperature. A disadvantage of the radiation method in general and coloring at low temperatures in particular is the variety of paramagnetic species generated in addition to the F centers. The crystals can be split to finished dimensions or even mounted in the cavity prior to irradiation. F centers are photosensitive and manipulations, particularly with irradiated crystals, are normally performed in the dark or in illumination outside the F band to avoid converting the F centers to other centers. Exposure arrangements can be very simple, particularly when coloring the less hygroscopic crystals at room temperature with x-rays and γ-rays. For example, if the source room can be darkened, the crystals can be exposed in air without benefit of a container. Figure 7.3-4a shows a simple hermetically sealed container suitable for use with soft x-rays or 1–2 MeV electrons when it is necessary to exclude light or provide a controlled atmosphere. A stream of gas can be used to cool the samples under electron bombardment. In most experiments dosimetry is not a problem because the number of F centers is determined subsequently by optical or chemical measurements. The current collected in the pill box is

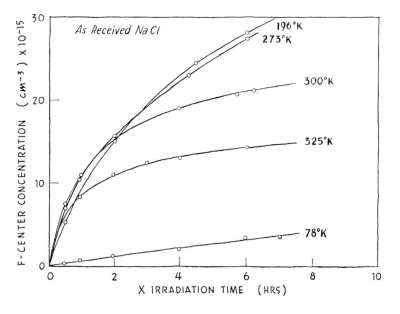

Fig. 7.3-3. Dependence of F-center growth rate on crystal temperature for production by x-ray irradiation. (Courtesy B-3.)

adequate for monitoring relative doses with electrons. Arrangements b and c are for coloring crystals at low temperatures with either electrons or x-rays. In arrangement c the float maintains the crystal just below the surface of the cooling liquid and the removable dewar top excludes light and room air. In arrangement d the crystal is irradiated in the cavity by electrons coming through the 0.002 in. thick window. A demountable cup containing the coolant surrounds the cavity and a stream of dry helium or nitrogen prevents moisture from condensing inside the cavity. After irradiation the cavity can be inverted and immersed in a conventional dewar for the EPR measurements.

7.3.3   Pertinent Properties of Color Centers

The F centers in alkali halide crystals have several well-established properties of pertinence to an EPR experiment. First, the position of the F band depends on the interatomic distance. Theoretically, Frohlich determined the peak of the F-band absorption as

$$\lambda_F = cd^2 16m/h \qquad (7.3\text{-}1)$$

and Ivey fitted empirical equations of the same type to measured bands and obtained

$$\lambda_F = 703d^{1.84} \qquad (7.3\text{-}2)$$

where d = interionic distance in centimeters, h = Planck's constant, m = electron mass, and c = the velocity of light.

These bell-shaped absorption bands appear in the visible and UV regions of the spectrum, as shown in Fig. 7.3-5 for some of the common alkali halides. About 10^{16} color centers are visible and can be detected by EPR. If the sample thickness is limited to about 1 mm, the concentration required is about $10^{17}/cm^3$. In most past experiments the number of F centers have been determined from optical measurements, but at the concentrations required for EPR experiments the optical density frequently is too high for measurements at the peak of the absorption curves. Smakula first used the classical dispersion equation to determine the color-center concentration as a function of the optical absorption data (S-13). When the half-band-width is small compared with the resonant frequency as in the case of color centers, the equation simplifies to (S-7)

$$N_0 f = 1.31 \times 10^{17}[\eta_0/(\eta_0^2 + 2)^2]KW \qquad (7.3\text{-}3)$$

where N_0 = F centers/cm^3; f = oscillator strength of the absorbing centers; η_0 = refractive index at absorption peak; K = maximum absorption coefficient in reciprocal centimeters; and W = half-width of the band in electron volts.

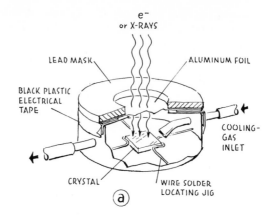

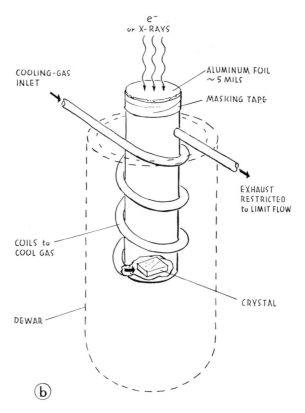

Fig. 7.3-4. Arrangements for producing F centers by ionizing irradiation. (*a*) Light-tight pillbox for irradiations near room temperature; (*b*) light-tight canister for irradiations down to 77°K.

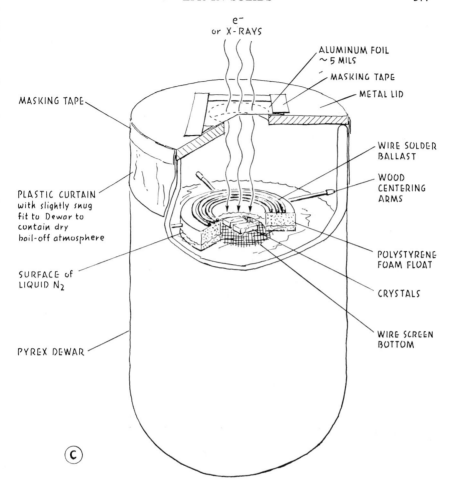

e^-
or X-RAYS

ALUMINUM FOIL
~ 5 MILS

MASKING TAPE

METAL LID

MASKING TAPE

WIRE SOLDER
BALLAST

WOOD
CENTERING
ARMS

PLASTIC CURTAIN
with slightly snug
fit to Dewar to
contain dry
boil-off atmosphere

SURFACE of
LIQUID N$_2$

POLYSTYRENE
FOAM FLOAT

CRYSTALS

PYREX DEWAR

WIRE SCREEN
BOTTOM

(c)

Fig. 7.3-4. (c) Simple float method for irradiations in liquid nitrogen.

When crystals are too dark for a direct measurement, K can be determined by proportionality from density measurements on the tails of the resonance peak. In many cases a classical oscillator strength of unity is assumed for f. However, f has been determined for a few of the alkali halides by chemical measurements of the stoichiometric excess of the alkali metal in additively colored crystals. Obviously quantitative EPR measurements provide another method of determining f if the number of spins can be measured by comparison to a suitable yardstick.

The F center electrons can be excited either optically by illumination in

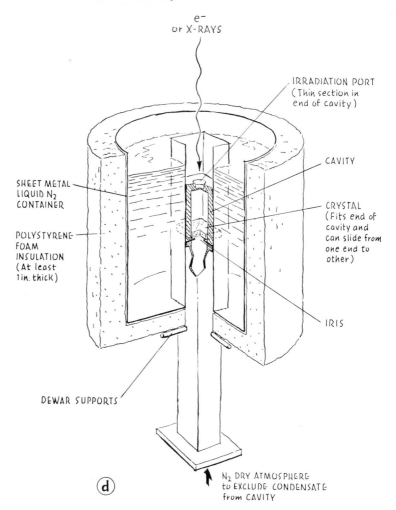

Fig. 7.3-4. (*d*) Irradiation in cavity at temperatures down to 77°K. Forced cooling is not required with x-ray irradiations or electron beams of 10 W energy or less but a positive dry gas pressure keeps moisture from condensing on the crystals. Circulating gas in (*a*) and (*b*) permits use of 50 W beams of 2 MeV electrons without undue heating.

the *F* band or thermally by heating up to about 400°C, depending on the material. Although we previously stated that all *F* centers are alike for physical and EPR spectral purposes, the results of bleaching do depend on the method of coloring. In chemically and electrolytically colored crystals *F* centers can be transformed into other centers but the number of excess electrons must be preserved so the total number of centers remains constant.

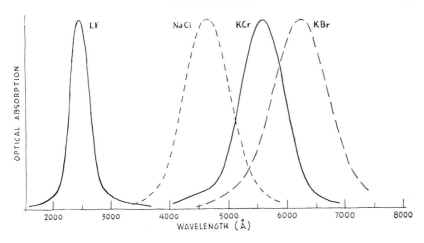

Fig. 7.3-5. F bands in LiF, NaCl, KCl, and KBr.

With irradiated crystals the F center electrons readily combine with holes to re-form the original lattice so these crystals can be bleached by optical or thermal excitation. In all cases some excitation will generate other centers which may confuse the EPR spectrum and its interpretation; therefore, a number of the references in Table 7.3-1 mention that as a precaution the crystals were handled in subdued light, frequently filtered to avoid the F band.

7.3.4 EPR Equipment and Techniques

Most of the color-center data have been obtained with "homemade" spectrometers, reflecting perhaps the early date of the work, a common academic atmosphere, or a rugged individualist; however, present commercial spectrometers are quite adequate for color-center studies. The common frequency is the X band and the availability of large samples with high F-center concentrations usually eliminates the need for higher frequencies. A considerable variety of both homodyne and superheterodyne spectrometers participated in gathering the data of Table 7.3-2. Early measurements of the g factor, ΔH, and the line shape were largely obtained with homodyne systems operating at modulation frequencies of 400 c or less. Since ΔH ranges from about 45 to 200 G for the unresolved F bands and the resolvable hf lines are several gauss wide, high-frequency modulation line broadening is no problem. The superheterodyne systems have been used, particularly in relaxation time measurements, studies of rf saturation, and in ENDOR measurements of the hf structure.

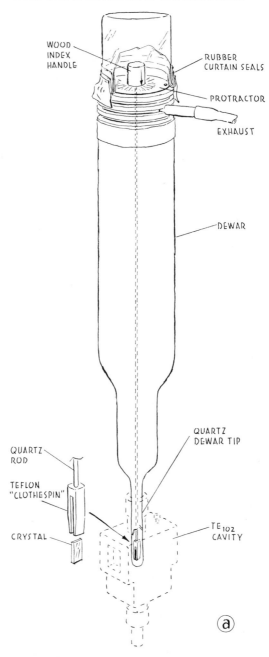

Fig. 7.3-6. Four cavity and sample arrangements used in EPR measurements on alkali halide crystals. [(*b*) After N-2; (*c*) courtesy H-14; (*d*) after 36.]

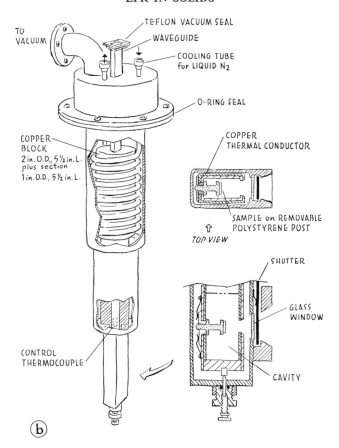

Fig. 7.3-6b.

Cavities and sample mounting procedures are generally straight-forward, and are complicated only by requirements to avoid F band illumination when installing the crystals for measurements at low temperatures. Rectangular cavities are used most often in the work reported to date. Both reflection and transmission systems appear, although reflection cavities are generally used at low temperatures. Figure 7.3-6 shows four cavity and sample arrangements used in measuring the F-center data included in this section. Arrangement a is a commercial TE_{102} rectangular cavity with an internal dewar. The crystal is supported and oriented with respect to the magnetic field by a Teflon "clothespin" on a quartz handle. Orientation is indicated by the pointer and dial on top of the dewar. Rubber gaskets and the glass lid prevent contamination of the liquid

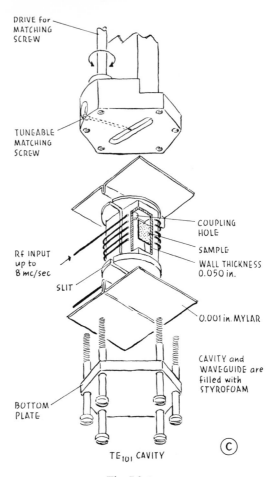

DRIVE for MATCHING SCREW

TUNEABLE MATCHING SCREW

RF INPUT up to 8 mc/sec

SLIT

BOTTOM PLATE

COUPLING HOLE

SAMPLE

WALL THICKNESS 0.050 in.

0.001 in. MYLAR

CAVITY and WAVEGUIDE are filled with STYROFOAM

TE_{101} CAVITY

(c)

Fig. 7.3-6c.

nitrogen by moisture from the room air. Black velvet cloths draped over the dewar reduce the light reaching the sample so that no F center bleaching was observed. Again the chief advantage of the internal dewar system is the ease of changing samples. Cavity b provides variable temperatures over the range from about 90 to 200°K with control to better than 0.1°. The sample supported on polystyrene post was cooled by conduction through a copper block of considerable thermal inertia whose temperature is controlled by the rate of nitrogen flow through the cooling coils. One of the most exhaustive F-center studies in terms of types of measurements and varieties of alkali halide crystals involved cavity c, which is suitable for both EPR and ENDOR experiments. Polystyrene foam holds the sample midway on

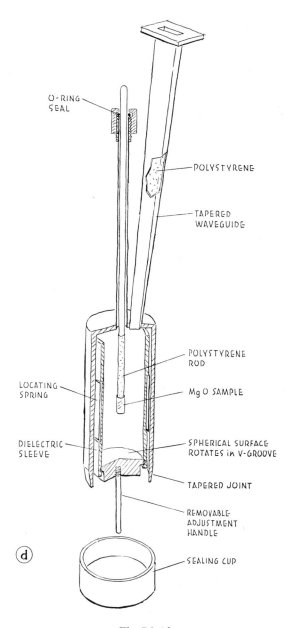

O-RING SEAL

POLYSTYRENE

TAPERED WAVEGUIDE

POLYSTYRENE ROD

LOCATING SPRING

Mg O SAMPLE

DIELECTRIC SLEEVE

SPHERICAL SURFACE ROTATES in V-GROOVE

TAPERED JOINT

REMOVABLE ADJUSTMENT HANDLE

(d)

SEALING CUP

Fig. 7.3-6d.

Table 7.3-2

Examples of Spectrometers and Parameters Involved in Studying EPR in Alkali Halides

Spectrometer type	Cavity and mode	Rf power	Measured parameters	Remarks	Ref.
RH1-X	Rectangular TE_{102}	40–50 mW	ΔH		B-33
RS1-X	TE_{102}		ENDOR vs. angle with H	ENDOR coil in cavity	D-8
RS-X	TE_{102}		$1/\tau$ vs. temp	Pulsed to 12 W for rapid passage	F-9
RH1-X	Rectangular TE_{101}		hfs		H-14
RH-X	TE_{101}	0.4 mW	hfs, g, ΔH		H-18
TS1-K	Rectangular TE_{101}	~0.1 G	T_1, g, line shape	23 and 400 c modulation	H-30
RH-X	Rectangular TE_{101}		g, ΔH	400 c modulation	J-3
R-X			g, hfs	8 c modulation	K-1
RH-X	Rectangular TE_{102}		g, ΔH	6 kc modulation	K-9
RS1-X	TE_{101}	0.01 G	T_1	500 c modulation	O-2
RH-X	TE_{102}		g, ΔH, saturation	6 kc modulation	P-14
RS-X	TE_{101}		g		W-20

the narrow side wall of the TE_{101} mode cavity and excludes liquid helium from the major volume of the cavity and the waveguide. The two halves of the cavity are electrically insulated from each other and from the waveguide by 0.001 in. Mylar films in order to establish the megacycle field at the sample. This field is generated by the surface currents on the interior cavity walls and this design is effective up to about 80 Mc/sec. The rf coil of from 4 to 8 turns is spaced about 10 mils away from the cavity walls. Cavity d was used with F centers in MgO, but is suitable for other materials. Here the feature of primary interest is the tilting bottom which is adjusted to maximize the cavity Q as one step in the tuning operation (36). After adjustment the tuning handle is removed to make room for the sealing cup. This adjustment corrects for any distortion in the rf field resulting from the sample and supports, which destroy the electrical parallelism of the cavity ends. Polystyrene in the waveguide permits the cross section to be reduced for convenience in attaching the dewar. In this case, the MgO samples were ground to a cylindrical geometry and cemented to the polystyrene support with Duco Cement. Since all the crystals introduced similar losses, it was not necessary to provide a variable coupler.

7.3.5   Typical EPR Data for F Centers in Alkali Halides

Figure 7.3-7 shows unaltered traces of F centers in four of the common alkali halides produced and measured under the same conditions, i.e., the F centers were produced by electron bombardment with the crystal at 300°K and the EPR spectra were obtained with the cavity arrangement Fig. 7.3-6a. In agreement with the literature cited in Table 7.3-2, partial resolution of the hf structure is observed in LiF; however, NaCl, KCl, and KBr exhibit only a single broad gaussian-shaped peak. Table 7.3-3 summarizes F center data for a number of the alkali halides and in all cases the g values are slightly less than that of a free electron. The variation from material to material is small ranging from 1.971 for KI to 2.002 or 2.008 for LiF. As previously indicated, the absorption bands are broad ranging from 45 G for KCl to about 200 G for KI.

Holton and Blum (H-14) measured the hf structure in LiF as a function of crystal orientation in the magnetic field and obtained the spectra in Fig. 7.3-8. In most orientations the splitting between lines is about 12–14 G.

Kip et al. (K-9) report the line shape and width are properties of the particular material and do not vary with the F-center concentration, method of generating the F center, or the temperature of the EPR measurement. Of course, the method of preparation can influence the spectra if other paramagnetic species are generated in the process. For example, the ΔH of 110 G reported in Table 7.3-3 for F centers generated by proton bombardment is almost twice the other values listed (J-3). Similarly, ΔH for KCl dropped from 45 to 34 G when centers such as the R and N centers were removed by thermal treatment (B-33).

When F centers are generated by irradiation or excited by illumination, the sample temperature is an important factor in controlling the sites where the electrons will be trapped. For example, the samples used to obtain Figs. 7.3-7 and 7.3-9 were split from adjacent positions in single crystals of the various materials and irradiated in the same manner except for the temperatures, which were 300 and 77°K, respectively. In Fig. 7.3-9 the typical F bands are lost in a welter of hf lines extending over an energy range much wider than the F band, thereby indicating unpaired electrons in a variety of environments. Since these spectra were obtained only for the purpose of illustrating the importance of sample temperature, no particular effort was expended in finding or resolving all the hf lines. The number of visible lines are 124 for KBr, 61 for KCl, 29 for NaCl, 4 for LiF and 81 for CaF_2. Apparently the responsible electrons are either in shallow traps or subject to interactions with electron deficiency centers because warming of the samples to 300°K is accompanied by extensive thermoluminescence, a visible change in color in some cases, and a substantial reduction in the

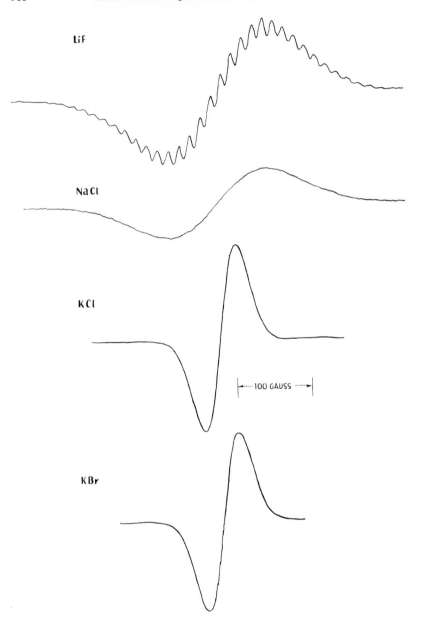

Fig. 7.3-7. EPR spectra of F centers in various alkali halide single crystals at room temperature. The hfs is resolved only in LiF. Spectrometer type RH4-X; H parallel to the [100] crystal axis; the F centers are produced by bombarding Harshaw crystals with 2 MeV electrons from a Van de Graaff generator.

Table 7.3-3 EPR Characteristics of Color Centers

Crystal	Color centers per cm^3	Temp, °K	g value	ΔH, G	T_1,[a] sec	Number of resolved hf lines	Hf splitting, G	Ref.
LiF		294	1.999 ±0.001	65				J-3
LiF[b]		296	2.002 ±0.001	110				J-3
LiF[b]		1.3	2.0005 ±0.0006					H-14
LiF[b]			2.008 ±0.001	77– 160				A-9
LiF[b]			1.999	65				P-14
LiF[b]	~3.4 ×10^{18}	300			1.5 ×10^{-4}	19	32	H-27
LiF[b]	~3.4 ×10^{18}	4			2.6 ×10^{-3}			H-27
LiCl	~10^{18}	1.3	1.9980 ±0.0008	57.2	9.2			H-14
NaF			2.0021 ±0.0001					A-9
NaF		1.3	2.0011 ±0.0008	220		19	37.7	H-14
NaCl		77	1.987	162				P-14
NaCl	~10^{18}	1.3		142	<3			H-14
NaBr	>5 × 10^{17}	1.3	1.994 ±0.005		43			H-14
KCl	5 × 10^{16}	1.3	1.9955 ±0.0014	49.5	216			H-14
KCl	2 × 10^{17}	1.3	1.9955 ±0.0014	49.5	72			H-14
KCl	10^{18}	1.3	1.9955 ±0.0014	49.5	<3			H-14
KCl			1.997 ±0.001	49.3				N-2
KCl			1.996 ±0.001	45				M-14
KCl	8 × 10^{16}	2			~450			O-6
KBr	>10^{18}	1.3	1.986 ±0.01		<1			H-14
KBr			1.98	152				H-27
KBr			1.986 ±0.001					N-2
KBr		77	1.980	146				P-14
KI			1.971 ±0.001	200				A-9
^{6}LiH		78	2.004 ±0.001	14.3				L-9
^{7}LiH		78		30.6				L-9
^{7}LiD		78		28.5				L-9
^{6}LiD				10.1				L-9

[a] Relaxation time by rapid passage inversion–recovery methods.

[b] Produced by proton bombardment.

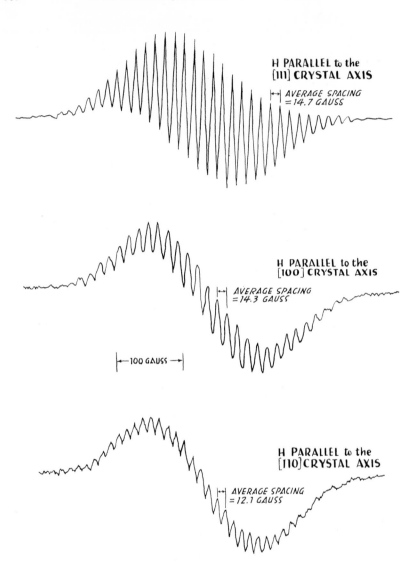

Fig. 7.3-8. Effect of crystal orientation in the magnetic field on the hfs of F centers in lithium fluoride: spectrometer type, RS7-X with additional microwave loops to control the primary and local klystron oscillators; cavity, rectangular TE_{101}; intermediate frequency, 35 Mc/sec; temperature 1.3°K. The F centers are produced at room temperature by exposure to 50 kV x-rays for times from $\frac{1}{2}$ to 15 hr, i.e., 10^{17}–10^{18} F centers/cm³. (Courtesy H-14.)

number of hf lines. Careful thermal annealing should permit some unfolding of the spectra in these materials.

Since the hyperfine field interaction determines the linewidth observed for F centers, the broadening is of the inhomogeneous type and, at least in KCl, the absorption line does not change shape on saturation. In fact, Portis (P-14) developed his general theory of saturation while working on KCl. Figure 7.3-10 shows normalized peak absorption and dispersion signals plotted as a function of the microwave power level. The absorption expression reaches a constant value while the dispersion shows no sign of saturation. For this reason many of the studies on relaxation time and line shape have been performed on dispersion curves where the larger signals were available.

F centers have been popular candidates for spin relaxation measurements because they have been extensively studied by optical techniques and their structure is rather well understood in comparison to other paramagnetic centers (F-9). Table 7.3-4 summarizes enough of the relaxation measurements to indicate the range of methods, variables, and results but makes no pretense at being a complete list of the available work.

Direct methods predominate the more recent work with the inversion-recovery technique in top billing, i.e., inversion by rapid passage. The

Table 7.3-4

Examples of Relaxation Time Measurements on Alkali Halide Crystals

Salt	Measuring technique	Spectrometer type	F-center concentration per cm^3	Temp, °K	T_1, sec	H_0, G	Ref.
LiF	Rapid passage	TS1-K	$\sim 3.4 \times 10^{18}$	300	1.5×10^{-4}	$\sim 10^4$	H-30
LiF	Rapid passage	TS1-K		4	2.6×10^{-3}	$\sim 10^4$	H-30
LiCl	Rapid passage	Similar to RH1-X	$\sim 10^{18}$	1.3	9.2	3500	H-14
NaCl	Rapid passage	Similar to RH1-X	$\sim 10^{18}$	1.3	< 3	3500	H-14
NaBr	Rapid passage	Similar to RH1-X	$> 5 \times 10^{17}$	1.3	43	3500	H-14
KCl	Rapid passage	Similar to RH1-X	5×10^{16}	1.3	216	3500	H-14
KCl	Rapid passage	Similar to RH1-X	2×10^{17}	1.3	72	3500	H-14
KCl	Rapid passage	Similar to RH1-X	10^{18}	1.3	< 3	3500	H-14
KCl	Saturation–recovery	RS1-X	8×10^{16}	2	450	3500	O-2
KBr	Rapid passage	Similar to RH1-X	$> 10^{18}$	1.3	< 1	3500	H-14

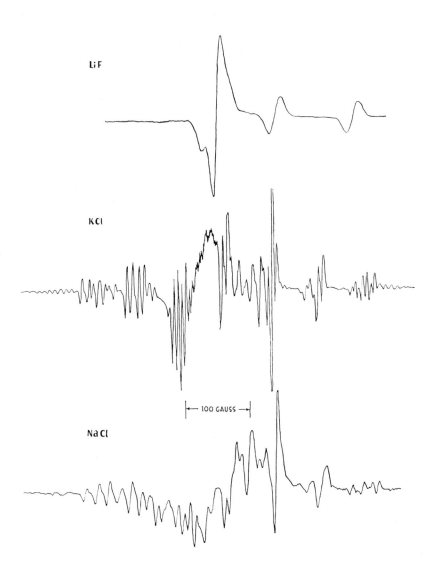

Fig. 7.3-9. EPR spectra for various alkali halide crystals bombarded with 2 MeV electrons. The temperature was maintained at 77°K throughout: H parallel to the [100] crystal axis; Spectrometer type, RH4-X.

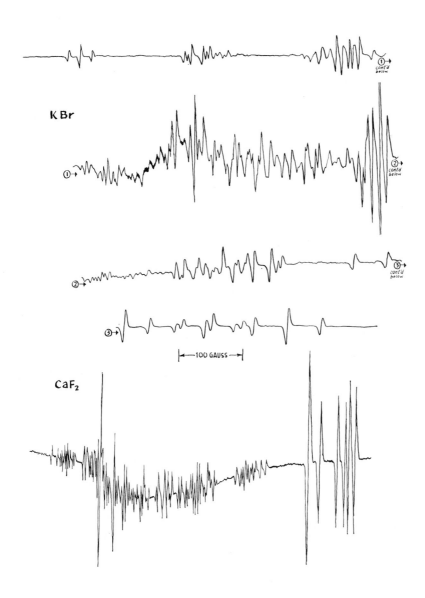

K Br

CaF₂

|← 100 GAUSS →|

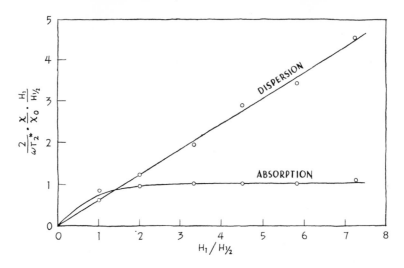

Fig. 7.3-10. Saturation behavior of F centers in KCl; $H_{1/2}$ = value of the micro-wave magnetic field where the saturation parameter $S(\omega_0 H_1) = 1/(1 + \frac{1}{4}\gamma^2 H_1{}^2 T_1 T_2)$ $= \frac{1}{2}$. In the absence of saturation x/x_0 is constant so that the curve is a straight line as for dispersion. In the constant part of the absorption curve the decrease in x/x_0 counteracts the increase $H_1/H_{1/2}$. Spectrometer, type RH1 X-band reflection homodyne with pound stabilizer, magic T, and crystal detection; cavity, rectangular TE_{102}; temperature, room temperature; rf power level, 250 mW max; modulation, fre-quency = 6 kc/sec, modulate rf power 100% with gyrator band pass, about 0.1 cps. (Courtesy P-14.)

parameters or factors influencing the recovery time fall into two categories: (*1*) extrinsic, involving defects in the host crystal which generally tend to shorten the time and (*2*) intrinsic, indicative properties of an F center in an ideal lattice (F-9).

Extrinsic factors:

1. Purity of the host crystal.

2. F-center concentration.

3. Past history of color centers, e.g., exposure to light.

Intrinsic behavior:

1. Temperature dependence.

2. Dependence on magnetic field strength.

τ is frequently used for the spin–relaxation time constant where both extrinsic and intrinsic factors influence the recovery rate. When the relaxa-tion is believed to be intrinsic, $\tau = T_1$. For example, in Ref. F-9 τ was "judged to be intrinsic when it is the longest time measured at a given T and H_R, and when it can be consistently observed with crystals having the 'best' sample preparation." T is the temperature and H_R the magnetic field intensity under which the spins were allowed to relax.

Most authors comment that their samples exhibited exponential recoveries as a function of time after inversion. Figure 2-26 illustrates the intrinsic curve behavior for the specimen containing about 8×10^{16} F centers per cubic centimeter. The curve for the sample containing 3×10^{18} F centers per cubic centimeter has a slight curvature, presumably indicating some extrinsic influence from the high color-center density.

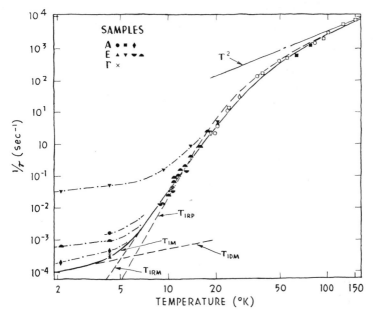

Fig. 7.3-11. Temperature dependence of $1/\tau$ at 3.2 kOe. The experimental points and labels on the curves have the following meaning: A = additively colored (chemical process); E = electrolytic coloring; Γ = irradiated by γ-ray; T_{ID} = relaxation by a direct process; T_{IRP} = Raman relaxation involving the crystal field and phonon mixing of states; T_{IRM} = Raman relaxation involving the magnetic hyperfine field; T_{IM} = Relaxation involving T_{IRM} and T_{ID}.

Solid points = data for crystal in cryogenic medium and uncertainty in temperature is less than the symbols size. Hollow points = data taken while sample temperature is drifting up or down and the absolute error is greater but the relative uncertainty is indicated by the symbol size (courtesy F-9).

Spectrometer, X-band superheterodyne with microwave power for rapid passage inversion provided by an auxiliary X-13 klystron; cavity, rectangular reflection TE_{102} silvered epoxy resin (Hysol 6000), $Q \sim 4000$ at $300°K$ and ~ 6000 at $4.2°K$; temperature, $2–150°K$; rf power level, monitoring klystron 10^{-8} W, inversion klystron up to 12 W; sweep field, external Helmholtz coils in liquid He allow sweep up to 120 G in less than 20 μsec.

Optical bleaching in the F band in both x-rayed and additively colored KCl has accelerated the relaxation process in crystals containing 10^{17}–10^{18} F centers per cubic centimeter (O-6). Thermal bleaching of M, R, and N bands restores the relaxation to its preoptical bleaching value, again suggesting extrinsic factors (O-6).

Figures 7.3-11 and 7.3-12 show the intrinsic behavior of KCl where the reciprocal of the relaxation time is plotted as a function of temperature and external magnetic field, respectively. The strong temperature dependence above about 5°K causes τ to vary over about 7 decades, i.e., 2000 to 10^{-4} sec in a 150°K interval. Feldman et al. (F-9) discuss the curve in terms of three temperature regions: "$T \geq 50°K$, where τ is approximately proportional to T^{-2}; $T \leq 5°K$, where $\tau \propto T^{-1}$; and $5°K < T < 50°K$," where the variation is much faster. Raman multiphonon processes control the relaxation in the two higher-temperature regions while direct (one-phonon) interactions dominate at the lowest temperatures.

The long recovery times associated with the low temperatures make it

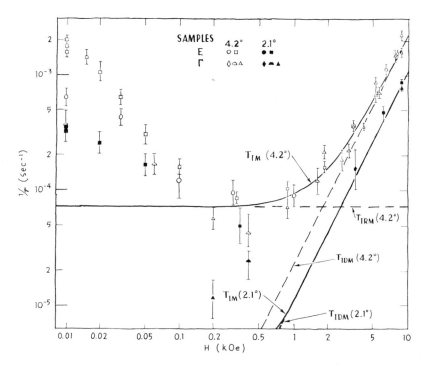

Fig. 7.3-12. Field dependence of $1/\tau$ at 4.2 and 2.1°K. The nomenclature follows the definition under Fig. 7.3-11 except for the open and solid points, which here designate temperature. (Courtesy F-9.)

possible to measure the magnetic field strength dependence of τ because there is sufficient time to adjust the field to the desired level for most of the recovery. Periodically the field is returned briefly to H_0 in order to monitor the extent of recovery. Figure 7.3-12 shows data obtained by this method at temperatures of 2.1 and 4.2°K. The substantial scatter between samples at low fields indicates an extrinsic behavior for recovery in this region.

7.3.6   *F* Centers in MgO

In some respects the oxides and sulfides of face centered cubic structure offer a simpler system for the EPR study of *F* centers than the traditional alkali halide systems. For example, MgO has the same structure as NaCl but a simple hfs is anticipated because the host crystal ions have essentially no magnetic moment. In the alkali halides ENDOR techniques were required to resolve many of the inhomogeneously broadened lines and the observed spectra indicated interactions with several successive shells of paramagnetic alkali and halide ions (W-12). The only isotopes with non-zero spin in MgO are the 10.11% abundant ^{25}Mg and a negligible fraction of ^{17}O; therefore, 53% of all magnesium ion octahedra should contain only ^{24}Mg and ^{26}Mg nuclei surrounding the *F*-center electron and the corresponding EPR spectrum should be a single narrow line (W-12). About 36 and 10%, respectively, of the *F* centers will encounter one and two ^{25}Mg nuclei ($I = \frac{5}{2}$) leading respectively to a 6- and 11-line hfs centered on the strong single component.

Experimentally the main problems involve sample preparation. First, impurity ions appear to be prevalent in the available MgO crystals and these ions undoubtedly effect the electronic properties of the crystals. Wertz et al. comment that "In the best specimen we have observed thus far, iron was present to the extent of 3 parts per million" (W-20). Second, the usual MgO crystal contains relatively few negative ion vacancies (less than $10^{13}/cm^3$) which can trap electrons to form *F* centers. Furthermore, the strong binding energy of MgO prevents the formation of such vacancies by methods effective with the alkali halides. Apparently positive ion vacancies, which can trap holes to generate competing EPR spectra, exist in appreciable numbers (up to $10^{17}/cm^3$). This is the reverse of the situation encountered in the alkali halides where *F*-center production predominates.

Two successful methods for producing detectable concentrations of *F* centers are (*1*) neutron irradiation and (*2*) grind-and-irradiate techniques. The first successful spectra were obtained with single crystals exposed to neutron irradiation in a nuclear reactor, e.g., exposures of 10^{19} to 3×10^{19} neutrons per square centimeter (W-12). Apparently this rather rugged treatment can generate the necessary negative ion vacancies. In the grind-and-irradiate ritual, extended grinding of high-purity MgO gives appreciable concentrations of F centers (W-20). After grinding, this concentration can be further enhanced by irradiation with x-rays, but x-rays alone are not effective. Apparently negative ion vacancies are left behind in the grinding process. Reference W-13 describes methods of preparing powdered samples of the other oxides, sulfides, and selenides used in companion measurements to MgO. The technique of successive annealing at progressively higher temperatures has been useful in unraveling spectra from the various centers, particularly in the more extensively studied MgO. Partially due to impurities and partially because of the early stage of the effort, the optical properties of the various centers remain to be established (W-13).

EPR spectrometer considerations are essentially the same as those for the alkali halides. Wertz and his associates have used an X-band reflection homodyne spectrometer (type RH3) extensively in measurements of MgO at room temperature and 77°K. The cylindrical TE_{011} cavity of Fig. 7.3-6d is typical of the cavities used with MgO.

Values of the spectroscopic splitting factor for MgO and other oxides, sulfides, and selenides are listed in Table 7.3-5 for F centers and F_2 centers. A tentative model for the F_2 center is an electron trapped at a negative-ion vacancy associated with a positive-ion vacancy. In single crystal MgO with

Table 7.3-5

g Values for F Centers and F_2 Centers in Powders
(W-13)

Powder	g (F center)	g (F_2 center)
MgO	2.0023	2.0008
CaO	2.0001	1.9995
SrO	1.9846	1.981_6[a]
BaO	1.936	
MgS	2.0062	2.0038
CaS	2.0033	
SrS	2.0036	2.0023
BaS	1.9641	
MgSe	2.0035	1.9981
CaSe	2.0030	
SrSe	2.003_2[a]	1.989_6[a]
BaSe	1.9670	

[a] Uncertainty in fourth decimal place indicated by displaced number.

H_0 perpendicular to the [100] crystal axis, g also equals 2.0023 $\pm$ 0.0001, i.e., the free electron g value. The other oxides listed have g values smaller than those for the free electron in contrast to most of the sulfides and selenides with their larger values.

Figure 7.3-13 shows an EPR spectrum for F centers in MgO with the hyperfine contributions from the various combinations of neighboring ^{25}Mg nuclei indicated below the curve. With H_0 perpendicular to a [100] axis, rotation of the crystal about this axis gives one set of six lines which

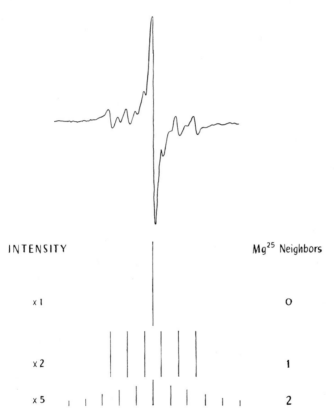

Fig. 7.3-13. Derivative spectrum for F centers in MgO when H_0 is along a [111] axis. The central component results from trapped electrons surrounded only by ^{24}Mg and ^{26}Mg ions while the sextet and eleven-line set correspond to interactions with one and two ^{25}Mg neighbors, respectively, as indicated by the lines below the spectrum (courtesy W-12).

Spectrometer, X-band reflection homodyne; cavity, rectangular; temperature, room; rf power levels, about 0.3 MW; modulation, 340 cps, external coils; magnet, 6 in. Varian; number of centers, about 1.2 $\times$ 10^{19} F centers/cm^3.

is stationary and two sets which vary in position. The extreme separations between the outermost of the six lines varied from 17.6 to 24.7 G. All three sextets coincide when H_0 is parallel to the [111] axis, as in Fig. 7.3-13. The linewidth between points of maximum slope varied from 0.7 to 0.9 G, depending on the crystal. All of the lines in Fig. 7.3-13 are easily saturated at room temperature in the purest crystal.

7.3.7   *U* Centers and Products of Photodecomposed *U* Centers

The *U* center is another of the elite centers with a fairly well documented pedigree established through numerous optical absorption measurements and chemical techniques. Assuming that the previously mentioned model is correct and the *U* center is a negative hydrogen ion trapped at a halogen ion vacancy, the $U \rightarrow F$-center transition should be written as *U* center + $h\nu \rightarrow F$ center + H where both the *F*-center and the H atom have unpaired electrons and should be susceptible to EPR techniques. Traditionally the homeless H atom has been relegated to an interstitial position in the crystalline lattice; therefore, the early EPR studies on *U*-center decomposition products focused largely on the state of the H atoms (D-5).

Sample preparation in KCl and KBr is relatively easy; however, little information is available on the other alkali halides. The chemical production of *U* centers was described in Section 7.3.2a. Here we will discuss only the photodisintegration step. When the *U* centers are converted in KCl or KBr at room temperature, the resulting EPR spectrum indicates only the presence of *F* centers, but when the conversion is performed at liquid nitrogen temperatures both H atoms and *F* centers appear in the spectra shown in Fig. 7.3-14. Apparently at the higher temperature the H atoms have sufficient mobility to move through the lattice until spins are paired up by forming hydrogen molecules. At 80°K the reduced mobility permits stabilization of the atoms for a detectable time.

Spectrometer requirements are essentially the same as those for *F* centers; however, in Ref. D-5 the dual-phase selective modulation technique was used to advantage in unraveling the hfs. Figures 7.3-14 and 7.3-15 show the preferential supression of the spectrum from the two species made possible by the marked difference in relaxation time.

While *g* values were not measured, the doublet in Fig. 7.3-14 is nearly centered on the *F* band resonance so the spectroscopic splitting factor is close to the free electron value. Any departure appears to be toward a smaller *g* value than for the *F* center.

Spectra were obtained for both KCl + KH and KCl + KD crystals irradiated according to the schedule indicated under Fig. 7.3-14. The doublet for hydrogen had a splitting of 500 ± 10 G and a linewidth of 68 ± 5 G. Deuterium had a splitting of 156 G between outer components

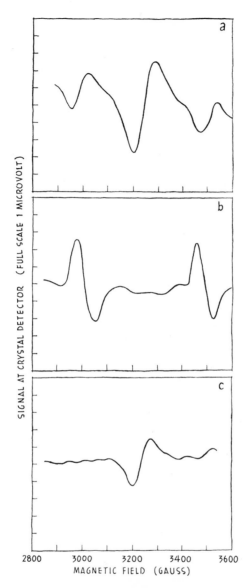

Fig. 7.3-14. *F* centers and hydrogen atom spectra in a KCl crystal containing *U* centers (KCl + KH) after 3 hr of exposure to an unfiltered AH-4 lamp followed by 8 min with the lamp filtered with a Corning 9863 filter, all with the crystal at 80°K. Phase discrimination permits some unfolding of the spectrum. (*a*) The composite spectra; (*b*) *F* center resonance suppressed; (*c*) hydrogen atom resonance suppressed.

Spectrometer, *X*-band, reflection, homodyne with AFC locked to the sample cavity, magic T bridge, and a dual modulation system; cavity, rectangular TE_{102}; temperature, 80°K; modulation, 2 kc/sec with coils on cavity, 25 cps with coils on magnet poles having a maximum sweep of 125 G; sample, about 3 × 3 × 12 mm; color center concentration, about 2×10^{18} *U* centers. (Courtesy D-5.)

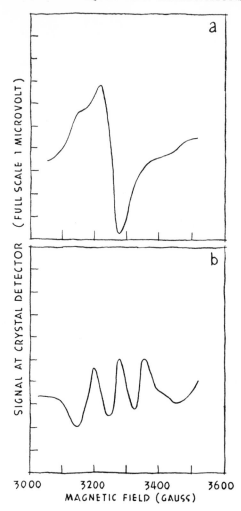

Fig. 7.3-15. *F*-center and deuterium atom spectra in KCl + KD crystal after the illumination recorded under Fig. 7.3-14: (*a*) has the deuterium resonance suppressed and (*b*) has the *F*-center resonance suppressed (spectrometer, see Fig. 7.3-14). (Courtesy D-5.)

of the triplet. These values are in good agreement with the splittings usually given for these atoms, i.e., 506 and 156 G, respectively.

Another property of considerable importance in performing successful measurements is the thermal stability of the hydrogen atoms. Figure 7.3-16 shows the results of a pulse annealing study in which the samples were annealed for 2 min at the indicated temperature then returned to 80°K

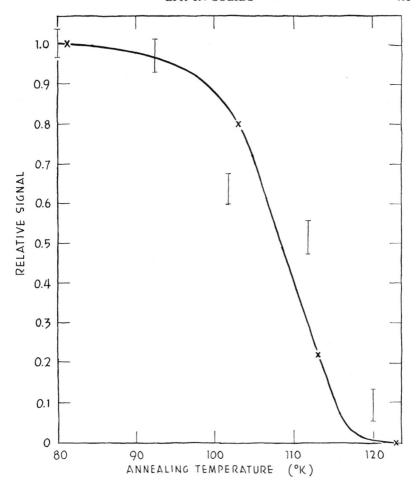

Fig. 7.3-16. Stability of hydrogen atoms as measured by the pulse annealing technique. The fraction of hydrogen atoms remaining after 2 min at the annealing temperature was measured by hydrogen atom resonance and by optical absorption of the U_2 band, all at 80°K (spectrometer, see Fig. 7.3-14). (Courtesy D-5.)

for the EPR or optical measurement. The hydrogen atom EPR signal disappears very rapidly above 100°K and similar results were also obtained with KCl and KD. No hydrogen atoms were found for annealing temperatures above 120°K in these potassium halides.

7.3.8   V Centers

Some of the numerous lines observed in Fig. 7.3-9 are due to V centers. In a study of radiation damage in LiF Känzig (K-1) mentions that about a dozen different paramagnetic defects could be found in crystals irradiated at low temperatures. He studied the four predominate centers described as follows:

1. Self-trapped hole: this *V* center is an electron deficiency not associated with other imperfections.

2. V_F center: believed to be the antimorphy of the *F* center; i.e., a hole trapped by a lithium ion vacancy.

3. V_t center: an unpaired electron located on three fluorine ions.

4. *H* center: an interstitial fluorine atom best described as a F_2^- molecule ion substituting for a fluorine ion.

Figure 7.3-17 shows suggested models for these centers in accordance with the above definitions.

V centers have been produced by the radiation method at low temperatures, e.g., in Ref. K-1 LiF crystals located 7.5 cm from the tube target were irradiated for 100 hr with 70 kV peak x-rays. The tube current was 8 mA and the filtration corresponded to 4 mm of Al. Crystal temperatures of 20 or 77°K made no change in the number of lines observed but the relative sizes of the lines were altered slightly. When the crystals were irradiated at 196°K, none of the above centers developed, although a complex new spectrum appeared. The lines were unfolded by the pulse

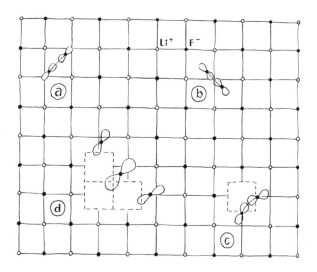

Fig. 7.3-17. Schematic representation of the four trapped-hole centers in LiF. The fluorine nuclei near the hole are connected with a heavy line. The 2*p* functions forming the main part of the linear combination of atomic orbitals for the hole are symbolized by figure eights: *a* = self-trapped hole; *b* = *H* center; *c* = V_f center; *d* = V_t center. (Courtesy K-1.)

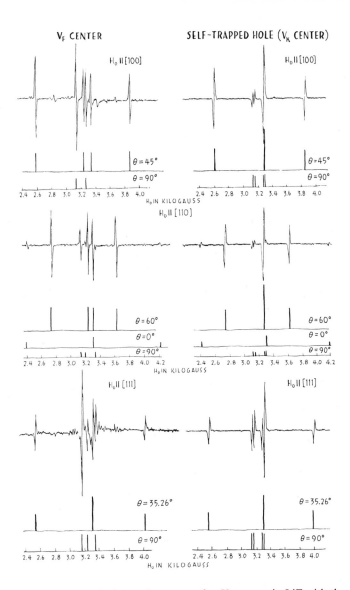

Fig. 7.3-18. Comparison of the EPR spectra for V_F centers in LiF with the corresponding spectra for self-trapped holes (V_K centers). The angle between the magnetic field H_0 and the orthorhombic axis z of the centers is designated by θ. The line drawings underneath the recordings represent the decomposition into basic spectra. Superposed upon the V_F spectra are a number of much weaker spectra belonging to unidentified centers. Conditions of experiment: X-band spectrometer, field modulation, several oersteds at 8 cps; power level, microwatts to milliwatts; temperature, 77°K, sample treatment for V_F spectra: x-ray irradiation at 77°K and subsequent annealing at 200°K. Sample treatment for V_K spectra: x-ray irradiation at 77°K. (Courtesy K-2.)

Table 7.3-6

EPR Characteristics of V_F Centers and the Self-Trapped Hole (K-1 and K-15)

Parameter	V_F Center	Self-trapped hole	Direction of H_0	Angle θ[a]
Spectroscopic splitting factor[b]				
g_x	2.023 ± 0.002	2.0227 ± 0.001		
g_y	2.023 ± 0.002	2.0234 ± 0.001		
g_z	2.001 ± 0.002	2.0031 ± 0.001		
Hf splitting constant[c]	(in gauss)			
A_1	688		(100)	45
A_1	741		(111)	35.26
A_1	913		(110)	0
A_1	483		(110)	6
A_2	589		(100)	45
A_2	741		(111)	35.26
A_2	913		(110)	0
A_2	415		(110)	6

[a] Angle between H_0 and crystal z axis.

[b] At 9.3 kMc.

[c] Contributions from two fluorine nuclei in the V_F center for various orientations of the magnetic field.

anneal technique, e.g., crystals were held for 30 min at various elevated temperatures then returned to 77°K for observation. Changes in the EPR spectrum occurred at temperatures where thermoluminescence and stimulated conductivity had been reported. Spectrometer requirements for observing V centers are the same as for the low-temperature measurements of F centers.

Typical g values, hf coefficients, and spectra are given in Table 7.3-6 and Fig. 7.3-18.

7.4. TRANSITION METAL IONS

Transition metal ions have been intimately linked with the development of EPR in physics, particularly the physics of crystalline fields where the unpaired electrons proved to be a very sensitive environmental indicator. Despite the importance of these ions we will discuss them only briefly in this volume. Two factors account for such brisk treatment: (*1*) the transition elements have been thoroughly considered in a number of books already present in every EPR library, (L-13,B-17,B-26,A-9,I-3,G-15, etc.) and (*2*) the experimental techniques are essentially the same as those already

Table 7.4-1

Atomic Structure of the Elements[a]

The Representative Elements (Differentiating electron in outermost shell)

Periods — n	s 1 (1)	s 2 (2)	p 1 (3)	p 2 (4)	p 3 (5)	p 4 (6)	p 5 (7)	p 6 (8)
$1s^2$ — 1	1 H 1.008 K 1	2 He 4.002 K 2						
$2s^2$, $2p^6$ — 2	3 Li 6.94 K L 2·1	4 Be 9.02 K L 2·2	5 B 10.82 K L 2·3	6 C 12.00 K L 2·4	7 N 14.008 K L 2·5	8 O 16.000 K L 2·6	9 F 19.00 K L 2·7	10 Ne 20.183 K L 2·8
$3s^2$, $3p^6$ — 3	11 Na 22.997 K L M 2·8·1	12 Mg 24.32 K L M 2·8·2	13 Al 26.97 K L M 2·8·3	14 Si 28.06 K L M 2·8·4	15 P 31.02 K L M 2·8·5	16 S 32.06 K L M 2·8·6	17 Cl 35.457 K L M 2·8·7	18 Ar 39.994 K L M 2·8·8
$4s^2$, $3d^{10}$, $4p^6$ — 4	19 K 39.096 L M N 8·8·1	20 Ca 40.08 L M N 8·8·2	31 Ga 69.72 L M N 8·18·3	32 Ge 72.60 L M N 8·18·4	33 As 74.91 L M N 8·18·5	34 Se 78.96 L M N 8·18·6	35 Br 79.916 L M N 8·18·7	36 Kr 83.7 L M N 8·18·8
$5s^2$, $4d^{10}$, $5p^6$ — 5	37 Rb 85.44 M N O 18·8·1	38 Sr 87.63 M N O 18·8·2	49 In 114.76 M N O 18·18·3	50 Sn 118.70 M N O 18·18·4	51 Sb 121.76 M N O 18·18·5	52 Te 127.61 M N O 18·18·6	53 I 126.92 M N O 18·18·7	54 Xe 131.3 M N O 18·18·8
$6s^2$, $5d^1$, $4f^{14}$, $5d^9$, $6p^6$ — 6	55 Cs 132.91 N O P 18·8·1	56 Ba 137.36 N O P 18·8·2	81 Tl 204.39 N O P 32·18·3	82 Pb 207.22 N O P 32·18·4	83 Bi 209.0 N O P 32·18·5	84 Po 210 N O P 32·18·6	85 At 210 N O P 32·18·7	86 Rn 222 N O P 32·18·8
$7s^2$, $6d^4$ — 7	87 Fr 223 O P Q 18·8·1	88 Ra 225.97 O P Q 18·8·2						

The Related Metals[b] (Differentiating electron in second from outermost shell)

n	d 1 (9)	d 2 (10)	d 3 (11)	d 4 (12)	d 5 (13)	d 6 (14)	d 7 (15)	d 8 (16)	d 9 (17)	d 10 (18)
3	21 Sc 45.10 L M N 8·9·2	22 Ti 47.90 L M N 8·10·2	23 V 50.95 L M N 8·11·2	24 Cr 52.01 L M N 8·13·1	25 Mn 54.93 L M N 8·13·2	26 Fe 55.84 L M N 8·14·2	27 Co 58.94 L M N 8·15·2	28 Ni 58.69 L M N 8·16·2	29 Cu 63.57 L M N 8·18·1	30 Zn 65.35 L M N 8·18·2
4	39 Y 88.92 M N O 18·9·2	40 Zr 91.22 M N O 18·10·2	41 Nb 93.3 M N O 18·12·1	42 Mo 96.0 M N O 18·13·1	43 Tc 99 M N O 18·13·2	44 Ru 101.7 M N O 18·15·1	45 Rh 102.91 M N O 18·16·1	46 Pd 106.7 M N O 18·18·0	47 Ag 107.88 M N O 18·18·1	48 Cd 112.41 M N O 18·18·2
5	57 La 138.92 N O P 18·9·2	72 Hf 178.6 N O P 32·10·2	73 Ta 181.4 N O P 32·11·2	74 W 184.0 N O P 32·12·2	75 Re 186.31 N O P 32·13·2	76 Os 191.3 N O P 32·14·2	77 Ir 193.1 N O P 32·15·2	78 Pt 193.3 N O P 32·16·2	79 Au 197.2 N O P 32·18·1	80 Hg 200.61 N O P 32·18·2
6	89 Ac 227 O P Q 19·9·2									

The Rare Earths[c] (Differentiating electron in third from outermost shell)

n	f 1 (19)	f 2 (20)	f 3 (21)	f 4 (22)	f 5 (23)	f 6 (24)	f 7 (25)	f 8 (26)	f 9 (27)	f 10 (28)	f 11 (29)	f 12 (30)	f 13 (31)	f 14 (32)
4	58 Ce 140.12 N O P 19·9·2	59 Pr 140.91 N O P 20·9·2	60 Nd 144.24 N O P 22·8·2	61 Pm (145) N O P 23·8·2	62 Sm 150.35 N O P 24·8·2	63 Eu 151.69 N O P 25·8·2	64 Gd 157.25 N O P 25·9·2	65 Tb 158.92 N O P 26·9·2	66 Dy 162.5 N O P 28·8·2	67 Ho 164.93 N O P 29·8·2	68 Er 167.2 N O P 30·8·2	69 Tm 168.93 N O P 31·8·2	70 Yb 173.04 N O P 32·8·2	71 Lu 174.97 N O P 32·9·2
5	90 Th 232.14 O P Q 19·9·2	91 Pa (231) O P Q 20·9·2	92 U 238.05 O P Q 21·9·2	93 Np (237) O P Q 22·9·2	94 Pu (242) O P Q 23·9·2	95 Am (243) O P Q 24·9·2	96 Cm (247) O P Q 25·9·2	97 Bk (249) O P Q 26·9·2	98 Cf (251) O P Q 27·9·2	99 Es (254) O P Q 28·8·2	100 Fm (252) O P Q 29·8·2	101 Md (256) O P Q 30·8·2	102 No (254) O P Q 31·8·2	103 Lw O P Q

[a] An extension of W. F. Luders compilation in *J. Chem. Educ.*, **20**, 21 (1943). [b] Iron group 22–29; Palladium group 40–47; Platinum group 72–79. [c] Rare earth group 58–71; Actinide group 90–103.

discussed in Sections 7.2 and 7.3. In the following paragraphs we will touch on a few properties of the ions, the EPR parameters of interest, sample preparation, and experimental considerations.

7.4.1   Ion Properties and EPR Parameters

Tabulating the elements according to the arrangement of Luder, Table 7.4-1 emphasizes the interesting electron structure of the five transition groups. Since the table is divided into groups according to the locations of partially filled electronic shells, all of the transition elements are in group 2 or group 3 where electrons are missing from the first and second shell, respectively inside the valence level. Chemical reactions cannot pair up odd electrons in these inner positions so they are permanently paramagnetic in marked contrast to electrons in the group 1 elements where heroic efforts are usually required to generate unpaired spins. When there are an even number of electrons in the transition elements, the constraints of Hund's rule and Pauli's exclusion principle still permit paramagnetism (L-13); therefore, altogether these paramagnetic species constitute a sizable fraction of the elements, i.e., nearly half.

When the transition elements are incorporated into crystalline compounds, the electrons outside the incomplete shell will provide some shielding from the crystalline fields and thus influence the interaction between the unpaired spin and the field from the neighboring ions. Where the unpaired electron is highly shielded as in the rare earth group, the coupling is weak and paramagnetic properties are close to that of free ions, e.g., the crystalline field does not break down the coupling between the orbital magnetic moment and the spin so that both contribute to the observed EPR. In contrast, the iron, palladium, platinum, and actinide groups exhibit medium to strong interactions with the crystalline field (B-26) because the unpaired spins are next to the outside shell. Consequently, the spins in these ions are sensitive to their neighbors, particularly highly polar molecules. Frequently the crystalline fields uncouple the spin from the orbital magnetic moment so that the EPR measurements detect only the spin.

All of the EPR parameters are of interest for the transition elements because the values do not converge on a trivial value such as the near free-electron value of the splitting factor encountered in many materials. Since the g values indicate the orbital contribution to the magnetic moment, the rare earth group would be expected to exhibit g values that depart substantially from the free-electron value and they do. Some ions exhibit a fine structure because the crystalline field has not separated the ground state levels beyond the quantum energy available from the rf field. When this is the case, constants D and E help determine the energy levels.

Hyperfine structure becomes important when the ion nucleus exhibits a spin and a magnetic moment. In several cases where the nuclear spin was not already known, the value was determined from EPR hf measurements. Examples of hfs are included in Fig. 2-14.

The dependence of the g value and linewidth on the crystal orientation in the magnetic field provides information about the symmetry of the ions surrounding the transition ions, including the nature and strength of binding to diamagnetic neighbors. Finally, the relaxation time which is associated with the linewidth provides additional insight into mechanisms for transferring energy from the spins to the crystal lattice.

7.4.2 Sample Preparation and Spectrometer Considerations

The main consideration in sample preparation is to find a suitable host crystal, i.e., a material that accepts a detectable quantity of the transition element, provides the desired field geometry, and contains no unwanted spins. Both the transition ion concentration and the sample temperature are used to control the linewidth and thus the observation of hfs. Concentrations are controlled by growing mixed crystals where the dilution by diamagnetic material typically is on the order of 200:1 to 1000:1 (I-3). Most of the crystals studied in early work were grown from solution and contained water of crystallization. Hydrogen has a strong magnetic moment so the presence of ordinary water can broaden narrow lines. When this source of line broadening is present, some reduction in the linewidth can be obtained by growing the crystal in heavy water. For example, the linewidth at half maximum for copper in $CuK(SO_4)_2 \cdot 6H_2O$ can be reduced to about 6 G by dilution with Zn or Mg which replaces the copper. Then a further reduction to about 2 G results from the use of heavy water (B-26). From this standpoint crystals that grow from the melt are ideal. Table 7.4-2 lists some examples of host materials and diluents used with the various groups. With the actinide group, crystal growing is sometimes a problem because of the strong radioactive nuclei. In addition, the internal radiation can produce other paramagnetic species such as radicals and unpaired electrons whose spectra may interfere with observations of the transition ion.

The spectrometer requirements for observing transition element ions have been met with a wide variety of spectrometers and cavities because sensitivity, resolution, and rf saturation have not been severe problems. There is no danger of line broadening by high-frequency modulation and either high-frequency modulated homodyne (TH2, RH1, etc.) or super-heterodyne (RS1, RS2, etc.) spectrometers are satisfactory. Physicists frequently use superheterodyne systems because the cryogenic cavity construction is simplified. Since most measurements on the transition

Table 7.4-2

Host Crystals for Transition Ions (B-26,L-13)

Crystal	Formula	Examples of ions	Symmetry	Transition ion group
Tutton salts	$M_2^{1+}M^{2+}(S^*O_4)_2 \cdot 6H_2O$	$M^{1+} = K, Rb, NH_4; M^{2+} = Mg, Zn; S^* = S, Se$	Octahedral	Iron group
Alums	$M^{1+}M^{3+}(S^*O_4)_2 \cdot 12H_2O$	$M^{3+} = Al$ or any trivalent ion of $3d$ group	Octahedral	Iron group
Double nitrates	$M_3^{2+}M_2^{3+}(NO_3)_2 \cdot 24H_2O$	$M^{2+} = Mg$ or any divalent $3d$ group ion; $M^{3+} = Bi$ or $4f$ group ion	Octahedral	Iron group / Rare earth group
Fluosilicates	$M^{2+}SiF_6 \cdot 6H_2O$	$M^{2+} = Zn$ or any divalent ion of the $3d$ group	Trigonal	Iron group
Bromates	$M^{2+}(BrO_3)_2 \cdot 6H_2O$	$M^{2+} = Zn$ or any divalent ion of the $3d$ group	Cubic	Iron group
Sulfates	$M^{2+}SO_4 \cdot 7H_2O$	$M^{2+} = Zn$ or any divalent ion of the $3d$ group	Orthorhombic	Iron group
Complex cyanides	$K_3M^{3+}(CN)_6$	$M^{3+} = Cr, Mn, Fe,$ or Co	Orthorhombic	Iron group
Complex cyanides	$K_4M^{2+}(CN)_6 \cdot 3H_2O$	$M^{2+} = V, Mn,$ or Fe	Tetragonal	Iron group
Complex halides	$M^{1+}M^{4+}X_6$	$M^{4+} = Ir, Pt; X = Cl, Br$	Cubic	Platinum group
	$Na_2M^{4+}X_6 \cdot 6H_2O$	$M^{4+} = Ir, Pt; X = Cl, Br$	Triclinic	Platinum group
Ethyl sulfates	$M^{3+}(C_2H_5SO_4)_3 \cdot 9H_2O$	$M^{3+} =$ trivalent rare earth ion	Hexagonal	Rare earth group
Uranyl-type rubidium nitrate	$M^{4+}O_2Rb(NO_3)_3$	$M^{4+} = U, Np, Pu,$ etc.	Hexagonal	Actinide group

elements are made at low temperatures, cryogenic considerations are important. Bleaney and Stevens (B-17) note that in the iron group relaxation times vary from 10^{-4} to 10^{-11} sec at $10°K$. With times longer than 10^{-7} sec line broadening is usually not a problem, but when the time exceeds 10^{-5} sec, rf saturation may occur.

Besides cooling, the cavity should permit various sample orientations in the magnetic field; consequently, the cylindrical cavities are generally favored for such measurements. When crystals are small, the TE_{011} mode gives the highest sensitivity. Where good thermal contact to the cavity is required, as in relaxation time measurements by saturation or inversion techniques, the TE_{111} cavity can be used to good advantage with the sample in intimate contact with the bottom.

Some results of EPR measurements on transition elements are found in Chapters II and V. For example, Figs. 2-11 to 2-14 show the fine structure characteristics of Ni^{2+} in nickel fluosilicate in various field orientations and the hfs of elements with various nuclear spins. Copper and manganese spectra are included in Figs. 5-7 and 5-9.

7.5   FREE RADICALS IN SOLIDS

The past two decades have witnessed the transition of trapped radicals from an experimental rarity to a very common occurrence, at times almost a universal nuisance.* Various factors have contributed to this development, including improved cryogenic and spectroscopic techniques. However the greatest impetus stems from the need to understand the role played by these reactive intermediates in many physical, chemical, and biological reactions. Minkoff (M-9) illustrates this growth in his monograph *Frozen Free Radicals* with a short historical survey that commences with the pioneering trapping experiments of Dewar at the turn of the century and follows developments through the major contributions of Vegard and Lewis to the present widespread activity associated with EPR techniques.

Most of his monograph and this section are concerned with matrix isolation techniques for stabilizing radicals produced by pyrolysis, electrical discharge, photolysis, and radiolysis. Stable free radicals are also included here because the EPR techniques are similar for all radicals in solids. Organic compounds are emphasized particularly in the examples but many of the methods are suitable for a wider variety of radicals.

In trapped radical studies, EPR observations have been concerned principally with measuring the hfs and the spin concentration in order to

---

* We say nuisance because in studies of irradiation effects, it is virtually impossible to find a dielectric container that does not develop unpaired spins under irradiation.

identify the radical species and to determine the G values, respectively. Simple detection is also useful in following radical reactions. The spectroscopic splitting factor for most radicals is very close to the free electron value; therefore, it is generally ignored as a vital source of information particularly in the many multicrystalline glassy, or plastic samples of chemical importance. Blois et al. (B-20) note that when the hfs fails to be resolved, the g value may be the only measurable quantity available for use in identifying the radical, and with precision measurement differences in g values frequently are detectable. These g values are always slightly higher than the free electron value of 2.0023 and generally fall between 2.0023 and 2.01 (H-4).

In the following paragraphs we will consider first the spectrometer requirements then techniques of sample preparation. Finally, typical results are grouped under each method of radical production.

7.5.1 Spectrometer Considerations

The spectrometer requirements vary considerably for the three general types of radical measurements: (1) detection or tracing, (2) identification, and (3) yield or G value. Enough radicals (concentrations of 10^{18}) can normally be stabilized to permit detection and tracing with the simplest spectrometers, e.g., a straight transmission system without automatic frequency control (AFC) (TH1). The linewidths range from about 1 to 20 G, as a result, resolution is not a problem. High-frequency modulation does not broaden the lines and modest magnets are adequate because a field that is uniform and stable over the sample volume to one part in several thousand is sufficient for hfs observations. It is the yield or G value measurements that can tax even the most elaborate instruments to the limit of their sensitivity. This problem results from two kinds of saturation phenomena. First, the yield frequently depends on the radical concentration, as shown in Fig. 7.5-1, where an equilibrium value is reached and the radicals are disappearing through back reactions or cross reactions as fast as they are generated. In this situation yield values have little meaning except at the beginning of the curve where the radical concentration is very small. Second, the isolation necessary to stabilize radicals frequently leads to a long relaxation time and the accompanying propensity for rf saturation, particularly in the dilute concentration situation in Fig. 7.5-2. One restriction frequently leads to another and the loss of signal sustained in avoiding these saturation effects increases the measuring time for an adequate signal-to-noise ratio thereby increasing the spectrometer stability requirements. Although the sweep times are still modest (15–30 min) compared with those for high resolution experiments, there is ample time for base-line drifts to distort the curve and thus the measured concentration of radicals.

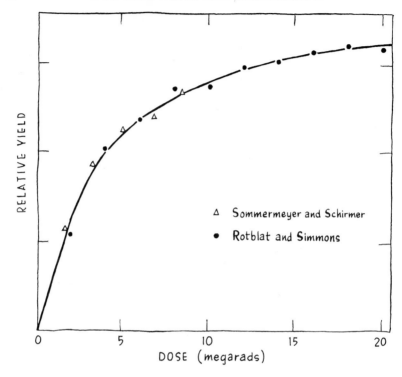

Fig. 7.5-1. Relative yield of radicals in glycine as a function of dose illustrating the onset of saturation in the concentration of free radicals. (Courtesy B-23.)

Currently most observations of radicals for identification or tracing purposes are made with type TH1 or RH1 homodyne spectrometers equipped with high-frequency modulation and with the automatic frequency control locked to the sample cavity. Stable AFC frequently requires enough power in the cavity to produce some rf saturation and this is accepted along with some spin concentration saturation for operating convenience and a large signal. Numerous G values determined under such conditions contain unknown errors. Caution dictates the determination of the operating conditions with respect to both types of saturation before yield measurements are attempted. In order to reduce the power level below rf saturation, it is frequently necessary to lock the AFC to an auxiliary cavity, e.g., a type RH2 spectrometer and to observe the other measures outlined for maximum sensitivity in Chapter III. Earlier in this chapter we encountered similar rf saturation problems in semiconductors with low spin concentrations. There the prevailing practice was to measure the dispersion which does not saturate as readily as the absorption curve. While this procedure

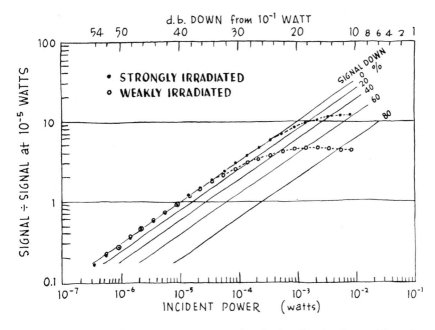

Fig. 7.5-2. Radiofrequency power saturation in irradiated toluene. Note the dependence on radical concentration as indicated by the strongly and weakly irradiated samples.

Spectrometer type, RH4-X; cavity, rectangular TE_{102}; temperature, 77°K; modulation, 100 kc; sample, slug irradiated with 2 MeV electrons in the apparatus of Fig. 7.5-18. (Courtesy M-3.)

apparently is not used with radicals, it should be considered when rf saturation is a serious problem.

A few superheterodyne spectrometers are involved in trapped radical measurements; however, those who use them generally prefer the simplicity of the high-frequency modulated homodyne spectrometer for most radical work. Where both types of spectrometers are available, it is convenient to use high-frequency modulation first and switch to a superheterodyne spectrometer only if needed.

A wide variety of rectangular TE_{1on} and cylindrical TE_{011} cavities are suitable for trapped radical work. For identification and tracer experiments, the main cavity requirements are provision for sample temperature control and slits for illumination. Observations down to 77°K are usually performed with internal dewars similar to Fig. 7.3-6a or with gas flow coolers, both of which are commercially available. Radical studies frequently involve numerous samples; therefore, sample accessibility is an important factor usually outweighing the slight improvement in Q achieved with only the sample in the cavity. When liquid helium is the refrigerant, the preference in dewars is not as unanimous and no one style is appropriate for all modes of radical production; therefore, the factors influencing the choice will be considered under each production technique.

Quantitative measurements of radical concentration and yield introduce the additional requirement of a standard or yardstick and rectangular TE_{104} cavities with two sets of modulation coils as shown in Fig. 4-30 are convenient for this purpose. Actually most of the G values reported in the following sections were measured in cavities with only one set of modulation coils.

7.5.2   Stable Free Radicals

In Section 6.2.2 we encountered a number of polyatomic radicals that were relatively long lived in appropriate solutions. Here we consider a few radicals that are compatible with their brethren in the solid state. Historically such free radicals attracted attention in the early days of EPR as promising subjects for resonance detection. For example, Wertz (W-11) reports that pentaphenylcyclopentadienyl was the first radical to be detected by EPR (1947), which was followed by Banfield and Kenyon's radical (1949), and 1,1-diphenyl-2-picrylhydrazyl (DPPH) (1950). DPPH attracted considerable attention because it had the narrowest linewidth for any solid observed in the early 1950s; consequently, it occupied a prominent position in the studies of exchange narrowing. Current interest in DPPH and similar radicals stems principally from their widespread use as g markers, yardsticks for measuring numbers of spins, and a scale for rating spectrometer sensitivity. The g values and linewidths of stable polycrystalline free radicals are tabulated in numerous references (A-9,C-13, E-7,I-2,W-11), which should be consulted for explanations of free radical

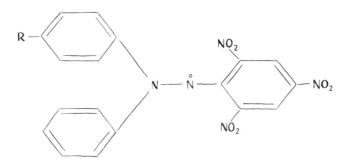

Fig. 7.5-3. Stable free radicals similar to DPPH. (Courtesy B-7.)

Table 7.5-1

Linewidths and Splitting Factors for some DPPH Derivatives
(Powder Samples) (B-7)

Compound[a]	R	Linewidth ΔH_{ms},[b] G	g Value
DPPH	H	1.9 ± 0.2	2.0036
I	Cl	1.1 ± 0.1	2.0038 ± 0.0002
II		2.2 ± 0.2	2.0036 ± 0.0002
III	CH₃	6.9 ± 0.4	2.0035 ± 0.0003

[a] See Figure 7.5-3 for structure.
[b] ΔH_{ms} = width at maximum slope.

behavior. The material which follows is limited to DPPH, some of its derivatives, and precautions pertinent to the use of these radicals as yardsticks. On the basis of the hfs for dilute solutions of DPPH in a solvent such as benzene, the unpaired electron is assigned to the nitrogen, as indicated in Fig. 7.5-3. Despite isolation, the unpaired electron is sensitive to members on the phenyl group at R and to impurities associated with the molecule. Table 7.5-1 shows the change in linewidth resulting from substituting various groups at R (B-7). Some of the dispersion in values reported for the width of the DPPH line results from the solvent used in growing the crystals. Table 7.5-2 shows the variations in observed linewidth for DPPH crystallized from eight commonly used solvents. DPPH is commercially available (Eastman, for example); consequently, it is no longer necessary to prepare your own radicals; however, it is pertinent to know the solvent used in the final crystallization. While the heading for this section is "Stable Radicals" stability is a relative matter. DPPH molecules tolerate each other, but they do react with many other radicals. For example, DPPH is frequently used as a scavenger for free radicals; therefore, stability implies a suitable degree of isolation from other species. According to Ref. A-9 DPPH crystallized from carbon disulfide or chloroform interacts with O_2 to broaden the absorption line, however, such broadening is negligible when benzene is the solvent. For the highest stability, DPPH standards should be crystallized from benzene and sealed in vacuum or in an inert gas. If stored in the dark, the decomposition can be reduced to less than several per cent per year (W-11).

Values of the published splitting factor show a dispersion beyond the limits of the measuring precision indicated by the number of reported

Table 7.5-2

Linewidth in DPPH Samples Crystallized from Various Solvents
(A-9)

| | ΔH, G | | |
| | $\nu = 300$ Mc | | $\nu = 9400$ Mc |
Solvent	295°K	90°K	295°K
Benzene	6.8	4.6	4.7
Toluene	2.9	2.6	2.6
Xylene (mixture)	2.5	2.2	2.3
Pyridine	5.3	5.0	5.0
Bromoform	2.2	2.5	2.5
Carbon tetrachloride	1.9	2.7	2.3
Chloroform	1.7	2.1	2.0
Carbon disulfide	1.3	1.3	1.5

significant figures. Table 7.5-3 shows that values for this widely used standard can range from about 2.0030 to 2.0041, depending on the orientation of single crystals. Polycrystalline samples have a g value very close to 2.0036.

Another source of uncertainty appears when DPPH is used as a standard of known spin concentration because the number of spins in a given mass may also depend on the solvent used in growing the crystals (W-9). Since fewer DPPH radicals are present than calculated from the mass, the concentration determined for the unknown may be too high by as much as 50%.

Table 7.5-3

Variation in g Values for DPPH at Room
Temperature and 77°K

Sample	g Value	Ref.
Single crystal[a]	2.0027–2.0039	V-2
Single crystal	2.0035–2.0041	W-11
Single crystal	2.0028–2.0038	I-2
Single crystal	2.0030–2.0040	A-9
Powder[a]	2.0037	V-2
Polycrystalline	2.0036 ± 0.0003	I-2
Polycrystalline	2.0037	P-12

[a] Sample at 77°K; others at room temperature.

Van Garven et al. (V-2) have examined the line shape, and relaxation times for DPPH in considerable detail over the temperature range from 293 to 1.7°K. At all temperatures the line shape is Lorentzian, as illustrated by Fig. 7.5-4.

Rf saturation is not a problem with DPPH because the usual klystrons in spectrometers do not generate enough rf power. Bloembergen and Wang

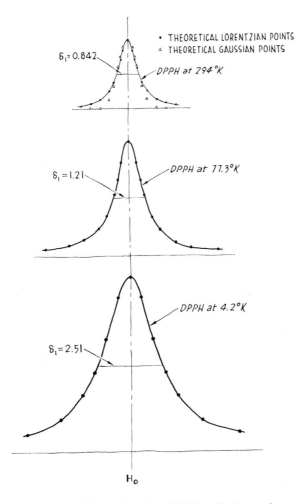

Fig. 7.5-4. Comparison of line shape for DPPH with Lorentzian and gaussian curves: Spectrometer, 27–29 Mc; temperatures 4.2–293°K; modulation, sweep field for oscilloscopic display—314 cycles; sample, DPPH is crystallized from CHCl₃, crushed to a very fine powder, and sealed in a small glass tube. (Courtesy V-2.)

(B-19) were able to produce about 50% saturation at 77°K with a pulsed magnetron which gave an H_1 of 2 G at the sample. They found a T_1 of 6.3×10^{-8} sec.

7.5.3 Radicals by Pyrolysis

In Chapter VI we encountered radicals in the gas and vapor products of pyrolysis. Now we turn to the radicals left behind in the solid residue. Actually, the examples considered here will include some radicals that originated without the benefit of pyrolysis but have properties and a behavior that have linked them to the literature of pyrolysis products. Historically, the spin resonance of pyrolyzed solids commenced with activated charcoals (I-4) and spread to various charred carbohydrates and carbonaceous fuels. It soon became apparent that two general categories of radicals were involved, those associated with low-temperature pyrolysis, i.e., below 900°C and those produced at high temperatures, above 1400°C. Apparently no radicals are generated in the intermediate range from 1000 to 1400°C; at least they have not been reported (I-2). Much of the activity in the low-temperature region concerns carbonaceous fuels of various ages and stages of development, i.e., peats, lignites, and soft and hard coals where the radicals normally present in these materials appear identical to those in carbohydrate chars. For example, Uebersfeld et al. (U-1) report that damage to carbohydrates—either by nature as in coals, by heating as in charcoals and pitch, or by irradiation of woods and sugars—produce the same EPR line. Questions about the origin and stability of these radicals in nature have led to investigations of botanical origin, generation by natural radioactivity, and geothermal possibilities (D-11). Another source of radicals with the low-temperature characteristics are the carbon blacks extensively used in rubbers, plastics, paints, and inks; therefore, considerable technological importance is attached to their properties. These blacks are different from the charred materials in that their formation temperature is from 1100 to 1750°C, i.e., extending from the high down into the intermediate temperature region; however, the reaction time is very short, apparently resulting in a mixture of both high- and low-temperature carbons (I-2), the latter EPR characteristics predominating (C-16). Finally, some of these radicals are important in experimental EPR as stable standards and yardsticks for quantitative measurements.*

High-temperature pyrolysis produces resonance centers that are more like defect centers than radicals. For example, in graphites and carbons, the electrons behave as if they were highly localized on a carbon atom and

---

* Pitch standards are commercially available from Varian Associates, Palo Alto, Calif.

do not interact appreciably with foreign atoms such as oxygen. Since the EPR requirements are comparable to those of semiconductors of similar conductivity, no further consideration will be given to these high-temperature carbons. Reference I-2 can be consulted for further details of the spins involved.

High concentrations of radicals have been obtained from all types of charred organic matter. Table 7.5-4 lists some of the materials used for chars and the temperature for production of maximum radical concentration. The carbonizing temperature has a substantial effect on the number of unpaired spins generated as indicated in Fig. 7.5-5. In all the material reported in Table 7.5-4, the peak concentrations also developed at temperatures of about 550–600°C and the spin centers disappeared frequently

Table 7.5-4

Production and Characteristics of Radicals in some Low-Temperature Chars

Material charred	g Value	ΔH, G	Temperature for peak radical production, °C	Ref.
Glucose and other sugars	2.0020 ± 0.0003	8 ± 2	550	B-6
Deposits from luminous flames	2.0020 ± 0.0003	8 ± 2	550	B-6
Natural or artificial cellulose	2.0020 ± 0.0003	8 ± 2	550	B-6
Anthracene and glycerine	2.0020 ± 0.0003	8 ± 2	550	B-6
Vegetable root and other complex natural organic materials	2.0020 ± 0.0003	8 ± 2	550	B-6
Charcoals formed below 600°C	2.0020 ± 0.0003	8 ± 2	550	B-6
Coals and coal derivatives formed below 600°C	2.0020 ± 0.0003	8 ± 2	550	B-6
Charcoals from pinewood and cocoanut				U-1
Saccharose and glucose				U-1
Pitches from crude oil distillation				U-1
Naphthalene	2.0024 ± 0.0003	1.	670	M-1
Anthracene	2.0024 ± 0.0030	1.5	640	M-1
Decalin	2.0024 ± 0.0003	1.5	600	M-1
Secondary butyl alcohol	2.0024 ± 0.0003	0.5	670	M-1
Anthracite coal[a]				U-1
Fossilized plants[a]	2.002			D-11
Peats[a]	2.002			D-11
Lignites[a]	2.002			D-11
Coals[a]	2.002			D-11
Carbonized coals	2.0030 ± 0.0003	7 ± 1	550	I-6
Donetz coal[a]	2.007 ± 0.001			V-9

[a] Radicals exist in these natural materials without heat treatment.

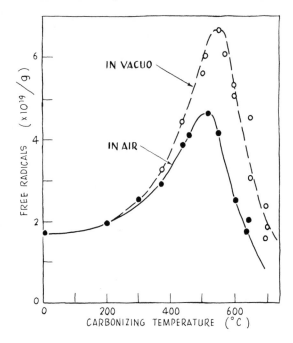

Fig. 7.5-5. Variation of radical concentration with temperature of carbonization. (Courtesy I-2.)

by 700°C and in all cases by 900°C. Heating schedules vary and frequently are not mentioned but several examples are given below.

A. In Ref. M-1 deposits formed by an electrical discharge in the vapor of the parent material were heat treated in steps of 100°C up to 1000°C. Each sample was heated from room temperature to the treatment temperature in 13 min, held at the treatment temperature for 2 min and quickly returned to room temperature.

B. The charred dextrose in Refs. H-17 and P-4 involved up to a week's preparation time with the following ritual:

1. Gradually heat analytical grade anhydrous dextrose under flowing 99% pure nitrogen so that the temperature reaches 200°C in a 2 day period. Halt at 200°C for about 2 or 3 days until tarry materials cease to distil over. Then increase the temperature at about 10°C per hour to 300°C and hold at 300°C for at least 12 hr.

2. Cool the material to room temperature, still under an atmosphere of nitrogen.

3. Grind in air to a fine powder and return to furnace in a container thoroughly flushed with nitrogen.

4. Gradually heat to treatment temperature (usually 560°C) and hold at this temperature for 12 hr.

5. Cool under nitrogen, grind to a fine powder in air, insert in a sample tube, connect to the vacuum manifold, submerge the sample bulb under liquid N_2, and outgas with a pressure of about 10^{-4} torr for about 2 days during which time the liquid N_2 is gradually removed. The point is to keep the capillary stem free of char particles in order to insure a vacuum tight seal off.

6. After about a week of outgassing the pressure reaches 10^{-7} torr, either hot (450°C) or cold (25°C), and the sample is sealed off. This procedure is recommended for preparing stable paramagnetic resonance standards (H-17).

C. Collins et al. (C-16) started with carbon black (channel black Spheron 6*) and heated the samples at the treatment temperature for 2 hr under a nonoxidizing atmosphere in an induction furnace.

Table 7.5-5

Relaxation Time T_1 at Various Temperatures for Radicals in Dextrose Charred by Recipe B (P-4)

Pyrolytic tempera- ture, °C	Composition of sample, % by weight					Relaxation time T_1,[a] μsec		
	Ash	C	H	N	O	77°K	4.2°K	1.4°K
250						2.0	40	40
300	0.13	80.63	3.35	0.09	15.8	0.50	1.6	2.0
350						0.07	0.12	0.28
400							0.04	0.08
450	0.00	86.57	3.10	0.04	10.3			< 0.03
550	0.00	93.38	2.79	0.12	3.7			

[a] T_1 measured by a direct-pulse method.

In materials such as the coals and carbon blacks, the radicals initially present are fairly stable up to 500 or 600°C but higher temperatures cause the spin concentration to decrease rapidly to a minimum in the vicinity of 1000–1400°C, depending on the material (C-16). According to Ingram (I-2) the concentration of trapped free radicals increases rapidly as the carbon content in the char increases from 80 to 94%. When the carbon content is low, long relaxation times are observed and the resonance signals readily saturate with rf power. Table 7.5-5 shows the dependence of T_1 on the carbon concentration as interpolated through the pyrolysis temperature scale. Apparently the measuring temperature has a negligible influence on T_1.

Oxygen effects both the yield of detectable radicals in the carbonizing process and the spectrum observed for the trapped radicals. Figure 7.5-5 shows the increase in radical yield for carbonizing in vacuum in contrast to air and Fig. 7.5-6 shows the effect of oxygen on the spectrum of radicals in carbon black. The linewidth of about 15 G for carbon black in air reduces

* Manufactured by Godfrey L. Cabot, Inc.

to about 7 G when the sample is evacuated and broadens to at least twice the air value when oxygen is introduced to the evacuated sample. In the sequence of Fig. 7.5-6, the concentration of radicals apparently remained constant; only the linewidth changed. Table 7.5-6 shows the influence of sample preparation environment on the linewidth for some commercial carbon blacks. Although the width varies considerably from one material to another, the effects of a vacuum or inert atmosphere environment are consistent throughout, i.e., treatment D (Table 7.5-6) always produces the narrowest line. While the detailed nature of these oxygen effects remains to be clarified, it is experimentally expedient to seal pitch standards either

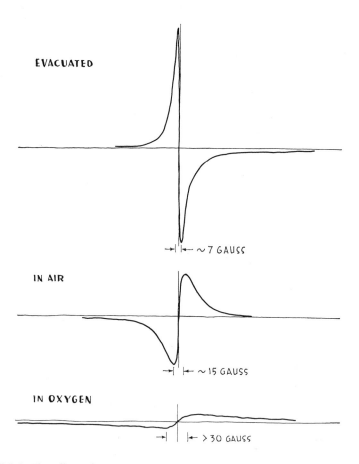

Fig. 7.5-6. The effect of atmosphere on the linewidth of carbon black. The total intensity of the line does not change. (After P-8.)

Table 7.5-6

Electron Spin Resonance Data on Commercial Carbon Blacks (C-16)

Sample	Preparation	$10^{-19} \times$ no. spins/g	ΔH, G	g Factor
Philblack A	A^a		28	2.0035
	B^b		16	2.0006
	C^c		15	
	D^d	10	15	
Philblack O	A		54	2.0031
	B		46	2.0043
	C		41	
	D	8.0	29	
Philblack I	A		92	2.000
	B		78	2.001
	C		60	
	D	9.2	41	
Philblack E	A		133	1.998
	B		94	2.001
	C^e		46	
	D	8.1	20	
Wyex	A		14	2.0023
	B		3.7	2.0026
	C		2.8	
	D	15	1.1	
Acetylene Black	A		4.8	2.0031
	B		3.8	2.0034
	C		3.7	
	D	3.8	3.3	
Thermal (P-33)	A		18	2.0019
	B		13	2.0033
	C		13	
	D	5.9	12	
Lampblack 888	C		4.2	
	D	5.8	4.1	
Spheron 6	A		31	2.0041
	B		11	2.0047
	C		5.3	
	D	13.9	1.5	2.0024

[a] A, crushed, in air.
[b] B, crushed, in benzene.
[c] C, crushed, in vacuum of 0.01 μ.
[d] D, crushed, evacuated to 0.01 μ at 250°C, with several helium flushes.
[e] Sample was inadvertently helium flushed during evacuation.

under vacuum or in an inert gas such as helium or nitrogen in order to insure stability.

With carbon blacks, the electrical conductivity may be sufficiently high in caked samples to limit the rf field penetration; therefore, powdered samples are commonly used. In Ref. C-16 pellets were crushed lightly between sheets of paper until further crushing made no change in the signal size.

7.5.4   Radicals by Electrical Discharge

Electrical discharge provides one of the oldest methods for producing radicals in gases and vapors as described in Chapter VI. Several modifications of the technique are also suitable for obtaining radicals in solids, i.e., either by self-trapping or by burying. Two examples will illustrate these methods. In the self-trapping technique used by Mangiaracina and Mrozowski (M-1) organic vapors were decomposed by a high-voltage low-frequency discharge in the apparatus shown in Fig. 7.5-7. Pressure in the glass discharge tube is controlled by the temperature of the sample at A, the pumping speed of the mercury diffusion pump, and the valve. Electrodes wrapped around the tube at points B and operated at 15 kV, 60 c, provide the field to ionize the vapor. Table 7.5-7 lists the temperatures and pressures used for several of the materials already encountered in the previous section on pyrolysis. After a deposit formed on the walls of the tube near the electrodes, the tube was opened, the deposit was scraped

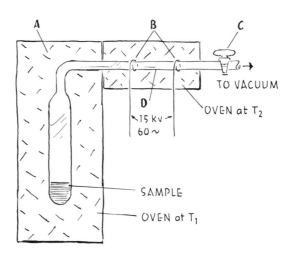

Fig. 7.5-7. Schematic diagram of apparatus for the production of radicals by the electrical discharge method. (After M-1.)

Table 7.5-7

Conditions for Radical Production by Electrical Discharge Method (M-1)

Material	T_1, °C	T_2, °C	Vapor pressure, mm Hg
Naphthalene	Warmed with bunsen flame	Room	—
Anthracene	150	170	1
Decalin	-70	Room	0.1
sec-Butyl alcohol	-70	Room	0.005

loose, and samples were transferred to quartz vials suitable for EPR measurements or further treatment by pyrolysis.

Foner et al. (F-14,J-2) have combined the high-frequency electrical discharge technique with the burying form of the matrix isolation method to successfully trap and detect a series of very reactive atomic and molecular free radicals. Their apparatus, which is illustrated in Fig. 7.5-8, consists of three interconnected chambers which accommodate the three steps in the experiment, namely, radical production, isolation in an inert matrix, and EPR measurement. Radicals are produced outside the dewar in a quartz tube between two external aluminum foil electrodes. Typical conditions for the discharge were as follows: pressure, about 0.1 mm Hg; frequency, 8 Mc/sec; power, up to 100 W when producing free atoms but usually considerably less for molecular radicals; tube diameter, 25 mm. A mercury diffusion pump pulls the discharge products past the connection to the dewar at a speed of about 1500 cm/sec. Some of these products pass into the dewar through the "glass slit" and deposit on a sapphire finger 2 mm in diameter and 50 mm long soldered into the bottom of the liquid helium container. Simultaneously, inert molecules enter through the matrix slits (see insert) deposit on the sapphire finger and bury the discharge product. In optimum cases, samples about 1 mm thick required 1 hr to deposit. Pertinent dimensions for the glass slits are 0.11 × 6 mm for most experiments, and 0.5 × 10 mm for H atoms. For EPR measurements the finger was lowered through a 5 mm diameter hole into the rectangular TE_{102} X-band cavity. Since the cavity is kept at liquid nitrogen temperatures, it serves as part of the radiation shield that completely surrounds the liquid helium system except for an opening opposite the slits and four radiation baffled pumping slots (not shown) which permit cryopumping by the liquid helium-cooled surfaces. The cavity was electroformed of copper, had a 4.9 mm diameter iris tapered as indicated and a quarter-wavelength

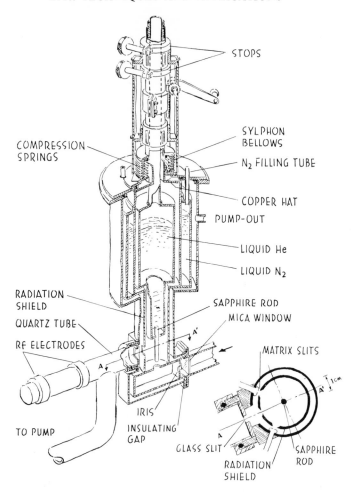

Fig. 7.5-8. The discharge system and low-temperature cell used to trap radicals in inert matrix. The insert shows the slit system in detail. (Courtesy J-2.)

extension of the waveguide beyond the iris to permit a vacuum gap between the cooled cavity and the room temperature waveguide. A mica window in the room temperature coupling flange seals the cavity and dewar. At 77°K the unloaded Q is about 18,000 and the 4.9 mm diameter iris reduced the Q by 60%.

Atomic and molecular free radicals generated by this technique include H, D, N, and CH_3 with the results shown in Fig. 7.5-9. Table 7.5-8 contains the g values and hyperfine coupling constants obtained from the spectra.

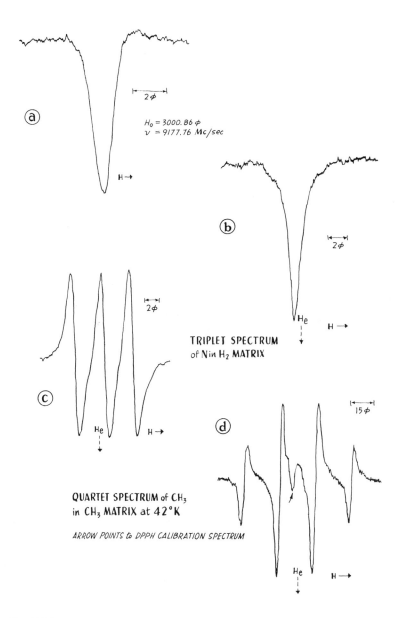

Fig. 7.5-9. Resonance spectra of trapped atomic free radicals: (*a*) Low field line of the *H* atom doublet in H_2 matrix. The line shape indicates fast passage conditions resulting from a long relaxation time and high modulation frequency. (*b*) Center line of deuterium atom triplet in D_2 matrix. The shape also shows fast passage effect. (*c*) Triplet spectrum of N atoms in N_2 matrix. (*d*) Quartet spectrum of CH_3 in CH_4 matrix. H_e stands for the free electron resonance field.

Spectrometer, type RH1-X; cavity, rectangular TE_{102} (see Fig. 7.5-8); temperature, 4.2°K; modulation, 400 cps. (Courtesy J-2.)

Table 7.5-8

Characteristics of Atomic and Molecular Free Radicals Produced by the Rf Discharge Technique of Fig. 7.5-8 (J-2)

Radical	Matrix	g Value	Separation between lines, Oe	hf coupling constant A, Mc/sec
H	H_2	2.00230	508.69	1417.11
D	D_2	2.00231	77.7	217.71
N	N_2	2.00200	4.31	12.08
CH_3	CH_4	2.00242	22.9	64.39

7.5.5 Radicals by Photolysis

Photolysis has been associated with much of the important progress in our understanding of radicals in solids, particularly in the classic experiments of Lewis and Lipkin (L-8) and Norman and Porter (N-3). EPR entered the picture in 1955 when Ingram et al. reported spin resonance in a series of materials prepared in the tradition of Norman and Porter (N-3). Now the technique is regularly used, particularly when radical identification is the principle concern. It has been pointed out in various papers (P-10,I-2) that photolysis provides the most delicate and controlled method of generating radicals *in situ*. The experimenter has at his disposal the mode of excitation, the energy of excitation, and the environment of the site of excitation; consequently, in principle, selected bonds can be ruptured. In contrast, radical production by electrical discharge or ionizing radiation is somewhat like cracking peanuts with a sledge hammer. Enough energy is present to break any bond so nature must be allowed to take its course. Actually, other factors intervene so that the high-energy particles do not generate a completely random assortment of radicals; however, the fine control observed in resonant photolysis is lost.

Photolysis techniques can be classified into three categories:

1. Direct:
$$M + h\nu \rightarrow R^{\cdot}_1 + R^{\cdot}_2$$

2. Indirect:
$$M + h\nu \rightarrow R^{\cdot}_1 + R^{\cdot}_2$$
$$R^{\cdot}_2 + M_1 \rightarrow R^{\cdot}_3 + M_2$$

3. Conversion:
$$R^{\cdot}_1 + h\nu \rightarrow R^{\cdot}_2 + M$$

In the direct method the molecules of interest are dissolved or dispersed in an inert matrix which is transparent to the light $h\nu$. When the photon ruptures the molecular bond, the matrix must exhibit sufficient flexibility to permit at least one of the radicals to escape; otherwise, the fragments will recombine. This cage effect can seriously limit the quantum yield. Another obvious limitation arises because only a limited number of materials can be decomposed photolytically in the available matrices (P-10). The indirect method extends photolysis to some molecules that are transparent throughout the same wavelength region as the inert matrix. In this technique the radicals formed from the small quantity of photosensitive constituent attack the matrix and produce the radical to be observed. When the primary radicals are chemically very active such as photolytically decomposed hydrogen peroxide, a good yield and high concentration of solvent radicals may be accumulated. The third procedure, conversion, involves changing one radical into another by illumination in an absorption band characteristic of the initial radical. This technique is used primarily to unfold overlapping spectra or follow radical reactions. Also this mechanism can be a special case of the direct and indirect processes.

A minor experimental question is whether to generate the radicals inside or outside of the cavity. Frequently the choice is a matter of necessity, e.g., when the cavity has no illumination slits or when working at 4°K where sample transfer becomes a bit involved. At liquid nitrogen temperature, samples are readily transferred so that the choice is primarily a matter of convenience.

(a) Direct Process. Pimentel (P-10) and Norman and Porter (N-3) list the following glasses as suitable matrices for *in situ* radical production at 77°K:

1. 3 MeP.P: 3 parts methylpentane, 2 parts isopentane.
2. P.MeH or M.P.: 3 parts isopentane, 2 parts methylcyclopentane.
3. E.P.A.: 5 parts ether, 5 parts isopentane, 2 parts ethyl alcohol.
4. Pure isopentane.
5. Pure 3-methylpentane.

Pure isopentane is not sufficiently rigid for efficient trapping at 77°K; therefore, it is usually used at lower temperatures. According to Norman and Porter (N-3) E.P.A. is superior from the diffusion standpoint but prone to react with the radicals. Other matrix materials suitable for radical production at liquid helium temperatures include inert gases and vapors such as N_2, Ar, Xe, CO_2, and CH_4.

In the initial paper Ingram et al. (I-5) used the photosensitive molecules, temperatures, and excitation energies listed in Table 7.5-9. After freezing in silica tubes, these samples were exposed to 2540 Å radiation in one dewar, then transferred at 77°K to a cold TE_{101} cavity for EPR measurements. The experiments of Foner et al. (F-14) on hydrogen atoms trapped

Table 7.5-9

Radical Production by the Direct Photolysis Method

Photosensitive material	Matrix	Sample temp, °K	UV Light, Å	Ref.
Ethyl iodide	P·MeH	77	2540	I-5
Toluene	P·MeH	77	2540	I-5
Benzylamine	P·MeH	77	2540	I-5
Benzyl chloride	P·MeH	77	2540	I-5
Benzene	P·MeH	77	2540	I-5
Toluene	E.P.A.	77	2540	I-5
Hydrogen peroxide	H_2O	77	2540	I-5
Hydrogen iodide, 1%	Neon	4.2	2537	F-14
Hydrogen iodide, 1%	Argon	4.2	2537	F-14
Hydrogen iodide, 1%	Krypton	4.2	2537	F-14
Hydrogen iodide, 1%	Xenon	4.2	2537	F-14
Nitromethane	Argon	20		P-10
Diazomethane	Nitrogen and argon	20		P-10

in matrices of neon, argon, krypton, and xenon illustrate the more elaborate requirements for these matrices. Using the apparatus already described in Fig. 7.5-8, a 1% mixture of HI in the matrix gas was deposited through the matrix slits onto the sapphire rod. In the photolytic experiments, the glass slits were replaced by a quartz or sapphire window to permit illuminating the sample with either light from a mercury (2537 Å) or hydrogen discharge. Samples about 0.5 mm thick required exposures ranging from 1 to 24 hr to generate an adequate concentration of radicals with a Hanovia SC-2537 mercury lamp. After sufficient radicals had been generated, the sapphire rod was lowered into the cavity for the EPR measurements as previously described. Figure 7.5-10 shows typical results for HI photolized in several matrices. Rapid passage effects are present in the two top curves; however, the most interesting feature of the spectra is the variety of satellite lines characteristic of the matrix. For example, the first line on the left of the argon matrix was observed also in the photolysis of H_2O and NH_3 in argon indicating the presence of several nonequivalent trapping sites for H atoms. The still more exotic structure for xenon presumably arises from interactions with the two isotopes ^{129}Xe ($I = \frac{1}{2}$) and ^{131}Xe ($I = \frac{3}{2}$). Nonmagnetic Ne, Ar, and the small abundance of ^{83}Kr favor simpler spectra in these matrices. Table 7.5-10 summarizes the results in Ref. F-14 for H atoms trapped in rare gas matrices. For purposes of

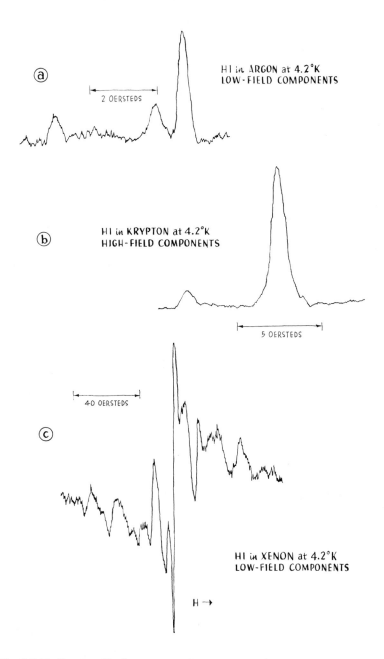

Fig. 7.5-10. Spectra of hydrogen atoms in rare gas matrices at 4.2°K: (*a*) produced by photolysis of HI in argon, low field component; (*b*) produced by photolysis of HI in krypton, high field component; (*c*) produced by photolysis of HI in xenon, low field component. The spectrometer and conditions are the same as those in Fig. 7.5-9. (Courtesy F-14.)

Table 7.5-10

Hyperfine Structure Constants and g Factors for H Atoms Produced by the
Photolysis of HI in Rare Gas Matrices (F-14)

Matrix	A, Mc/sec	$\Delta A/A_f$, %[a]	g	$-\Delta g$
Free state	1420.40573 (5)		2.002256 (24)	
Neon	1426.56 (20)	$+0.43$	2.00207 (8)	19×10^{-5}
Argon[b]	1413.82 (40)	-0.46	2.00220 (8)	6×10^{-5}
Argon	1413.82 (40)	-0.46	2.00220 (8)	6×10^{-5}
Argon	1416.30 (80)	-0.29	2.00224 (12)	2×10^{-5}
Argon	1436.24 (40)	$+1.15$	2.00161 (8)	65×10^{-5}
Krypton[b]	1411.79 (30)	-0.59	2.00179 (8)	47×10^{-5}
Krypton	1411.79 (30)	-0.59	2.00179 (8)	47×10^{-5}
Krypton	1427.06 (280)	$+0.47$	1.99967 (31)	259×10^{-5}
Xenon[b]	1404.99 (28)	-1.09	2.00170 (8)	56×10^{-5}
Xenon	1405.57 (34)	-1.04	2.00057 (8)	169×10^{-5}

[a] $\Delta A/A_f = (A_{\text{matrix}} - A_{\text{free state}})/A_{\text{free state}}$.
[b] Prepared by electrical discharge technique; numbers in parenthesis indicate experimental and/or conversion errors in the last figures of the associated values.

comparison, results for atoms deposited by the electrical discharge technique are listed along with values for the photolysis of HI. Argon has been used most extensively as the matrix and an impressive list of radicals have been studied with this system, e.g., Fig. 7.5-11 shows spectra for alkyl, formyl, and cyanogen free radicals. In each case, the solid matrix contained about 1% of the photosensitive base for the radical.

Other experimental arrangements suitable for photolyzing specimens both at 77 and 4.2°K are described in Section 7.6, for example, Fig. 7.6-4a to e.

(b) Indirect Process. Experimentally, the details of illumination and the EPR measurement are the same as those for direct photolyses. The only change involves selecting a matrix that will be attacked by the primary radicals to generate the species of interest. Because of its versatility, this process has been used more extensively in EPR studies than the direct process. Hydrogen peroxide and hydrogen iodide are convenient photosensitive materials as indicated by Table 7.5-11. Figure 7.5-12 shows the spectra for several of the alcohols listed in Table 7.5-11. These samples (5 mm diam × 10 mm long) initially contained about 10^{18}–10^{19} hydrogen peroxide molecules and about the same concentration of free radicals

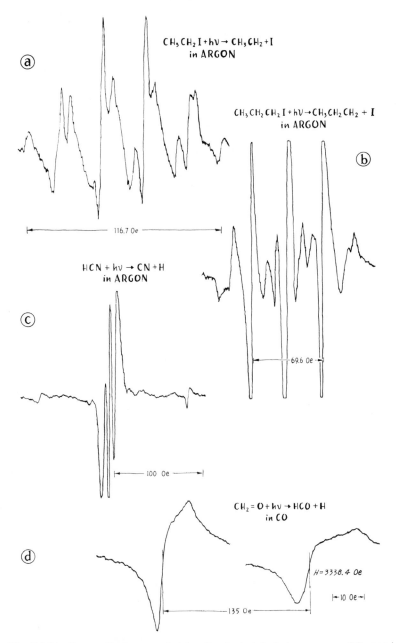

Fig. 7.5-11. Free radicals generated by direct photolysis in argon or CO matrix at 4.2°K: (a) ethyl iodide in argon matrix (courtesy C-15); (b) n-propyl iodide in argon matrix (courtesy C-15); (c) HCN in argon matrix (courtesy C-14); (d) CH_2O in CO matrix (courtesy A-3). The spectrometer and conditions are the same as those in Fig. 7.5-9.

Table 7.5-11

Preparation of Radicals by Indirect Photolysis

Glass	Photosensitive ingredient and amount	Temp, °K	Exciting wave-length, Å	Time, hr	Ref.
Methanol (50%); water (50%)	H_2O_2, 10^{-1} to $10^{-2}M$	77	3650	6	G-4
Ethanol (90%); phosphoric acid (10%)	H_2O_2, 10^{-1} to $10^{-2}M$	77	3650	6	G-4
n-Propanol	H_2O_2, 10^{-1} to $10^{-2}M$	77	3650	6	G-4
Allyl alcohol	H_2O_2, 10^{-1} to $10^{-2}M$	77	3650	6	G-4
Cyclohexanol	H_2O_2, 10^{-1} to $10^{-2}M$	77	3650	6	G-4
Ethylene glycol (50%); water (50%)	H_2O_2, 10^{-1} to $10^{-2}M$	77	3650	6	G-4
Propylene glycol (50%); water (50%)	H_2O_2, 10^{-1} to $10^{-2}M$	77	3560	6	G-4
Glycerol (50%); water (50%)	H_2O_2, 10^{-1} to $10^{-2}M$	77	3650	6	G-4
Diethyl ether (50%); phosphoric acid (50%)	H_2O_2, 10^{-1} to $10^{-2}M$	77	3650	6	G-4
n-, sec-, and tert-Butyl alcohol		90	3650		F-15
tert-Amyl alcohol		90	3650		F-15
Isopropanol		77	3650		F-15
HCO_2H	H_2O_2, $0.4M$	77	2537 3130 3650		B-32
HI	CO	4.2	2537		B-32
CH_3CHO	H_2O_2, $0.4M$	77	2537 3130 3650		B-32

developed under long irradiation (F-15). In Ref. C-14 HCO radicals were produced by three reactions:

(a) $HI \xrightarrow{h\nu} I + H$ CO matrix

                $H + CO \longrightarrow HCO$

(b) $CH_2O \xrightarrow{h\nu} HCO + H$ Argon matrix

(c) $CH_3OH \xrightarrow{3h\nu} HCO + 3H$ Argon matrix

The observed spectra were very similar to Fig. 7.5-11; however, the indirect process a gave a substantially better signal to noise ratio. Brivati et al. (B-32) summarize a variety of experiments which give rise to trapped formyl radicals.

(c) Conversion. Reaction (c) above is an example of the conversion process involving multiple photon absorption and bond rupture in a single

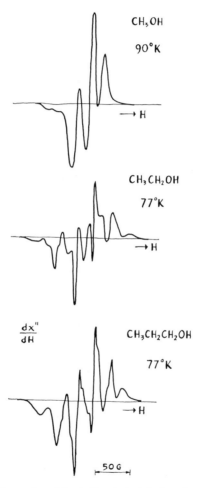

Fig. 7.5-12. Radicals produced by indirect photolysis using 3650 Å illumination to decompose hydrogen peroxide in solid alcohols: spectrometer type, TH1-X; cavity, rectangular TE_{104}, entire cavity cooled; temperature, 77 and 90°K; modulation, 100 kc, internal hairpin loop; samples illuminated in quartz tubes through a hole in the bottom of the cavity. (Courtesy F-15.)

molecule. The first photon removes a hydrogen to produce a radical with the three-line spectrum shown for CH_3OH in Fig. 7.5-12. This radical has an absorption peak in the ultraviolet and additional illumination removes additional hydrogen atoms, leaving the HCO radical of Fig. 7.5-11. Conversion is not limited to radicals produced by photolysis and frequently the products of ionizing radiation can be converted either optically or thermally—a procedure which may assist in clarifying the spectrum and identifying the radical.

7.5.6   Radicals by Radiolysis

Two factors contribute to the extensive use of ionizing radiation in the production of radicals for EPR observations. First, there is inherent interest in radicals of this origin because of their prominent role in radiation effects and radiation chemistry. Second, the method is convenient and almost universally effective, i.e., radicals can be produced in detectable quantities in virtually any solid dielectric. Fortunately all finesse is not lost in going from the specific excitation of photolysis to the random ionization of radiolysis. As previously mentioned we are saved from a conceivably hopeless mess of an infinite variety of radicals by mechanisms which usually limit the products to one or two species. These mechanisms are the Franck-Condon principle which describes how electronic transitions occur before the associated nuclei have time to move and the Franck-Rabinowitch cage which confines the decomposition fragments in a rigid network of neighboring molecules (A-5). The rapid electronic transitions reduce the importance of the particular electron and electronic state involved in the initial excitation because the electrons can adjust so quickly that essentially all molecules can rupture while in the same electronic state. The cage will favor the recombination of reactive fragments and will restore the original molecule or form another stable molecule unless one of the radicals can escape from the cage. Under these conditions small fragments such as hydrogen atoms have a better opportunity to escape, and experience with organic chemicals subjected to ionizing irradiation shows that hydrogen atoms are the predominant escapees. In designing an experiment it is important to consider how escape proof the cage is going to be for the materials and temperature involved. The cage must have sufficient rigidity to trap radicals long enough for observation yet be flexible enough for their initial formation. Obviously, the qualities which make it possible for small fragments to escape from the parent molecule also interfere with trapping before they react to form stable molecules. For example, hydrogen molecules are commonly observed in irradiated aliphatic compounds but trapped hydrogen atoms are a rarity, requiring either a matrix with a low affinity for hydrogen atoms or the rigidity possible only at very low temperatures. Control of the cage rigidity then is one of the important experimental variables. Usually the molecules under investigation provide their own matrix; therefore, once this selection is made, the remaining control of rigidity is achieved with temperature. Within the almost unlimited variations of organic compounds it is frequently possible to generate the same radical from a variety of starting points. Thus, the material is undoubtedly the most versatile variable. Sometimes as in energy transfer experiments it is not only practical but necessary to mix the test molecules with inert matrix molecules. The other main experimental parameters are the radiation characteristics, i.e., particle, dose rate, and total dose.

(a) Sample Preparation. The decision whether to generate the radicals in the cavity or to transfer them to the cavity after production outside is common to all methods of generation; however, in radiolysis experiments the choice becomes more involved because radicals develop in all dielectric containers suitable for external preparation. Some of the factors to be considered are as follows:

1. Sample characteristics: the melting point, structure—single crystal or glassy, desired sample purity, and the thermal and optical stability of the unpaired spins. Obviously the transfer technique is simplified when the sample material is solid at room temperature, the radicals generated are stable, and no complications arise from exposure to the atmosphere.

2. Irradiation source: the type of particle, source strength, and accessibility. Normally more irradiation time is required to prepare a number of samples when they are irradiated one at a time in the cavity than to expose a group of vials simultaneously.

3. Sample temperature: sample manipulation is relatively simple and straightforward down to liquid nitrogen temperature but transfer operations are considerably more difficult at liquid helium temperature.

4. EPR parameters to be measured, e.g., spin detection, hfs and g values, are easily satisfied with either type of sample; however, G values* require high precision in dosimetry and exposure, and the choice between internal and external preparation is not always obvious.

In most laboratories studying radicals down to 77°K the radicals are generated externally and transferred to the cavity dewar for the EPR measurement. Early commercial cavities as well as many homemade models were designed to accommodate internal dewars and samples mounted in simple vials. Frequently free radical studies involve numerous samples; therefore, the ease and speed of sample change associated with external irradiation are attractive features, provided all the advantages are

---

* The G value equals the number of radicals produced per 100 eV of energy absorbed.

not lost in correcting for the spins induced in the sample container. At lower temperatures it is usually advisable to irradiate the sample in the cavity, or at least the cavity dewar, to minimize manipulations.

(b) Quick and Dirty Techniques. "Quick" and "dirty" are both relative terms in need of further clarification but unfortunately the literature seldom provides information about the effects of small amounts of contamination on the EPR spectra. Normally samples consist of the purest material readily available and aside from scavenger experiments little attention goes to intentional adulteration. In samples "out of the bottle" the foreign atoms are statistically greatly outnumbered so that unless they are particularly good scavengers for radicals, electrons, or energy, their small contribution to the EPR spectrum will be negligible, particularly in detection and identification experiments. Scavengers are known to effect radical yields; therefore, more attention to such impurities is important in G-value measurements. Here we will classify as quick and dirty those techniques where materials are used as they come out of the bottle or chunk without degassing and where contact with the air is involved.

Materials that are solid at room temperatures, crystals, plastics, or glasses are readily irradiated by using the techniques described in Section 7.3. The arrangements of Fig. 7.3-4 are suitable for low-voltage x-rays, up to 50 kV, and electrons accelerated to several MeV. Pill box a is for room temperature exposures and containers b or c are for irradiations at 77°K.

Many compounds that are liquid at room temperature readily stabilize radicals at 77°K and samples are conveniently prepared as small balls by freezing drops of the sample in liquid nitrogen. Figure 7.5-13 shows several arrangements for ball production. At a drops regulated in size by the medicine dropper tip fall on the surface of the liquid nitrogen. Rapid localized boiling in the nitrogen buoys up the drop so that many liquids will float on the surface until frozen, then they sink to the bottom out of the way. Usually, it is best to have only one ball on the surface at a time because two or more balls are prone to stick together as an oversized ball or a dumbbell. When a large number of balls are desired, glass beakers make satisfactory dividers so that several balls can freeze simultaneously as indicated at b. Oxygen is easily excluded with a plastic bag tent as shown at c where the nitrogen boiloff keeps the bag inflated against the masking tape seal. When manufacturing balls wholesale the added visibility through a small window of clear plastic taped into the polyethylene bag is worth the slight taping effort. A hypodermic syringe is ideal for dispensing drops through the plastic bag. Black plastic electrical insulation tape is convenient for patching syringe holes and other leaks.

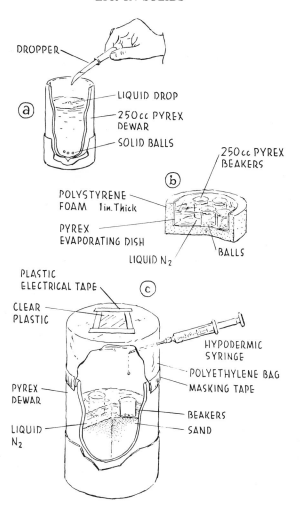

Fig. 7.5-13. Three simple arrangements for freezing ball samples of organic materials.

Several handy tools for manipulating the balls are indicated in Fig. 7.5-14. Balls are inserted and recovered from internal cavity dewars with the grapplers which also provide the necessary restraint to prevent excessive sample bounce due to the bubbling nitrogen. In the quartz four-prong design both the spherical tips and the prongs should be of uniform size otherwise the sample is prone to escape past the weaker prong. Also, the quartz is quite fragile and easily broken. The Teflon arrangement is not as fragile but it shields the sample and interferes with illumination of the ball

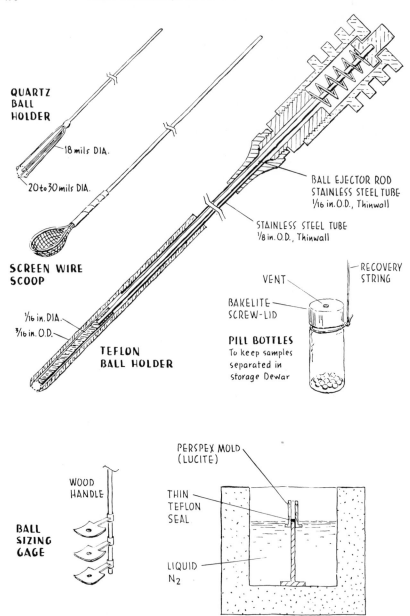

QUARTZ
BALL
HOLDER

18 mils DIA.

20 to 30 mils DIA.

SCREEN WIRE
SCOOP

1/16 in. DIA.

3/16 in. O.D.

TEFLON
BALL HOLDER

BALL EJECTOR ROD
STAINLESS STEEL TUBE
1/16 in. O.D., Thinwall

STAINLESS STEEL TUBE
1/8 in. O.D., Thinwall

VENT

RECOVERY
STRING

BAKELITE
SCREW-LID

PILL BOTTLES
To keep samples
separated in
storage Dewar

BALL
SIZING
GAGE

WOOD
HANDLE

PERSPEX MOLD
(LUCITE)

THIN
TEFLON
SEAL

LIQUID
N_2

Fig. 7.5-14. Simple tools for manipulating ball samples, i.e., grapples, scoop, sizing gage, and storage bottles. Materials that do not form good balls in liquid N_2 can be solidified in the slug mold (21).

in the cavity. For comparative measurements the sample balls should be the same size and since there is normally some variation in drop size, a size gage is convenient for finding matched samples. The screen scoops and storage bottle along with a few wooden sticks, some twine, and masking tape complete the tool kit for ball handling.

Many compounds become colored under ionizing irradiation and some of these color centers are photosensitive; therefore, it may be desirable to work in subdued colored light to avoid converting the color centers. Also many radicals are sufficiently stable under liquid nitrogen storage to last for years; we still have a few bottles of 1956 vintage radicals in irradiated ethanol. All materials do not form sound balls directly in liquid nitrogen in which case it may be necessary to freeze slugs in a refrigerated mold. Table 7.5-12 lists the freezing characteristics of a few common compounds

Table 7.5-12

Freezing Characteristics of Some Organic Materials Prepared as Ball Samples

Compound	Grade[a]	Melting point, °K	Mechanical soundness of balls	Transparency	Remarks
Hydrocarbons					
n-Pentane	P-research	143	Very poor	White	Full of N_2 bubbles
n-Heptane	P-research	182	Very poor	White	Full of N_2 bubbles
n-Octane	P-research	216	Poor	White	Full of N_2 bubbles
n-Nonane	P-research	219	Fair	White	Multicrystalline
n-Decane	P-pure	243	Fair	White	Multicrystalline
n-Undecane	P-tech.	247	Fair	White	Multicrystalline
Alcohols					
Methyl		175	Good	Mostly cloudy	Multicrystalline
Ethyl		159	Good	Clear	Glassy
n-Propyl	E-Red	146	Good	Clear	Glassy
n-Butyl	M-Ar	183	Good	Clear	Glassy
isoPropyl	E-Red	184	Good	Clear	Glassy
isoButyl	M-Ar	165	Fair	Mostly cloudy	
n-Amyl	B-Ar	194	Good	Clear	Glassy
isoAmyl	M-Ar	156	Good	Clear	Glassy
Ketones					
Acetone	B-Ar	254	Poor	White	Frequently broke
Methyl ethyl	Tech.	186	Fair	White	
Diethyl	Tech.	233	Fair	White	
isopropyl	Tech.		Very poor	White	Multicrystalline
Ethers					
Dimethyl		135			
Diethyl		157			
n-Propyl			Good	Clear	Glassy
Isopropyl			Good	Clear	Glassy
n-Butyl			Good	Clear	Glassy

(continued)

Table 7.5-12 (*continued*)

Compound	Grade[a]	Melting point, °K	Mechanical soundness of balls	Trans- parency	Remarks
Esters					
Methyl formate		174			
Ethyl formate	E-Red	194	Fair	White	N_2 bubbles
Methyl acetate	E-Pract.	174	Good	Clear	
Ethyl acetate	M-Ar	189	Good	Clear	
Amyl acetate	B	202	Good	Clear	
Alkyl halides					
Chloroform	B-Ar	210	Fair	White	Irregular, small
Methylene chloride	Tech.	176	Fair	White	Irregular, small
Ethylene chloride	MCB-Red	104	Fair	White	Irregular, small
Carbon tetra- chloride	M-Ar	250	Fair	White	Irregular, small
Ethyl iodide	E-Red	162	Poor		Stuck to container
Miscellaneous					
Ethylene glycol	E-Red	257	Fair		
Glacial acetic acid	Me-USP		Fair		
Acetic anhydride	E-Red	200	Good	Clear	
Pyruvic acid	E-Red	287	Poor	Opaque	Many N_2 bubbles
CS_2	9.9%	162	Poor	Opaque	Fragile
Glycerol	MCB-R	291	Good	Clear	Glassy

[a] B = Baker; E = Eastman; M = Mallenckrodt; MCB = Matheson, Colman, and Bell; Me = Merck; P = Phillips; Red = red label; Ar = analytical reagent; VSP = 99.5%; R = reagent grade.

and Fig. 7.5-14 shows a simple slug maker used successfully by Henriksen (21).

(c) **Vial Techniques.** Despite the complication of spins generated in the container the customary procedure for protecting chemical compounds from the atmosphere and associated contaminants is to seal the samples in glass or quartz vials. Various practices have evolved for dealing with the undesired spins induced in the vial during irradiation experiments. In fortunate cases the container spins do not interfere with the sample spectrum either because they resonate at a different magnetic field or because their amplitude is too small to distort appreciably the total curve. Figure 7.5-15*a* is an example of this second situation where the quartz line in the spectrum of irradiated acetonitrile not only produced little inter-

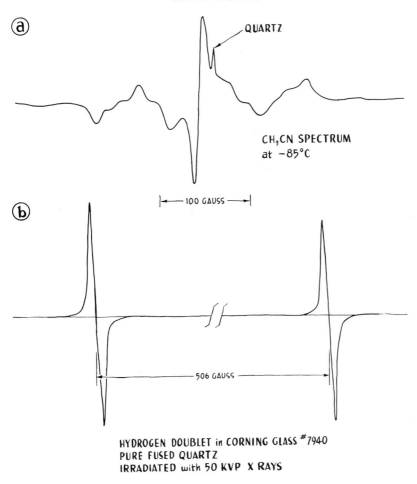

Fig. 7.5-15. Spectra of unpaired spins generated in quartz vials by γ-rays or x-rays. (a) The single quartz line in irradiated acetonitrile does not interfere seriously (courtesy H-2). However, hydrogen atoms would be hard to study in samples enclosed in the pure quartz responsible for the spectra at (b).

ference but proved useful as a secondary standard for indicating the magnetic field. In contrast, quartz containers should be avoided or at least used with extreme caution when looking for hydrogen atoms in samples irradiated at low temperatures. For example, pure silica quartz produced by burning silane gas is favored for optical experiments in radiation environments because of its low coloring rate; however, the hydrogen doublet shown in Fig. 7.5-15*b* develops when the quartz is irradiated at 77°K. Other grades of quartz do not have such a high yield of hydrogen atoms but the vials should be checked for spins before looking for radicals in the samples.

When container spins are a problem, the vials can be prepared in matched pairs so that one can be exposed empty to provide the container correction. This procedure is practical only when the irradiation source generates penetrating particles or rays that will produce essentially the same ionization in the full and empty vial.

The sliding slug technique is probably the most reliable arrangement for avoiding container spins and it certainly has the largest following of practitioners. As the name implies the sample is irradiated in one end of the vial and the EPR measurements are made in the other end which is shielded during the irradiation. Sometimes with large doses of penetrating particles, spins will develop throughout the vial but this can be corrected by annealing the measuring end with a torch while the sample end is cooled in an appropriate bath, e.g., H_2O, liquid nitrogen. The sliding slug is ideal for samples that are solid at room temperature. If the sample is a powder, it may be desirable to pelletize the material to avoid the possibility of fine powder clinging to the wrong end of the vial. Slug preparation can become a full blown ceremony for materials with very low freezing points and a propensity to pick up impurities from the atmosphere or coolant. The slug maker of Fig. 7.5-14 is adequate when the nitrogen and its boiloff provides sufficient protection, otherwise a truly dry "dry" box may be required. Figure 7.5-16 shows an elaborate apparatus for freezing slugs at liquid nitrogen temperature in a dry helium atmosphere. The ritual begins with drying the box after it has been stocked with tools and sealed vials of sample materials. Alternate evacuation and flushing with dry helium is continued until no dew freezes on the polished copper top of the freezing well at liquid nitrogen temperature. Slugs are (*1*) frozen in Teflon molds inserted in the freezing well; (*2*) sheared to length, thereby removing the Teflon stopper; (*3*) transferred to the vacuum lock position; and (*4*) extruded into the refrigerated sample tube. Next the vacuum lock is closed, the helium pressure in the sample tube is reduced with a mechanical pump to approximately 10^{-3} torr, and the sample tube is sealed off. Sufficient helium is left in the sample tube to provide good heat transfer between the slug and the walls. The vacuum lock allows the next sample tube to be attached and evacuated without disturbing the dry box atmosphere so that slug production can continue until the supply of Teflon molds, sample tubes, or patience is depleted. One complication was the moisture which apparently diffused through the gloves from moist hands—hence the ventilated double glove arrangement.

Exposure arrangements vary from simple at room temperature to

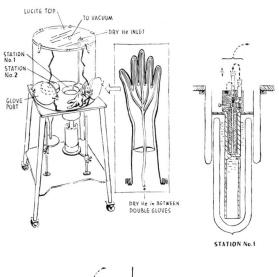

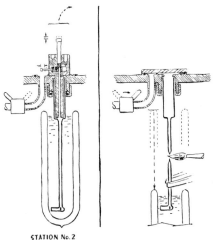

Fig. 7.5-16. Details of dry box, ventilated double glove, and plug making ritual. Dry helium gas flows between the double gloves and carries away perspiration so it will not diffuse through the rubber into the box. Plug molding procedure: (*a*) Insert the copper freezing block into the liquid nitrogen cooled socket at station 1. (*b*) Place the mold in the freezing block, fill it with sample material, and freeze the liquid. These molds are hollow Teflon cylinders 2.5 mm i.d. plugged at the bottom with a Teflon stopper. (*c*) Transfer mold to center hole, insert the prechilled driver above the mold and force the sample down until the stopper is within the horizontal shear block. (*d*) Move the freezing block to station 2. (*e*) Slide shear block horizontally to remove stopper so it will not go into "duck" along with sample. (*f*) Force the driver down to eject sample from mold into the precooled glass "duck." (*g*) Return freezing block to station 1 after dumping the stopper out of the shear block onto the bottom of the dry box. (*h*) Install the glass cover on station 2 O-ring seal and evacuate the glass duck. (*i*) Lower the dewar at station 2 and seal off the "duck." (Courtesy M-3.)

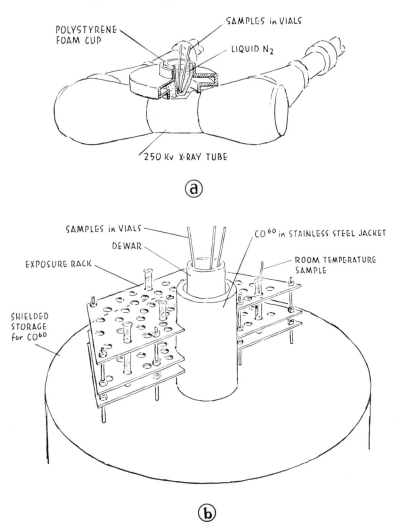

Fig. 7.5-17. Three arrangements for exposing samples in vials to x-ray or γ-ray irradiation. (*a*) Maximization of the irradiation rate with a conventional 250 kV x-ray tube (21). (*b*) Exposures at various temperatures and dose rates with a ^{60}Co source (12).

involved at 4°K. Figure 7.5-17 shows *a* a conventional x-ray tube source where it is desirable to locate the samples close to the target for maximum exposure rates, *b* a convenient ^{60}Co source which generates 3×10^6 rads/hr at the center of the cylinder, and *c* a submersible Au target on a 2 MeV Van de Graaff generator capable of generating about 5×10^6 R/hr at the

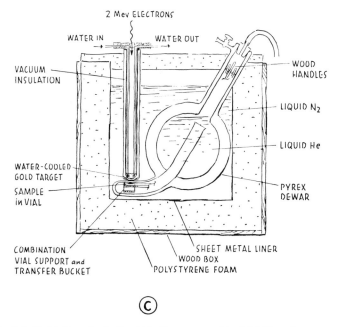

2 Mev ELECTRONS

WATER IN → ← WATER OUT

VACUUM INSULATION

WOOD HANDLES

LIQUID N₂

LIQUID He

WATER-COOLED GOLD TARGET

SAMPLE in VIAL

PYREX DEWAR

COMBINATION VIAL SUPPORT and TRANSFER BUCKET

SHEET METAL LINER

WOOD BOX

POLYSTYRENE FOAM

ⓒ

Fig. 7.5-17. (c) Samples in liquid helium exposed to 2 MeV peak x-rays.

samples. The float systems (Fig. 7.3-4c) used with the ball samples are practical for samples in tubes; however, a fine control of the liquid level is required for reliable dosages. Sealed vials are also suitable for irradiation with electron sources, provided the glass wall is thin enough to admit the electrons without undue loss of energy. Figure 7.5-18 shows a carrousel for rotating sample tubes "ducks" under a 2 MeV electron beam. The thin window, approximately 0.020 in. thick, always rests above the liquid nitrogen level so that the impedence in the electron's path is constant. Aluminum is used for the star shaped "duck" support, Faraday cup, and beam-limiting iris in order to minimize Bremsstrahlung production and the attendant irradiation of the measurement ends of the vials. Lead shields provide further protection but the Pyrex stems frequently require annealing because some spins form despite these precautions. The fog shield and overlapping sleeves maintain a dry atmosphere over the samples so that the duck heads remain free from frost and the fog generated during the periodic liquid nitrogen replenishments cannot interfere with the electron beam. Wave, splashing, and fog problems are further reduced by making all nitrogen additions in the outer channel, which in turn fills the sample chamber through small holes at the bottom of the wave baffle. With the rotation speed of 1 rpm and a 2 MeV electron beam spread over the 1 in.

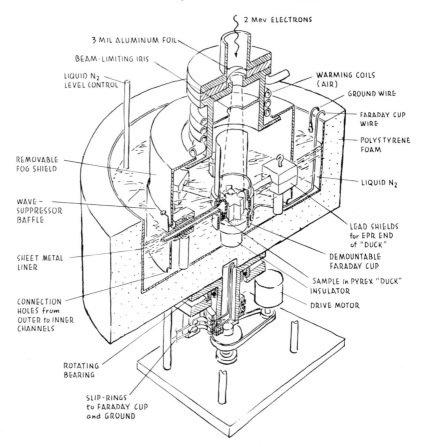

Fig. 7.5-18. Carrousel for exposing 6 vials simultaneously to the same average dose of 2 MeV electrons. (Courtesy M-3.)

diameter sample area, a power input of 7 W generated a barely detectable temperature increase in samples monitored with thermocouples, but cooled with the usual partial pressure of helium; however, exposures were generally limited to 0.5 W. Typical exposure times ranged from 1 to 30 hr so that nonuniformities in the electron beam distribution were averaged out by the sample rotation. After exposure the duck is transferred to a 250 cm^3 dewar where the spins in the measuring end are removed by heating, then the sample is transferred to the narrow end by suitable tapping and incantations while the whole duck is submerged.

Figure 7.5-19 shows an irradiation system and cavity dewar used with quartz vials at 4.2°K. The 2000 curie ^{60}Co source is shielded by water. Therefore, the dewars are sealed in a submersible water-tight container

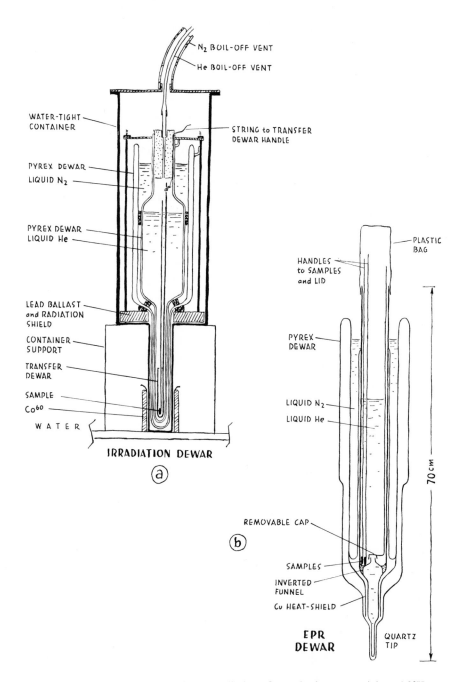

Fig. 7.5-19. (*a*) Dewar system for γ-irradiation of samples in quartz vials at 4.2°K. The ⁶⁰Co source is shielded in a pool of water. (*b*) Liquid helium dewar for EPR measurements at 4.2°K. (Courtesy W-2.)

equipped with vent tubes which conduct the boiloff gases to the surface where two gas meters monitor the consumption of the refrigerants. Plastic hoses are superior to rubber tubing for this application because radiation damage causes the rubber to disintegrate very quickly. A combination lead ballast and shield sinks the container and reduces λ-ray heating of the refrigerants. One 5.5 liter charge of helium last more than 48 hr; however, the 6 liter nitrogen container required filling at 12 hr intervals. Seven samples of about $3 \times 10^{-3}M$ in 3.5 mm o.d. high-purity quartz vials can be irradiated simultaneously. After irradiation the samples are transferred to the EPR cavity dewar with the aid of the small transfer dewar. The fog and snow generated in this maneuver are little short of spectacular and quantities of unwanted frozen air accumulate here and there; therefore, an inverted funnel and cap are incorporated in the design to keep the solid air and ice out of the EPR dewar tip. After the transfer the samples are arranged around the walls, always keeping the vials under the liquid helium; the transfer dewar is removed; and the polyethylene bag is installed. All subsequent manipulations, removing the cap, inserting samples in the tip, etc., are performed with the bag in place. Considerable ability is required to examine a series of samples without getting enough air particles into the tip to interfere either mechanically or thermally by blocking circulation of the liquid helium in the narrow tip. One way to avoid the air problem is to make the original transfer in a helium atmosphere, e.g., in a large polyethylene bag sealed to the necks of the dewars and inflated with helium gas. Incidentally the bag should contain an exhaust vent to accommodate the helium boiloff from the transfer dewar.

(d) Irradiations in the Cavity. Again there is no "best" arrangement for all experiments. Therefore, we will consider three alternatives: (1) simultaneous irradiation and EPR measurements; (2) irradiation followed by EPR measurements without moving the dewar; and (3) irradiation and EPR measurements in different locations. The first two possibilities are convenient from a manipulation standpoint, particularly when liquid helium is the refrigerant; however, they require exclusive use of the radiation source. For simultaneous irradiations and measurements the spectrometer control position must be shielded from the intense irradiation which involves remote control from outside the target room of electron accelerators. Alternatives (1) and (2) are most convenient and efficient when a series of exposures are slated for a single sample as when measuring radical yields (G values), radical concentration saturation, or unstable short-lived radicals (numerous irradiations and short EPR measurements on the same sample). When only one irradiation is required per sample and the time is short compared with the EPR study, the third procedure permits more efficient use of the source. When the irradiation and measurement times are about equal, several cavities permit both devices to run continuously.

As always, samples that are solid at room temperature allow more selection in cavity styles and greater freedom in mounting than liquid samples. To avoid the generation of extraneous spins, cements and dielectric supports should be avoided or confined to regions of the cavity where H_1 is essentially zero. When liquids are to be frozen in the cavity, a rectangular TE_{10n} or cylindrical TE_{111} mode satisfies the gravitational requirements with a suitable H_1 field at the bottom of the cavity. Cavities at the bottom of long dewars are conveniently filled through the coupling hole by using a hypodermic syringe equipped with a 2 or 3 ft needle as required to reach the cavity. Stainless steel and other noncorrosive tubing is available with outside diameters ranging down to 0.003 in. and 0.0005 in. wall thickness.* When working with fixed cavity dewar systems a collection of thin-walled $\frac{1}{8}$ and $\frac{3}{16}$ in. diameter stainless steel or brass tubes are useful for removing spent samples by vacuum, introducing washing solutions, and drying the cavity with warm air.

Figure 7.5-20 indicates two arrangements at 300 Mc for either simultaneous or consecutive irradiations and EPR measurements. Both systems involve similar coaxial cavities and solenoid magnets but the samples in *a* are cooled with crushed ice and irradiated with ^{60}Co γ-rays while at *b* they are cooled with liquid helium and irradiated with 2 MeV electrons. A technique for irradiating liquid samples in an X-band cavity was described in connection with Fig. 6.2-6 where the electrons reached the cavity through a coaxial hole in the magnet pole. A similar arrangement for radical production in solids is illustrated in Fig. 7.5-21 where 2 MeV electrons pass through a 6 mm hole in the pole, leave the vacuum through a 50 μ thick aluminum foil, and enter the TE_{102} cavity through a hole in the broad face to irradiate the sample. Inhomogeneities in the magnetic field at the sample location because of the hole in the magnet were about 0.8 Oe/mm along the path of the electron beam so that the line broadening for the typical spectra from samples 1–2 mm thick was negligible, i.e., the lines are typically 10 Oe wide. Exposure times were controlled by the shutter and a pancake-type ionization chamber monitored the electron beam, both to determine the dose rate and to permit control of the uniformity of the electron beam. This chamber consisted of two 5 μ foils separated by a 5 mm gap. With 160 V between the electrodes the current was approximately ten times the current measured on the shutter. The nitrogen boiler cooling system could maintain the sample at any temperature between -150 and $+150°C$ to within $\pm 1°C$ for exposure rates of up to 3×10^6 rads/sec.

---

* One source is Uniform Tubes, Inc., Collegeville, Pa.

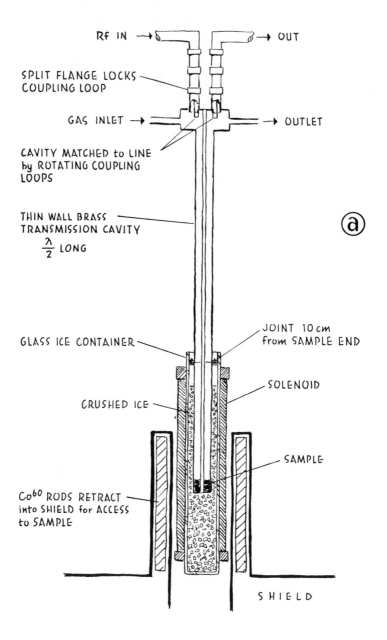

Fig. 7.5-20. Two arrangements for irradiating samples directly in cavities suitable for 300 Mc spectrometers. (a) The coaxial cavity is immersed in the cooling liquid and surrounded by the ^{60}Co source (12).

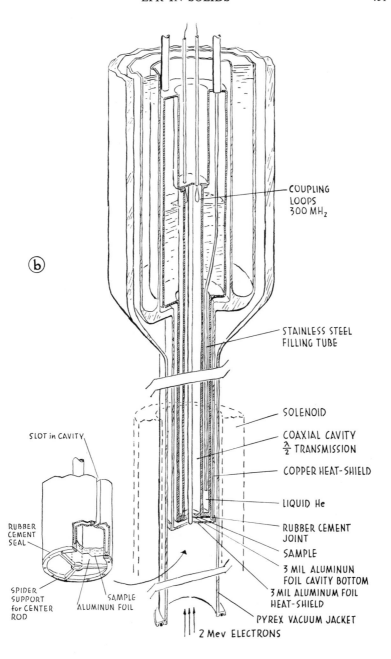

COUPLING
LOOPS
300 MH$_z$

STAINLESS STEEL
FILLING TUBE

SOLENOID

COAXIAL CAVITY
$\frac{\lambda}{2}$ TRANSMISSION

COPPER HEAT-SHIELD

LIQUID He

RUBBER CEMENT
JOINT

SAMPLE

3 MIL ALUMINUN
FOIL CAVITY BOTTOM

3 MIL ALUMINUM FOIL
HEAT-SHIELD

PYREX VACUUM JACKET

2 Mev ELECTRONS

SLOT in CAVITY

RUBBER
CEMENT
SEAL

SPIDER
SUPPORT
for CENTER
ROD

SAMPLE
ALUMINUN FOIL

Fig. 7.5-20. (b) The sample at 4.2°K is irradiated with 2 MeV electrons entering the
bottom of the cavity through a foil window.

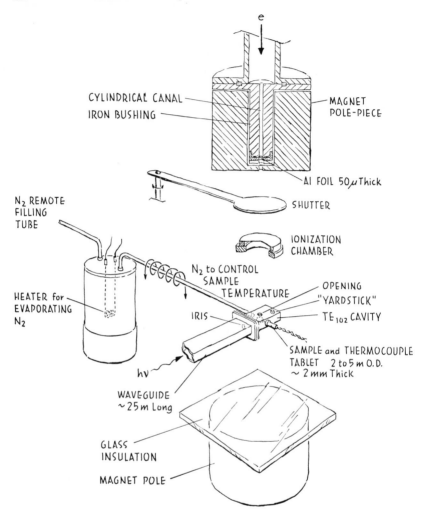

Fig. 7.5-21. Arrangement for EPR measurements on solid samples during irradiation with 2 MeV electrons. (After M-11.)

When exposures are made with the magnetic field turned off, electrons can be shot into the cavity along any accessible path, e.g., through the coupling iris or through a hole or thin section in the bottom or side of the cavity.

Irradiations with x-ray tubes and γ-ray sources are usually performed outside the magnet because of space limitations. Furthermore, the magnetic field would interfere with operation of the x-ray tube by deflecting the electrons emitted at the cathode.

The third category, radiations and measurements in different locations, embraces a host of variations ranging from moving the dewar to the edge of the magnet to transportation measured in terms of rooms or even miles. Low-voltage x-ray tubes of the 50 kV, 50 mA beryllium window variety can be used adjacent to the spectrometer either by moving the magnet away from the cavity or vice versa as discussed in Section 4.2.

Aluminum or beryllium foil windows are convenient for admitting the low-energy x-rays and a simple lead shield $\frac{1}{4}$ in. thick will provide sufficient protection with these 50 or 60 kV x-rays.

Figure 7.5-22 shows a dewar and cavity arrangement used in a series of studies involving hydrogen atoms and energy transfer in various rigid matrices, irradiated at 4.2°K with ^{60}Co γ-rays. Samples of CH_4, H_2O, HF, H_2, and mixtures in argon or krypton were deposited directly on the cavity

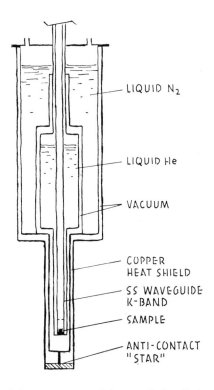

Fig. 7.5-22. Cavity and dewar system used for sample irradiation and EPR measurements, all at 4.2°K. The source was ^{60}Co (37).

walls, cooled to 4.2°K, transported to the ^{60}Co source, irradiated, and returned to the spectrometer, all steps taking place in the metal dewar. Forming the deposit in the cavity proved to be a considerable problem because the material tended to freeze out all over the inside of the cold waveguide. In addition the small iris hole further restricted the material getting into the cavity so that some of the measurements were made in a terminated waveguide without a cavity. Two preparation rituals were used: (1) The cavity was attached to the vacuum system, evacuated, closed off from the pump, filled with gas or a mixture of gases at the desired pressure (mixtures were allowed to mix for times ranging from a few minutes to an hour), cooled to 77°K until the sample froze, detached from the gas handling line, and finally cooled to 4.2°K in the helium dewar. (2) The evacuation and filling procedure were the same as above but the cavity was detached and inserted directly into the liquid helium bath to freeze the sample. When the freezing point of the sample is above 77°K, the case for most samples, the first procedure is most convenient for handling and permits closer control of the sample location because the cavity can be cooled while the waveguide is maintained above the freezing temperature. The all-metal dewar is similar in design to a number of commercial liquid helium dewars.

7.5.7 Radiation Sources and Doses

Here we consider a few characteristics of radiation sources pertinent to radical production. Aside from a very few experiments where the specific ionization of heavy particles is an important parameter in the study, radicals are virtually universally generated with light particles such as x-ray and γ-ray photons or electrons. The relative advantages of the various light particle sources depend on the nature of the EPR investigation. In qualitative or relative measurements such as hfs studies for radical identification or simple detection to follow radical reaction processes, the main requirement is a good signal-to-noise ratio, the distribution of the spins in the sample is usually unimportant, and any source of x-ray, γ-ray or electrons is satisfactory. Conversely, quantitative measurements of yield (G value) require uniform spin distributions and accurate dosimetry; therefore, penetrating γ-rays are preferred. Furthermore, ^{60}Co γ-rays readily penetrate the dewars, cavities, and sample holders so that no special access windows or ports are required as in the case of electrons or low-voltage x-rays. Of course, as a result of this penetration most of the energy is absorbed at extraneous locations in the system so that intense sources or lengthy exposures are required to get sufficient energy into the sample. Where access is available, electrons or high-intensity x-ray sources permit the shortest exposures, limited only by sample heating in the case of electrons.

At this point a precaution should be mentioned that may save an occasional accelerator tube window when radicals are generated with electrons. Some materials have a tendency to explode with considerable vigor when irradiated in liquid nitrogen exposed to the atmosphere, e.g., the ketones, particularly heptanone. Such difficulties are not encountered when the samples are in vacuum or an inert atmosphere such as helium or nitrogen. Radioactive isotopes such as tritium and carbon-13 can be incorporated either in the sample molecules or in mixtures to form an internal source of β-rays. According to Kroh and Spinks (K-16) the advantages of this arrangement are uniform ionization throughout the sample volume and minimum spin production in dielectric sample containers. When the contents are miscible with water, about 10% T_2O added to the sample provided adequate radiation. The extra precaution in handling the radioactive materials either in preparation or in disposing of the spent samples reduces the attraction of this method for most "quick" and "dirty" experiments.

Table 7.5-13 lists typical exposure data from various laboratories for a variety of sources and sample materials. In general, the total exposures are about 10^6 rads and this dose is useful in planning experiments; however, differences in radical yield for various molecules and temperatures can change this number by an order of magnitude so that a preliminary observation with one of the quick and dirty arrangements is often advisable before designing an elaborate dewar system where the required helium capacity will depend on the exposure time. Also the radical saturation concentration curve, Fig. 7.5-1, should be established for each material and temperature before commencing quantitative yield measurements.

7.5.8 Typical Results

As expected radicals generated by radiolysis also have spectroscopic splitting factors within the range from 2.0023 to 2.01 and little attention is given to the g factor. Table 7.5-14 illustrates the range with g values from the relatively few scattered sources where such measurements were made. In contrast G values (yield values) play an important role in radiolysis and numerous measurements are reported in the literature. Unfortunately, spin concentration measurements are beset with problems of rf saturation, filling factors, cavity Q's, reliable yardsticks, and other complications mentioned in Chapter V. When these complications are coupled with the uncertainties frequently encountered in determining the energy absorbed, i.e., dosimetry, it is not surprising that G values reported from various laboratories may exhibit considerable dispersion. Relative accuracies can be quite good for a series of similar molecules irradiated and measured under identical conditions; however, absolute yields may easily contain errors of 50–100%. When confronted with such dispersion, the experimental

Table 7.5-13
Typical Irradiation Conditions

Materials	Source	Dose rate	Total doses	Temp, °K	Ref.
H_2O, D_2O, H_2S, HF, HCl, H_2, CH_4, NaH, LiH, CD_4 in N_2	^{60}Co	4000 R/min	10^6 R	4.2	R-3
Sodium formate	Spent fuel elements, approx. 1 MeV	Not given	10^6–5×10^6 rads	300	O-6
Na_2HPO_3 $5H_2O$	^{60}Co	1900 curies	6.5×10^6 rads	77	A-14
Acetonitrile	^{60}Co	26.8×10^{19} eV/g-hr	1, 2, 4, 6 hr	78	H-2
	^{60}Co, 2000 curies	3×10^6 rads/hr		195	C-21
Nylon	^{60}Co, 2000 curies	6×10^5 rads/hr	10^7 rads	77	G-17
Polyethylene	2 MeV electrons	3×10^3–3×10^6 rads/sec	Simultaneous IRR and EPR measurements	123–423	M-11
Saturated hydrocarbons, alcohol, aromatic compounds	2 MeV electrons	2×10^4–10^6 rads/sec	2×10^6–10^8 rads		V-10
Aqueous solutions of sulfur compounds	220 kV x-rays	4000 R/min	4.15×10^5 R	77	H-8
Amino acids	14.3 MeV electrons 15 MeV electron linear accelerator	130,000 rads/sec	10^6–2×10^8 rads		R-5

Alkyl halides	^{60}Co, 1750 curies	7×10^{17} eV/ml-min	10^{20} eV/ml	77	A-15
H_2SO_4, $HClO_4$, H_3PO_4	^{60}Co, 1000 curies	3000 R/min	Very rough, $\sim 10^7$ R	77	L-10
2,2-Polystyrene, 2,3-poly-ethylene, 2,4-polytetra-fluoroethylene	200 kV x-rays	2000 R/min 8000 R/min	10^7 R	300 and 77	S-2
CH_4, H_2, D_2, N_2 in Xe, A, Ne, H_2	^{60}Co, 2000 curies	0.68×10^6 R/hr	2–60×10^6 R	4.2	W-2
T_2O + alcohols	Tritium	~ 0.1 W	4×10^{19} eV/ml	77	K-16
Alcohols, ethers, aromatic esters, ketones	2 MeV electrons 2 MeV x-rays 50-kV x-rays		180 W sec	77 4.2	A-6

Table 7.5-14

g Values for some Irradiation-Produced Radicals

Irradiated material	g Value	Ref.
Ascorbic acid	2.0043	B-21
CH_4 (H atom spectrum)	2.002	R-3
H_2O (H atom spectrum)	2.0025	R-3
D_2O (D atom spectrum)	2.0030	R-3
HF (H atom spectrum)	2.0018	R-3
H_2 (H atom spectrum)	2.0020	R-3
Paraformaldehyde	2.0038	B-32
Glyoxal monohydrate	2.0035	B-32
$C \cdot H(COOH)_2$	2.0026, 2.0035, 2.0033	W-18
$C \cdot H(OH)COOH$	2.0017, 2.0053, 2.0038	W-18
$C \cdot H(OH)CO_2^-$	2.0021, 2.0054, 2.0039	W-18

conditions may suggest a bias favoring one set of data. Both radical concentration saturation and rf power saturation reduce the G value observed; therefore, if the largest G value corresponds to minimum dose and minimum rf power, it would be favored on this score. Before undue significance becomes attached to models or interpretations based on G values, it should be recalled that both the efficiency of production and trapping are involved in this number; therefore, the observed value is always a minimum value for production, i.e., large G values represent both

Table 7.5-15

Examples of Yields for Radicals Produced by Irradiation

Starting material	Radiation	Temp, °K	Yardstick	G value	Ref.
Methane	^{60}Co γ-rays	4.2	DPPH	1.4	W-2
Hydrogen	^{60}Co γ-rays	4.2	DPPH	0.02	W-2
Deuterium	^{60}Co γ-rays	4.2	DPPH	0.02	W-2
Alcohols					
Methanol	2 MeV e^-	103–163	$CuCl_2 \cdot 2H_2O$	12	V-10
	2 MeV e^-	77	DPPH	5.5	A-6
Ethanol	2 MeV e^-	77	DPPH	8.3	A-6
Propanol	2 MeV e^-	103–163	$CuCl_2 \cdot 2H_2O$	8.4	V-10
Octanol	2 MeV e^-	103–163	$CuCl_2 \cdot 2H_2O$	5.4	V-10

(continued)

Table 7.5-15 (*continued*)

Starting material	Radiation	Temp, °K	Yardstick	G value	Ref.
Aromatic compounds					
Benzene	2 MeV e^-	103–163	$CuCl_2 \cdot 2H_2O$	0.2	V-10
	2 MeV e^-	77	Irradiated methanol	0.32	M-3
Toluene	2 MeV e^-	103–163	$CuCl_2 \cdot 2H_2O$	0.3	V-10
	2 MeV e^-	77	Irradiated methanol	0.53	M-3
Diphenyl	2 MeV e^-	103–163	$CuCl_2 \cdot 2H_2O$	0.045	V-10
	2 MeV e^-	77	Irradiated methanol	0.10	M-3
Naphthalene	2 MeV e^-	77	Irradiated methanol	0.10	M-3
Alkyl halides					
Ethyl iodide	^{60}Co γ-rays	77	DPPH	2.0	A-15
n-Propyl chloride	^{60}Co γ-rays	77	DPPH	2.7	A-15
n-Butyl chloride	^{60}Co γ-rays	77	DPPH	2.0	A-15
n-Butyl bromide	^{60}Co γ-rays	77	DPPH	1.1	A-15
n-Butyl iodide	^{60}Co γ-rays	77	DPPH	1.0	A-15
Amino acids					
Glycine	14.3 MeV e^-	Room	DPPH	3.7	R-5
Glycine	150 kV x-ray	Room	DPPH	2.9	M-16 K-13
β-Alanine	150 kV x-ray	Room	DPPH	1.4	K-13
Alanine	14.3 MeV e^-	Room	DPPH	2.0	R-5
Valine	14.3 MeV e^-	Room	DPPH	1.9	R-5
L-Valine	150 kV x-rays	Room	DPPH	2.4	M-16 K-13
Glutamic acid	150 kV x-rays	Room	DPPH	4.3	M-16 K-13
Glutamic acid	14.3 MeV e^-	Room	DPPH	1.6	R-5
Carbohydrates					
Sucrose	^{60}Co γ-rays	Room	Irradiated cholesterol	2	E-5
Trehalose	^{60}Co γ-rays	Room	Irradiated cholesterol	3.7	E-5
α-Glucose	^{60}Co γ-rays	Room	Irradiated cholesterol	3.0	E-5
β-Glucose	^{60}Co γ-rays	Room	Irradiated cholesterol	3.1	E-5
Polyamides					
Nylon	^{60}Co γ-rays	77	DPPH and molybdenum disulfide	0.7–1.4	G-17

efficient production and trapping but small values may indicate only poor trapping.

Table 7.5-15 is a composite of several tabulations of G values arranged loosely by material classification. If the aromatic compounds are excluded, a large majority of the values fall between 1 and 5, i.e., 100 and 20 eV per spin, respectively. The value for hydrogen is a minimum estimate and may well indicate an inefficiency in trapping this species. In contrast, the G values for aromatic compounds are lower than this general range by one or two orders of magnitude, illustrating the well-known stability of the benzene ring. Where several G values are listed for a single material, they are intended as an illustration of the typical spread in data from various sources. G values above 10 are rare and if encountered in the course of a measurement, should be examined carefully to make sure they are real, e.g., by comparison with a material previously examined by several other groups. Unfortunately the present art of predicting radiation stability is still in a primitive state so that little assistance is available for anticipating yields on the basis of molecular architecture. Such factors as bond strength, side groups or branches, the chemical nature, multiple bonds, and number of aromatic rings presumably influence radical production but only qualitative indications are currently possible.

Table 7.5-15 illustrates several general behavior patterns, particularly with regard to the benzene ring. For example, two or three benzene rings are more stable than one and it seems to make little difference whether they are arranged as biphenyl or naphthalene. Less significant is the substitution of groups such as methyl, ethylene, etc. for the hydrogens on the ring, but slightly higher G values are obtained for ⬡Cl and ⬡CH$_3$ than for benzene. Some of the data for alcohols suggest molecular size may be related to stability; however, the results are not uniformly consistent on this point. Taking another approach Voevodskii and Molin (V-10) attempt to connect the observed regularities to the first excited state of the molecule and the magnitude of this excitation energy compared to the energy of bond dissassociation. Sufficient data are not available at this time to establish the generality of this concept.

(a) Hyperfine Structure and Identification. The hyperfine structure observed in examples of radiolysis is similar and frequently identical to spectra of radicals generated by the other methods of this section; however, the differences that do exist and the greater probability of multiple species place additional requirements on the experimental techniques to unravel and simplify the spectra. Usually, the most instructive spectra are obtained when samples are available as single crystals because it may be possible to remove the line broadening due to anisotropic interaction by suitable

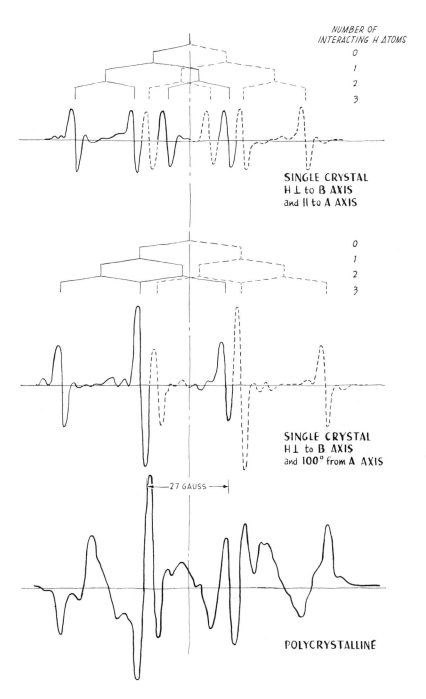

Fig. 7.5-23. Comparison of EPR hyperfine structures in single and polycrystalline samples of x-ray irradiated succinic acid. (After H-5.)

orientation in the magnetic field.* Figure 7.5-23 shows a good example of this improved resolution in the case of irradiated polycrystalline and single-crystal succinic acid. Identification is virtually impossible with the poly-crystalline spectrum but the two single crystal spectra readily resolve, as indicated in the diagram, into lines resulting from interactions with three hydrogen nuclei. When the A axis is parallel to the magnetic field, the contributions from the magnetic nuclei are all slightly different so 2^3 equal-intensity lines appear. The bottom spectrum consists of two triplets with intensity ratios of $1:2:1$, indicating that two of the hydrogen nuclei make the same contribution in this orientation. Both spectra require three hydrogen atoms and can be related to the portion of the molecule inclosed in the dashed line $CO_2H \vdots CH_2CH \vdots CO_2H$; however, the triplet spectra are most obviously related.

Many of the organic materials either are not available in suitable single crystals or they derive their importance from their noncrystalline struc-tures; therefore, other techniques must be used in resolving their hfs, e.g., suitable control of the temperature, atmosphere, and illumination. Some improvement in the resolution frequently results from thermally annealing a sample as illustrated in Fig. 7.5-24, which shows some sharpening of the lines in irradiated methane by annealing. In discussing this data, Wall et al. (W-2) noted that while the spin concentration was reduced by the anneal-ing, the sharper lines were not simply related to the average population because the linewidth was independent of spin concentration in unannealed samples. Other possibilities suggested were preferential reactions to elimin-ate closely associated radical pairs or clusters which would exhibit a strong spin–spin interaction because of close proximity, lattice adjustments to provide more uniform sites with the possibility of improved room for molecular rotation (motional narrowing), and the destruction of other types of radicals which exhibit interfering superimposed spectra.

Line distortion due to the sample atmosphere usually involves reactions with oxygen, and may result in line broadening, destruction of resonant species, or in one case the development of an undetectable species into a paramagnetic radical. Such line distortions have appeared already in the spectra of radicals produced by other methods. For example Fig. 6.2-12 and 7.5-6 show line broadening induced by oxygen in Wursters blue and carbon black, respectively. Unscheduled oxygen effects are most apt to creep into the quick and dirty type experiments where samples are exposed

---

* In Chapter II the anisotropic hyperfine splitting arising from dipolar interactions was given by a term $M_i g_n \beta_n [(3 \cos^2 \theta - 1)/r^3] g\beta/I$. If the molecular orientation is uniform throughout a single crystal, the magnitude of the anisotropic term can be controlled by the angle θ, i.e., the orientation in the magnetic field.

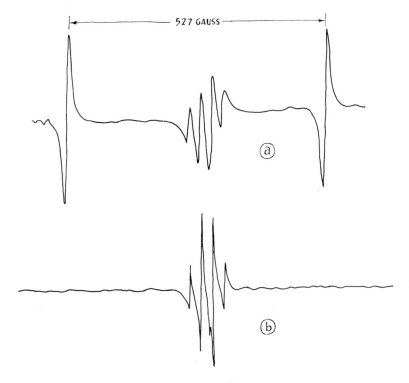

Fig. 7.5-24. EPR spectra of irradiated methane; (*a*) at 4.2°K; (*b*) after partial warmup the hydrogen doublet has disappeared and the quartet is considerably sharper.

Spectrometer type, RHI *X*-band; cavity, rectangular TE_{102} with internal dewar (Fig. 7.5-19); rf power, about 1 mW; sample 99.63% pure. (Courtesy W-2.)

to the air during irradiation and handling or when liquid samples are not deaerated.

Some radical species are photosensitive and can be modified by illumination in their optical absorption bands, thereby altering the EPR hfs and in some cases removing overlapping spectra. While irradiation colors most organic solids, the alcohols have been favored subjects for bleaching experiments. Figure 7.5-25 illustrates this technique with the optical absorption bands for several of the alcohols and the changes in the EPR spectrum of methanol produced by optically bleaching the color centers. Since the optical absorption peaks at about 5200 Å the samples are purple in color and bleach readily under white light or under mercury 5460 Å illumination. The species responsible for the color centers has not been identified but considerable evidence links the three lines remaining after

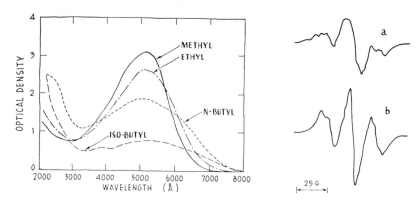

Fig. 7.5-25. Optical absorption bands in irradiated alcohols: the EPR spectrum of freshly irradiated methanol before bleaching (*a*) and after bleaching (*b*).

bleaching to the $\overline{C}H_2\overline{O}H$ radical where the 1:2:1 intensity ratio indicates equal interactions with the two hydrogens.

Many times the best available experimental spectrum is not sufficiently definitive to establish the identity of a radical and additional evidence is required. In order to overcome such EPR limitations as line broadening, overlapping spectra, and the inability to see the entire radical, it has been necessary to establish proof of identity by correlative experiments.

Preparation of the Radical by Unambiguous Methods. The formyl radical provides a classical example of this technique. Originally the distinctive hfs of this radical, i.e., a doublet with about 136 G splitting appeared in formic acid irradiated at 77°K and warmed to 190°K (G-12). Later it was found in irradiated methanol, methyl ethers and methyl esters after bleaching with 2537 UV light, or occasionally in embyonic form after the x-ray exposure (A-6). Finally the radical was generated in a series of photolysis experiments which established the identity (A-3):

(*a*) $HI \xrightarrow[\substack{\lambda = 2537 \\ +1849}]{h\nu} (I) + H \xrightarrow{CO} HCO$ in CO matrix

(*b*) $CH_2{=}O \xrightarrow[\substack{\lambda = 2537 \\ +1849}]{h\nu} HCO + H$ in argon matrix

(*c*) $CH_3OH \xrightarrow[\substack{\lambda > 1450}]{3h\nu} HCO + 3H$ in argon matrix

The spectrum for the first reaction is included in Fig. 7.5-11. Frequently, the "unambiguous methods" involve controlled photochemical reactions.

Tracer Techniques Using Isotopes that Have a Unique Nuclear Spin: Deuterium or Carbon-13. Figure 7.5-26 illustrates the use of deuterium labeling in establishing the identity of the radicals formed by irradiating

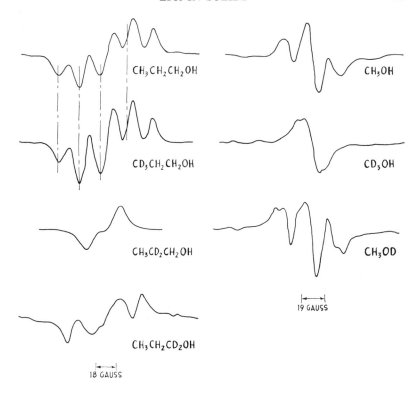

Fig. 7.5-26. Effect of deuterium labeling on the hfs of irradiated methanol and propanol.

methanol or propanol. Because deuterium has a spin of 1 and a smaller magnetic moment than hydrogen, the hfs due to deuterium is not resolved; however, the effect on the spectrum can be quite pronounced. Implicit in this technique is the assumption that the tagging and regular isotopes are equivalent and will not alter the radicals generated. Hydrogen and deuterium are not always equivalent but no inconsistencies are apparent in the alcohol spectra. The suggested radicals are therefore $\dot{C}H_2OH$ previously mentioned for methanol and $CH_3CH_2\dot{C}H OH$ for propanol because the deuterium only effected these positions. Only the enclosed portion of the molecule is detected.

Production of Identical Hyperfine Structure in Suitably Related Molecules, e.g., in Methanol and Dimethyl Ether. While not as definitive as unambiguous preparation or tracer techniques, the production of the same hf spectrum in a variety of materials containing a particular functional group in common can provide a clue to identification of the responsible radical. Two examples already encountered are the rather unique doublet with 135 G splitting in Figure 7.5-11d and the triplet in Figure 7.5-26. Although final identification of the doublet as the formyl radical came through the photolysis experiments, considerable evidence for the HCO structure had accumulated from the common spectra observed during the radiolysis of formic acid, methanol, methyl ethers, and methyl esters and from molecules containing the methyl group which did develop the doublet. Similarly, various molecules with ethyl groups developed a five-line structure similar to that of Figure 7.5-12.

(b) Line Shape, Linewidths, and Hf Splittings. In many of the irradiated solids the line shape is obscured by overlapping spectra and lack of resolutions but generally the shape is closer to a gaussian than to a Lorentzian curve. Since the observed spectrum depends strongly on the ratio of the linewidth to separation, several authors have tabulated constructed curves for a variety of width to splitting ratios and numbers of interacting protons as an aid to identification, as in Fig. 2-19. References L-2 and L-3 are extensive compilations filling two volumes which include examples where all the protons are not interacting equally. A familiarity with such constructed curves may help relieve that first shock when the spectrometer spins out an ungainly spectrum even after all experimental perturbations and distortions have been removed. In a series of irradiated alcohols, ketones, ethers, esters, acids, paraffins, and alkyl halides—over 50 different compounds in all—a majority of the spectra had an odd number of lines and the splitting ranged from about 18 to 30 G. Reference M-15 tabulates the hyperfine interactions for a number of single crystal specimens containing radicals of the type HCR_1R_2. Table 7.5-16 shows both the isotropic and anisotropic hyperfine interactions involving the α-protons indicated in the π-electron radicals by italics. All of the isotropic splittings are very close to 60 Mc/sec although the two examples with the electron centered on the nitrogen, possibly exhibiting a slightly stronger interaction. According to McConnell and Chesnut (M-5) the isotropic proton hf interaction α_H is proportional to the spin density on the central atom (ρ), i.e., $\alpha_H = Q\rho$ where Q is a constant approximately equal to -60 Mc/sec. The minus sign signifies a negative spin density at the hydrogen, i.e., it points oppositely to the electron spin density on the carbon (G-11). The anisotropic interactions have been related to the bond and π-orbital orientations indicated at the top of each column and it is apparent that the interaction approaches zero for the middle orientation (M-15).

For radicals such as those in Table 7.5-17 the β-proton interactions are

Table 7.5-16

Hyperfine Interactions with α Protons (M-15)

Radical	Original crystal	Isotropic	$\overset{\uparrow}{\underset{H\ \uparrow H_0}{\bigcirc}}$ C	$\overset{\uparrow\uparrow}{\underset{\uparrow H_0}{C}}$—H	$\uparrow C$—H $\uparrow H_0$
				Anisotropic	
HC(CO$_2$H)$_2$	H$_2$C(CO$_2$H)$_2$	−59	+31	+1	−32
H_2C(CO$_2$H)	H$_2$C(CO$_2$H)$_2$	−59	+29	+4	−33
		−63	+26	+4	−30
HCCH$_3$(CO$_2^-$)	CH$_3$NH$_3^+$CH(CO$_2^-$)	−54	+30	+6	−36
HCNH$_3^+$(CO$_2^-$)	NH$_3^+$CH$_2$(CO$_2^-$)	−62	+35	−5	−30
HCOH(CO$_2$H)	CH$_2$OH(CO$_2$H)	−57	+27	+2	−29
HCF(CONH$_2$)	CH$_2$F(CONH$_2$)	−63	+32	0	−32
HC(CO$_2$H) $\|$ CH$_2$(CO$_2$H)	CH$_2$(CO$_2$H) $\|$ CH$_2$(CO$_2$H)	−60	+30	+1	−31
HC(SO$_3^-$)$_2$	CH$_2$(SO$_3$K)$_2$	−60	+32	+3	−35
HN$^+$<	(NH$_4$)$_2$HPO$_4$	−65	+34	+2	−36
HN(SO$_3^-$)	NH$_2$(SO$_3$K)	−64	+39	+4	−34

almost isotropic; therefore, only one set of interactions is listed. When the β-protons are on a methyl group that is free to rotate the three protons are equivalent and have a hf interaction of approximately 70 Mc/sec which appears to be independent of the host crystal and the radical (M-15). In

Table 7.5-17

Isotropic Hyperfine Interactions with β Protons (Mc/sec) (M-15)

Radical	Crystal	β_1	β_2	β_3
CH$_3$C(CO$_2$H)$_2$	CH$_3$CH(CO$_2$H)$_2$	71	71	71
CH$_3$CH(CO$_2^-$)	CH$_3$CH(CO$_2^-$) $\|$ NH$_3^+$	70	70	70
		120	76	14
CH(CO$_2$H) $\|$ CH$_2$(CO$_2$H)	CH$_2$(CO$_2$H) $\|$ CH$_2$(CO$_2$H)	100	80	
CH(CO$_2$H) $\|$ (CH$_2$)$_3$(CO$_2$H)	CH$_2$CH$_2$(CO$_2$H) $\|$ CH$_2$CH$_2$(CO$_2$H)	112	74	
CH$_2$C(CO$_2$H)$_2$ $\|$ CH$_3$	CH$_2$CH(CO$_2$H)$_2$ $\|$ CH$_3$	70	57	
NH$_3^+$CH(CO$_2^-$)	NH$_3^+$CH$_2$(CO$_2^-$)	53	53	53
N(CH$_3$)$_3^+$	N(CH$_3$)$_4$Cl	75	75	75

fact, it may be possible to identify methylene groups in the radical by this distinctive β-proton hf splitting. This equivalence of the CH_3 protons due to fast rotation was illustrated beyond doubt in irradiated alanine which was cooled until the CH_3 rotation ceased and the protons exhibited different couplings (G-11). In the absence of a methyl group the splitting in Table 7.5-17 ranged from 14 to 120 Mc/sec, i.e., from about 7 to 60 G, a range which includes most of the splitting involving C—H bonds. References I-2 and W-11 list the hf pattern and overall splitting for 28 irradiated materials, ranging from simple alcohols to long-chain polymers. While illustrative of the spectra commonly encountered, these examples represent only a smattering of the many spectra published in the literature.

(c) **Radical Concentrations and the Missing Spin.** Two additional questions of concern to the experimentalist pertain to the missing spin and to the maximum concentration of radicals than can be stabilized. Spins still come in pairs but we seldom find equal concentrations of both radical species. In commenting on this situation Zeldes and Livingston (Z-1) offer the following four reasons for not observing the spins and note that with so many possibilities rationalization is not difficult:

1. The spins vanish through chemical reaction.

2. The missing electron has a broad, low absorption band which escapes detection under experimental conditions appropriate for the observed species.

3. Nonmagnetic electronic states prohibit detection.

4. Forbidden electronic transitions prohibit detection.

The first alternative is very appealing in the many compounds where radicals apparently form by the loss of hydrogen. The observation of hydrogen atom spectra in certain matrix materials and their escape under slight annealing substantiates this rationalization (W-2).

Saturation concentrations are discussed in Refs. P-10 and P-17 where the tabulated values extend over a decade from about 0.01 to 0.6 mole % radicals. Both the molecular species and the temperature exert a strong influence on this concentration.

7.6 THE TRIPLET STATE IN ORGANIC SOLIDS

Probably the most exciting search by EPR techniques involved electrons in the triplet state. These elusive electrons thwarted numerous attempts at detection during the years between the birth of EPR and the successful experiments of Hutchison and Mangum (H-23) on triplet naphthalene. In general the interest in triplet states stems from their role in the following:

1. Optical excitation and decay processes responsible for fluorescence and phosphorescence.

2. Energy transfer and storage mechanisms in solids.

3. Chemical reactions involving reactive intermediates.

4. Applications to optical masers.

More specifically from the EPR viewpoint the detection of resonance gives additional conformation to the Lewis and Kasha (L-7) model of excited states, and provides an ideal method for following these states in their interactions within and with the host material.

When EPR arrived on the scene, the impressive array of existing information included (*1*) absorption spectra for excitation to the metastable states, (*2*) phosphorescence emission spectra, (*3*) measurements of life times in the metastable state, (*4*) confirmation that this state was paramagnetic (L-6), and (*5*) a diagram of the energy levels. With this background we may well be curious why such an apparently ideal system repeatedly rebuffed detection by EPR techniques. In retrospect there is no overwhelming reason for these failures. Indeed the failures were achieved with samples and spectrometers comparable to current equipment. Early samples were of the glass variety common to the optical experiments and the anisotropically broadened lines for the randomly oriented molecules escaped detection during the allowed $\Delta M_s = 1$ transitions. Success required a dilute sample of triplet molecules in a compatible single crystal host. Later the glassy samples were found to be satisfactory, particularly for observations of the forbidden $\Delta M_s = 2$ transitions. Other factors influencing these early experiments were uncertainties of the magnitudes expected for the zero field splitting and the width of the lines; however, after Hutchison and Mangum achieved a suitable combination of sample and measuring conditions, the discovery of the triplet spins was promptly confirmed by observations in other laboratories. In the remainder of this section we will first indicate the nature of the triplet state and the associated transitions then consider in detail the experimental requirements and results for EPR measurements.

7.6.1 Properties of the Triplet State (W-1)

(a) Energy Levels and Transitions. In Chapter II we found that most atoms and molecules have singlet ground states where all the electron spins are paired and the resultant spin (S) is zero.

If one of the electrons is raised to an excited state, two spin orientations are possible: (*1*) the spins remain antiparallel to form an excited singlet state or (*2*) two spins line up parallel to form a triplet state, i.e., $S = \frac{1}{2} + \frac{1}{2}$ so that the ($2S + 1$) values of the angular momentum (J) can be identified as three different electronic states hence the term triplet. In general it is not easy to determine which transition will predominate for polyatomic molecules; however, certain selection rules provide some guidance. For example, the spin conservation rule $\Delta S = 0$ applies to small molecules in the absence of perturbations caused by the magnetic field of heavy atoms, surfaces, or inhomogeneities in the external magnetic field. If all the atoms in the molecule are light, e.g., H, C, N, and O, transitions between the ground singlet and the excited state will be very infrequent (W-14). When field perturbations cause the spin conservation rule to break down, the $\Delta S = 1$ transitions to the triplet state become allowed. Since the probability of the $\Delta S = 1$ transitions increases rapidly with atomic number, both the number of molecules excited to the triplet state and their lifetime in the state are dependent on the atomic number. Table 7.6-1 shows how the phosphorescence lifetime for a series of α- and β-naphthalene compounds decreases with increasing atomic weight.

The energy level diagram in Fig. 7.6-1 illustrates the various competing reactions involved in absorption, fluorescence, and phosphorescence. Historically Jablonski was the first to indicate that at least three states (S_0, S_1, and T_1) were involved in the phosphorescence process (W-1) and Lewis and Kasha identified the metastable state (T_1) as a triplet state. For every excited singlet level S_1 there is a corresponding triplet level T_1 usually of lower energy. The antiparallel and parallel spins are indicated schematically by the small arrows opposite each energy level. Transitions of primary concern in the production of triplet states are shown in bold arrows while light arrows indicate other competing reactions. In conventional photoexcitation the transition $S_0 \rightarrow S_1$ represents an electron being raised to an excited singlet state by the absorption of a photon. After the molecule drops to the lowest excited level S_1 by losing energy through collisions with other molecules, i.e., radiationless transitions. It can return to the ground state S_0 by three alternative routes:

1. Fluorescence: a radiating transition $S_1 \rightarrow S_0$.

Table 7.6-1

Effect of Heavy-Atom Substituents on Phosphorescence Lifetimes of Monosubstituents of α- and β-Naphthalene Compounds in Triplet–Singlet Emission (W-2)

Substituent	Lifetime in triplet state, sec	
	α Isomer	β Isomer
F	1.5	—
Cl	0.30	0.47
Br	0.018	0.0021
I	0.0025	0.0025

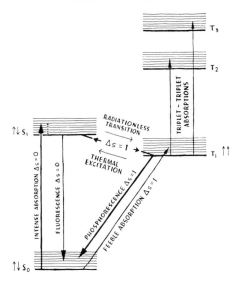

Fig. 7.6-1. Energy level diagram for the triplet state showing the competing reactions involved in absorption, fluorescence, and phosphorescence (W-14).

2. Phosphorescence: a radiationless transition $S_1 \to T_1$ followed by a radiating transition $T_1 \to S_0$.

3. Thermalization: a radiationless transition back to S_0 through collisions with other molecules.

Similarly, a molecule in the triplet state T_1 has three alternatives:

1. Phosphorescence: a radiative transition $T_1 \to S_0$.

2. Slow fluorescence: a thermal excitation back to the excited singlet state followed by the radiative transition $S_1 \to S_0$.

3. A radiationless transition back to S_0.

EPR techniques can detect the parallel spins only during the time the molecule is in the triplet state, i.e., T_1, T_2, or T_3 but normally T_1. Two factors are involved in obtaining a detectable concentration of molecules in this state: (1) the number of transitions $S_1 \to T_1$ and (2) the lifetime of the metastable molecule. The subsequent discussion of sample selection and preparation will be concerned with the optimum solution to these requirements.

(b) Habitat. Thus far our definition of the triplet state requires only that the molecule contain two electrons with parallel spins; however, biradicals also have this spin arrangement so that an additional distinction is desirable. This distinction is usually based on the degree of interaction between the two unpaired electrons. In the triplet state the interaction is strong and the EPR absorption is split to give two lines. Conversely, in biradicals the

Table 7.6-2

Some Organic Molecules Studied in the Triplet State by EPR Techniques

Molecule	Concentration	Host	Lifetime τ, sec		Absorption peaks, Å	Ref.
			77°K	Other temp		
Naphthalene	2M% in melt	Durene			2200, 2750, 3140	H-21
		Biphenyl			2200, 2750, 3140	H-19
	0.02M%	Durene			2200, 2750, 3140	V-1
	1.5M%	Durene	2.14	2.16 at 4°K	2200, 2750, 3140	H-15
	0.0154M/10³g	Alphanol	3.0		2200, 2750, 3140	D-3
	0.0083M/10³g	Cyclohexane, 1 part; decalin, 3 parts by vol.	2.7	5.0 at 20°K	2200, 2750, 3140	D-2
Dueteronaphthalene		Durene	2.1		2000, 2750, 3140	H-22
	0.0074M/10³g	Cyclohexane, 1 part; decalin 3 parts by vol.	20.3	20.5 at 20°K		D-2
Deuteronaphthalene		Durene	2.1			H-22
Phenanthrene		Biphenyl			2100, [2500, 2750, 2800, 2930], [3160, 3230, 3300, 3380, 3460]	H-19
Phenanthrene		Fluorene			2100, [2500, 2750, 2800, 2930], [3160, 3230, 3300, 3380, 3460]	H-19

Compound	Concentration	Solvent				Ref.
Fluorene		Biphenyl				H-19
Triphenylene	$0.0043\,M/10^3$g	Alphanol	13.3			D-3
1,3,5-Triphenyl-benzene	$0.0018\,M/10^3$g	Alphanol	5.1			D-3
Coronene	$0.0008\,M/10^3$g	Alphanol	7.9			D-3
Benzene	$0.0517\,M/10^3$g	Cyclohexane, 1 part, decalin, 3 parts by Vol.	4.2	11.7 at 20°K	2000, 2550	D-2
Benzene		EPA	0.02		2000, 2550	S-15
Deuterobenzene		EPA	0.15			S-15
Toluene	$0.0528\,M/10^3$g	Cyclohexane, 1 part; decalin, 3 parts by Vol.	7.7	11.2 at 20°K	2625	D-2
Triptycene	$0.0083\,M/10^3$g	Cyclohexane, 1 part; decalin, 3 parts by Vol.	12.3	5.0		D-2
Tribenzotriptycene	$0.0026\,M/10^3$g	Cyclohexane, 1 part; decalin, 3 parts by Vol.	4.6	4.9		D-2
Diphenyl		EPA	11.2		2460[a]	S-15
Anthracene					2500, 3800	S-15
Terphenyl					2515[b], 2760[a]	S-15
Chrysene					2200, 2570, 3060, 3600	S-15

[a] In hexane.
[b] In chloroform.

interaction is very weak and the spins behave independently as if isolated in two parts of the molecule. Usually biradicals involve large molecules and their EPR absorption approaches the free electron value. Although our attention here is limited to the triplet state, a considerable variation in the strength of the interaction will be observed.

Organic molecules with triplet states suitable for EPR detection generally contain unsaturated bonds and essentially all of the studies to date have involved aromatic compounds. Maximizing the triplet state population requires a dilute solution of the triplet molecule in an inert solid host where restricted molecular motion favors the transition $S_1 \rightarrow T_1$ in Fig. 7.6-1 and the dilution reduces the probability of deactivating triplet molecules by collisions between molecules of the same type. Finally, low temperatures may increase the lifetime in the triplet state.

Table 7.6-2 lists a number of compounds that have been successfully observed in the triplet state by EPR techniques. Also listed are the host materials, sample compositions, and information about the optical properties of the triplet molecules. All of these examples contain double bonds, frequently in a cyclic structure such as a benzene ring. Where concentrations are shown, the small number of phosphorescent molecules obviously permits complete entrapment by host molecules.

(c) Optical Properties. The optical properties of both the fluorescent molecule and the host are important in a triplet-state experiment. Since phosphorescence is produced in molecules by the absorption of energy within the normal absorption band of the molecule, this band should fall within the range of strong sources of radiant energy—usually the ultraviolet region of the spectrum. Conversely, the host material should be transparent throughout both the absorption and emission band. The absorption peaks listed in Table 7.6-2 are for molecules in such solvents as hexane or alcohol. While the peaks are scattered throughout the ultraviolet spectrum, the bandwidths are usually several hundred angstroms and readily excitable with light from a high-pressure mercury lamp. In Fig. 7.6-2 the spectra for naphthalene, anthracene, and benzene illustrate the broad bands typical of these molecules. Here the main absorption bands match the several hundred angstrom widths mentioned; however, some of the fine structure is narrower. Since the solvent has a slight influence on the position of the absorption peak, the wavelengths listed in Table 7.6-2 are precise only for the liquid solvents indicated; however, precise knowledge of the peak position is not needed with the UV lamps normally used.

(d) Lifetime in the Excited State (τ). Successful EPR spectra have been obtained for molecules with lifetimes in the excited state ranging from 0.15 to 20 sec, a variation of over two decades. Table 7.6-2 illustrates several factors controlling τ. Molecular structure and composition exercise the

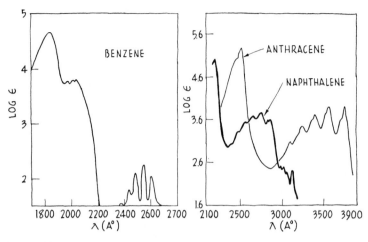

Fig. 7.6-2. Absorption spectra of benzene (courtesy K-15) and anthracene and naphthalene (courtesy G-5); ϵ is the molecular extinction coefficient.

main influence. Another factor is isotope substitution, for example, substituting deuterium for hydrogen increases τ for benzene and naphthalene more than sevenfold. While the data in Table 7.6-2 pertaining to host effects on τ are sparce and involve interlaboratory comparisons, some of the differences in times listed for benzene and naphthalene are probably due to the hosts. Finally the sample temperature may influence τ but the meager data indicate this effect depends on the molecule. In naphthalene, both $C_{10}H_8$ and $C_{10}D_8$, and tribenzotriptycene, τ is the same at 4, 20, and 77°K while benzene and toulene decay more slowly at low temperatures. Triptycene exhibits an anomalous temperature dependence of the lifetime. Deuteration has provided the principal experimental control over τ. In addition to increased lifetime, deuteration provides an additional advantage when the signal is weak because line broadening due to the hyperfine interaction is reduced.

7.6.2 EPR Parameters of Interest and Experimental Problems

Most EPR measurements on molecules in the triplet state have been concerned with establishing the energy levels for the state. Since the observed fine structure can be described for the case of spin $S = 1$ in an orthorhombic field by the Hamiltonian $\mathscr{H} = g\beta H \cdot S + DS_z^2 + E(S_x^2 - S_y^2)$, the principal parameters of interest have been the splitting factor g and the fine structure parameters D and E. Other parameters that have been measured are hyperfine anisotropy; the electron spin density at various molecular sites; ΔH, the linewidth; and τ, the lifetime in the triplet state.

Common experimental problems include the following:

1. Obtaining a suitable sample: This applies particularly to single crystal specimens because a host crystal that is inert, transparent to both the exciting illumination and emitted radiation, and compatible with the triplet molecule can prove to be hard to find. De Groot and van der Waals' "forbidden transition" technique (V-1) greatly simplifies the host problem by incorporating a ridged glassy matrix as the host; however, the anisotropic hfs is lost in this procedure.

2. Adequate concentration of molecules in the triplet state: Two factors are involved here: first, producing the triplets and second, avoiding large concentrations of stable photochemically produced radicals.

3. Overabundance of absorption lines in single-crystal experiments: If the triplet molecules can enter the host crystal in various orientations, each orientation will produce a pair of absorption lines and the resulting spectrum may require considerable unraveling.

7.6.3 Sample Preparation

Fluorescent and phosphorescent transitions are frequently extremely sensitive to the presence of foreign molecules. Therefore, both the triplet molecules and the host matrix deserve careful purification in order to maximize the population and lifetime of molecules in the triplet state. Satisfactory concentrations are indicated in Table 7.6-2. In single-crystal hosts an excess concentration usually is not a problem because the crystal will seldom accommodate more than about 2% of the foreign material (41). The durene–naphthalene mixed crystals used in the first successful EPR triplet experiments were grown by lowering a melt containing 2 mole % naphthalene through a temperature gradient (H-21). Glassy samples are easier to prepare. Since most of the hosts are liquid at room temperature, it is only necessary to freeze the mixture in a sealed quartz tube. Several satisfactory glasses are:

1. EPA (S-14), ether five parts; isopentane, five parts; and ethyl alcohol, two parts by volume.

2. Spectrograde cyclohexane, one part; and very pure decalin, three parts by volume (D-2).

3. Glycerol (V-1).

4. Alphanol 79, a commercially available mixture of primary alkanols containing 7–9 carbon atoms (D-3). Hydrogenation of the solvent at 100°C with Raney nickel as a catalyst reduced somewhat the UV light absorption which is normally small down to 2500 Å.

5. Methanol (S-14): UV illumination of methanol can generate radicals which are stable at 77°K, exhibit an EPR absorption spectrum with a g of about 2, and have a linewidth of about 60 G which usually falls between the lines for the triplet state and can generally be ignored.

Boric acid glass is not suitable as a matrix for aromatic hydrocarbons because UV illumination produces colored products (G-11).

Thin-walled quartz tubes 3 or 4 mm o.d. are commonly used to hold the glassy samples because they will fit in the simple dewars used in X-band cavities. Single-crystal samples normally require an adhesive and an alignment jig for mounting. Several adhesives currently in use in triplet experiments are Apiezon N vacuum grease (H-21), Dow-Corning vacuum grease (H-15), and glycerine. UV irradiation of the Dow-Corning grease at 77°K produces a resonance absorption at a g of about 2; however, this normally does not interfere with the triplet lines (H-15). Orientation can be achieved either with a goniometric device or with polystyrene wedges cut for the particular host crystal (H-21).

The main problem in exciting molecules to the triplet state involves getting sufficiently intense irradiation into the sample within the confining limitations of the cavity and dewar systems. High-pressure mercury lamps are generally used with quartz lenses and windows and aluminum-front surface mirrors. These lamps have the moderately small emitting volumes required for efficient optics and broad intense emission spectra covering

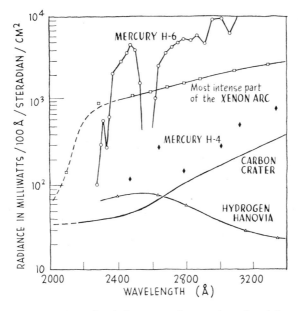

Fig. 7.6-3. Comparison of emission spectra from various ultraviolet sources. (Courtesy B-4.)

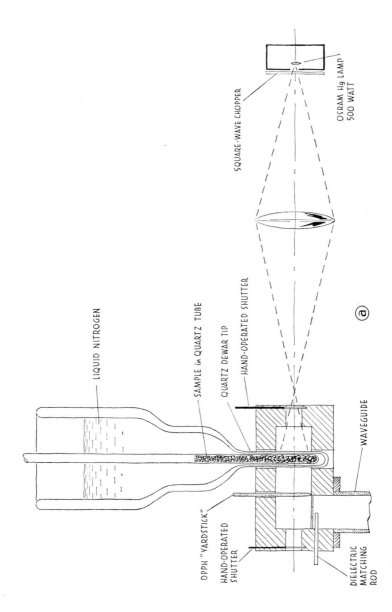

Fig. 7.6-4. Five arrangements for exciting samples to the triplet state in preparation for EPR observations. In all cases the samples are illuminated in the EPR cavity at low temperatures. (a) A glassy sample at 77°K in a rectangular cavity with an external dewar. UV light enters the cavity through a section of waveguide operated beyond cutoff for the cavity resonant frequency (40).

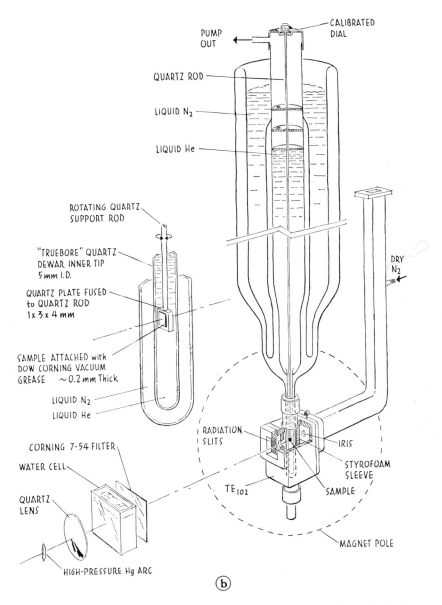

PUMP OUT

CALIBRATED DIAL

QUARTZ ROD

LIQUID N$_2$

LIQUID He

DRY N$_2$

ROTATING QUARTZ SUPPORT ROD

"TRUEBORE" QUARTZ DEWAR INNER TIP 5 mm I.D.

QUARTZ PLATE FUSED to QUARTZ ROD 1 x 3 x 4 mm

SAMPLE ATTACHED with DOW CORNING VACUUM GREASE ~ 0.2 mm Thick

LIQUID N$_2$
LIQUID He

CORNING 7-54 FILTER
WATER CELL
QUARTZ LENS
HIGH-PRESSURE Hg ARC

RADIATION SLITS
IRIS
STYROFOAM SLEEVE
TE$_{102}$
SAMPLE
MAGNET POLE

(b)

Fig. 7.6-4. (*b*) A commercial rectangular TE$_{102}$ cavity with internal dewar for liquid helium operation. The crystal rotates on the end of a long quartz rod and light enters the cavity through slits in the end of the cavity (after H-15).

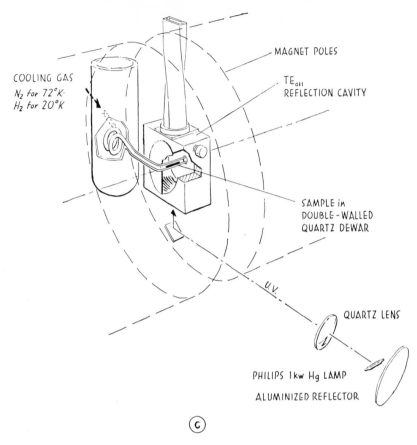

Fig. 7.6-4. (c) Cylindrical TE_{011} cavity with sample arranged for observing $\Delta M = \pm 2$ transitions. The UV light comes through slits in the cylindrical wall (26).

the entire UV spectrum, as shown in Fig. 7.6-3. Typical lamps in use are the AH-6, Osram HBO 500, 1 KW Philips, and the PEK Laboratories high-pressure mercury arc. Silver mirrors are not as efficient as aluminum for reflecting in the UV region because silver has a transmission window at about 3100 Å, which is the wavelength for exciting naphthalene. Figure 7.6-4 shows irradiation arrangements used successfully with various cavity and sample geometries. Parts a and b involve rectangular cavities with internal dewars and conventional illumination ports. In A the glassy sample in the quartz tube is immersed in liquid nitrogen while in B the single crystal on the quartz plate (see insert) can rotate as desired under liquid helium. Although filters are employed to limit the heat input into the

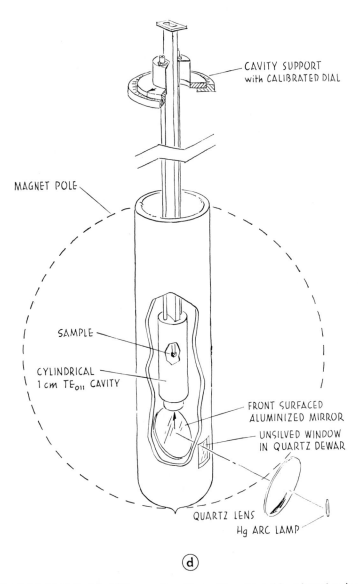

CAVITY SUPPORT
with CALIBRATED DIAL

MAGNET POLE

SAMPLE

CYLINDRICAL
1 cm TE_{011} CAVITY

FRONT SURFACED
ALUMINIZED MIRROR

UNSILVED WINDOW
IN QUARTZ DEWAR

QUARTZ LENS
Hg ARC LAMP

(d)

Fig. 7.6-4. (d) Cylindrical TE_{011} cavity with sample arranged for observing $\Delta m = \pm 1$ transitions at 77°K. The UV light enters through a hole in the bottom of the cavity (after H-21).

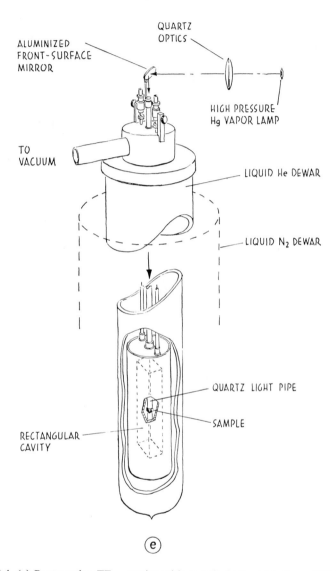

Fig. 7.6-4. (e) Rectangular TE_{102} cavity with sample in liquid helium. UV light comes down a quartz light pipe to the sample (41). Note that the optics are indicated schematically. For the most efficient illumination, locate the lens as close to the sample as complete illumination will permit.

dewar thereby reducing the consumption of liquid helium, it is not necessary to limit the spectrum because of the triplet state considerations.
Arrangement c is designed specifically for observing $\Delta M = \pm 2$ transitions;
therefore, H_1 of the cavity and the sample are parallel to H_0. A stream of
cold gas cools the sample and the UV light enters the cavity through
peripheral slots. Arrangements d and e are designed for single crystals in
cavities with external dewars. In d the light enters the dewar through an
unsilvered spot in the coating, reflects from the front surface mirror, and
enters the bottom of the cavity through a window. The entire cavity
rotates to align the crystal with the magnetic field. Arrangements a–d are
suitable for stationary magnets but e is designed for a rotating magnet system. A quartz light pipe transmits the UV light vertically along the axis of
magnet rotation so that the magnet poles will not intercept the light.

7.6.4   EPR Equipment and Techniques

(a) Spectrometer Considerations. The spectrometer requirements for
triplet state measurements are readily met by commercial instruments
although homemade cavities are frequently employed. Linewidths and rf
power saturation levels permit operation of high-frequency modulation
homodyne spectrometers in the range where their sensitivity is competitive
with superheterodyne systems; here the narrowest hf linewidths generally
exceed 1 G and saturation limits operation to between 0.1 and 1.0 mW (41).

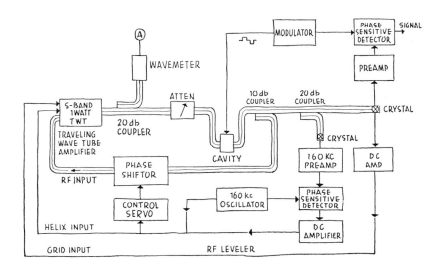

Fig. 7.6-5. Schematic diagram of a variable-frequency (1.5–4.5 kMc) zero magnetic
field spectrometer. (After 41.)

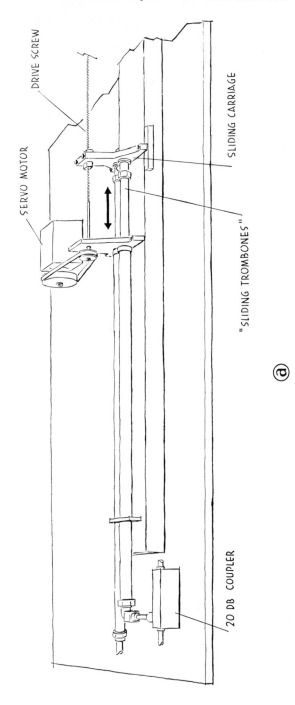

Fig. 7.6-6. (a) Construction of automatic phase shifter which keeps oscillation frequency from traveling wave tube locked to the variable-frequency cavity.

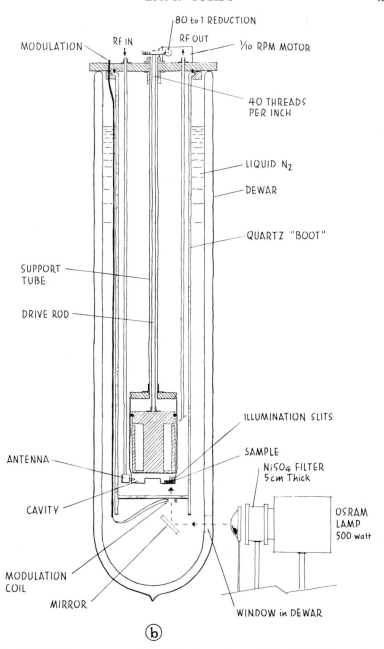

Fig. 7.6-6. (b) Arrangement of a variable-frequency cavity in a liquid nitrogen dewar showing the drive mechanism for varying the cavity length and provisions for illuminating the sample with UV light. (After 41.)

All of the materials listed in Table 7.6-2 were measured at X-band frequencies with 100–125 kc modulation.

One rather specialized instrument, the zero-field spectrometer, is uniquely suited to triplet state studies because it measures the zero-field splitting parameters directly. Since no external field is involved, this instrument scans the spectrum by varying the frequency, a neat trick at microwave frequencies. Figure 7.6-5 is a schematic diagram of a variable-frequency spectrometer used in triplet state measurements at the University of Chicago (41). A motor driven plunger gradually changes the transmission cavity length, thereby varying the resonant frequency. The feedback loop starting at the 10 db coupler goes through a phase shifter back to the microwave amplifier to lock the generator frequency to the resonance frequency of the cavity. As the frequency shifts, the motor driven phase shifter adjusts the physical length of this feed back circuit to maintain the electrical length constant. A second loop coming off at the 20 db coupler contains the 160 kc frequency modulation oscillator preamplifier and phase sensitive detector used to control the selsyn drive for the phase shifter. Automatic control to hold the rf power level constant as the frequency changes involved a third feedback loop labeled rf leveler. The last loop contains the magnetic modulation for the sample and the detector system, i.e., the crystal, preamplifier, and phase sensitive detector. Some characteristics of this spectrometer are as follows: frequency range, 1500–4500 Mc; power of traveling-wave tube, 1 W; phase stability, 20 or 30 kc; cavity Q, $\sim$ 1000. Figure 7.6-6 shows the drive mechanisms for the phase shifter (a) and the cavity (b). One factor in selecting a variable frequency cavity involves minimizing the change in sample filling factor as the cavity volume changes. In the more conventional coaxial, cylindrical, or rectangular cavities the volume change for a given frequency shift is substantially larger than in the reentrant cavity.

(b) Cavity Considerations and Arrangements. Obvious cavity requirements for triplet measurements are windows for illumination, provisions for cooling the samples, and for single crystals, sample orientation in the magnetic field. Other considerations that may affect the choice of cavity are provisions for measuring g or the signal amplitudes with internal yardsticks. Figure 7.6-7 shows how these requirements are met in four cavities responsible for many of the data in Table 7.6-2 and in the variable-frequency cavity.

Cavity and dewar arrangements a and b work well with glassy samples where orientation is not a problem but the relatively large number of specimens that can be handled by the $\Delta M_s = 2$ technique makes ease of sample change a definite advantage. Arrangements c, d, and e require cooling the cavity; however, these cavities are particularly suited for measurements on single crystals where the large number of measurements on each crystal means that the somewhat involved mounting procedures occupy a relatively small fraction of the total experimental time. Interesting features are:

Cavity a. (*1*) A length of $\frac{3}{2}\lambda$ which permits a port for a yardstick to mark the *g* value and indicate the concentration of spins.

(*2*) Thick walls on the four sides containing holes to provide cutoff waveguide sections, thereby minimizing the escape of rf power.

(*3*) A dielectric matching device which eliminates electrical contact problems.

(*4*) Printed circuit board walls under the modulation coils to transmit the 100 kc signal.

Cavity b. (*1*) Parallel orientation of the modulation field, H_0, and H_1.

(*2*) A spring loaded tuning screw to reduce variability of contact between screw thread and guide wall.

Cavity c. (*1*) A quartz window in the cavity-sealing cap. Joints between dissimilar materials in this case are of the housekeeper style held together with Epoxy cement, i.e., the window support is thinned to a feather edge at the joint with the quartz and the support is thinned for the joint to the brass. Rubber cement with kerosene as the solvent seals the tapered joint between the cap and lid.

(*2*) Thinning of the cavity walls next to the modulation coils permits the 125 kc modulation field to enter the cavity.

(*3*) A generous hole in the adjustable cavity bottom admits the light to the sample.

Cavity d. (*1*) An Amersil quartz light pipe conducts the UV light through the dewar lid and down to the sample in the cavity without interfering with the magnet rotation.

(*2*) The entrance and exit coupling antennas rotate and move up and down to permit adjustment of the coupling and matching of the load.

(*3*) A silver (plated or painted) Epoxy cavity and a Nylon sealing cup transmit the 125 kc modulation field from external coils which can rotate with the magnet.

(*4*) A (AuFe–Chromel) thermocouple permits temperature measurements from 4 to 300°K.

(*5*) A Lucalox sample support post (General Electric trade name for sapphire powder sintered together) provides good heat transfer, particularly at very low temperatures.

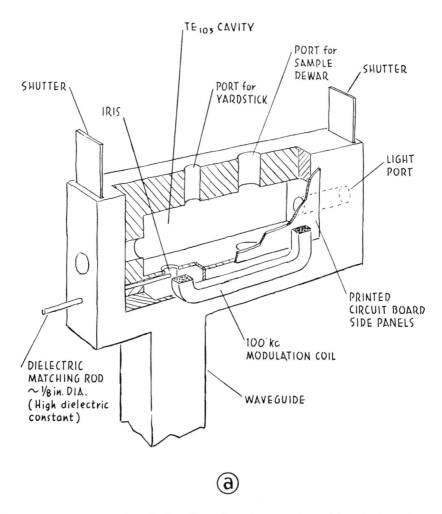

Fig. 7.6-7. Construction details of the four home made cavities of Fig. 7.6-4.
[(*a*) Ref. 40; (*b*) Ref. 26; (*c*) courtesy H-2; and (*d*) Ref. 41.]

Cavity e. (*1*) Motor driven, variable length; typical speed, $\frac{1}{10}$ rpm,
which moves the plunger 0.0025 in. per minute.

(*2*) The light and the modulation field enter the sample through slots
in the bottom of cavity.

(*3*) Highly polished aluminum surface in the cavity proper; slight roughness to generate losses where field may escape at the top of the movable
plunger.

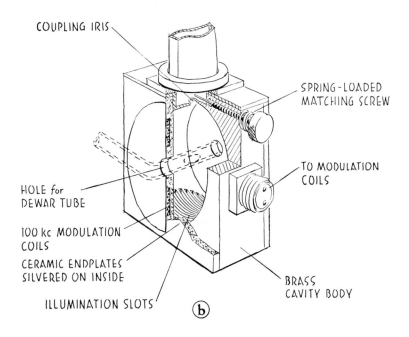

COUPLING IRIS

SPRING-LOADED
MATCHING SCREW

TO MODULATION
COILS

HOLE for
DEWAR TUBE

100 kc MODULATION
COILS

CERAMIC ENDPLATES
SILVERED ON INSIDE

ILLUMINATION SLOTS

BRASS
CAVITY BODY

(b)

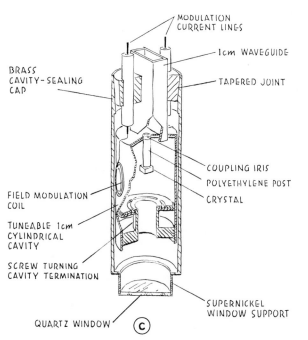

MODULATION
CURRENT LINES

1cm WAVEGUIDE

BRASS
CAVITY-SEALING
CAP

TAPERED JOINT

COUPLING IRIS

POLYETHYLENE POST

CRYSTAL

FIELD MODULATION
COIL

TUNEABLE 1cm
CYLINDRICAL
CAVITY

SCREW TURNING
CAVITY TERMINATION

SUPERNICKEL
WINDOW SUPPORT

QUARTZ WINDOW

(c)

Fig. 7.6-7b and c.

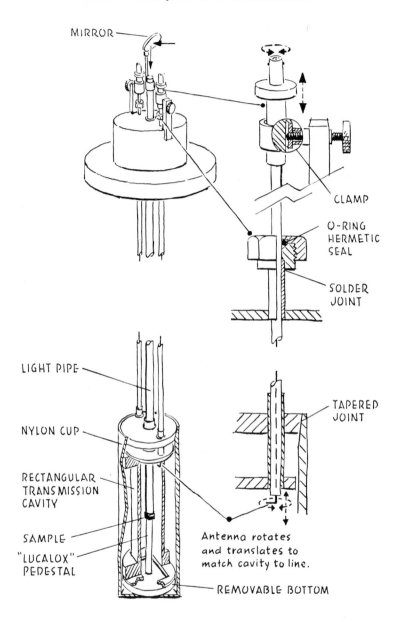

MIRROR

CLAMP

O-RING
HERMETIC
SEAL

SOLDER
JOINT

LIGHT PIPE

TAPERED
JOINT

NYLON CUP

RECTANGULAR
TRANSMISSION
CAVITY

SAMPLE

"LUCALOX"
PEDESTAL

Antenna rotates
and translates to
match cavity to line.

REMOVABLE BOTTOM

(d)

Fig. 7.6-7d.

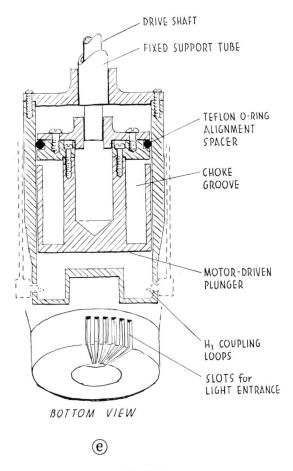

DRIVE SHAFT

FIXED SUPPORT TUBE

TEFLON O-RING
ALIGNMENT
SPACER

CHOKE
GROOVE

MOTOR-DRIVEN
PLUNGER

H_1 COUPLING
LOOPS

SLOTS for
LIGHT ENTRANCE

BOTTOM VIEW

(e)

Fig. 7.6-7e.

(4) A quartz tube with a clear flat end window keeps the refrigerant out of the cavity.

7.6.5 Examples of Experimental Results

We will use naphthalene as the principal example partially for historical reasons because it was studied in the first successful experiments but largely because of the abundance of information on this material.

(a) Naphthalene, $\Delta M_s = 1$ Transitions: $H_1 \perp H_0$. The number of fine structure lines anticipated will depend on the host material. In durene,

naphthalene molecules fit into the lattice in two crystallographic orientations which are not equivalent to each other. Therefore, four lines will
normally appear—two for each of the two molecular orientations. Figure
7.6-8a shows such a four-line spectrum for triplet naphthalene in a durene

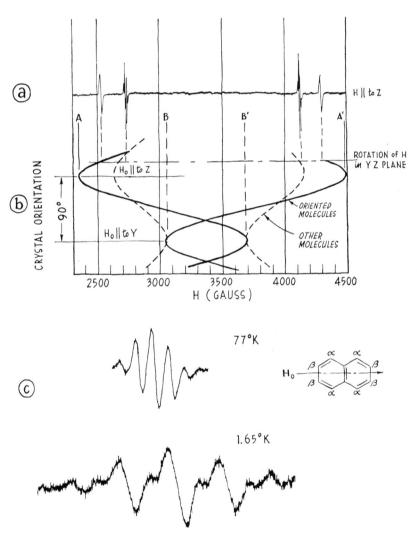

Fig. 7.6-8. (a) Four-line spectrum for triplet naphthalene in durene at 77°K
(after V-6). (b) Variation in H_0 as crystal in Fig. 7.6-4d is rotated in the magnetic
field in the YZ plane (after H-21). (c) Hyperfine structure for naphthalene in durene
at two temperatures and with H_0 parallel to the long axis of naphthalene (after H-15).

crystal at 77°K. Here the high and low field lines arise from molecules with the magnetic field H_0 perpendicular to the molecular plane, i.e., z axis $\parallel H_0$. The other molecules have their long axis parallel to the magnetic field ($H_0 \parallel x$ axis) and these molecules produce the two lines that exhibit hfs. In durene the y axes of the two naphthalene molecule orientations are almost parallel to each other while the x axes are nearly perpendicular. If the magnetic field is rotated in the yz plane for one of the molecular orientations the splitting exhibits the orientation dependence shown by the solid curve in Fig. 7.6-8b and reaches a maximum of 2150 G for $H_0 \parallel z$ and

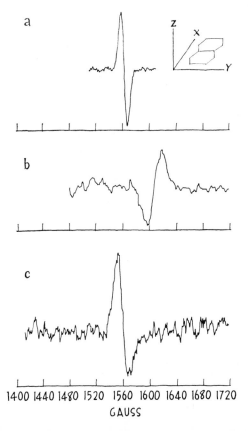

1400 1440 1480 1520 1560 1600 1640 1680 1720
GAUSS

Fig. 7.6-9. Spectra of $\Delta M_s = 2$ transitions in naphthalene: (a) A single durene crystal containing 0.02% naphthalene, H_0 and H_1 parallel to Y axis; (b) crystal with H_0 and H_1 approximately parallel to the x axis for half the naphthalene molecules and parallel to the z axis for the other half; (c) half-field spectrum for a ridged glass solution of 0.012 mole % naphthalene in glycerol. These spectra are mainly of historical interest since substanialy larger signal-to-noise ratios are now available. Microwave frequency, 9.425 kMc. (Courtesy V-1.)

a minimum of 650 G for $H_0 \parallel y$. The molecules with the other orientation are responsible for the splitting indicated by the dashed line (H-21). At certain field orientations lines from the two groups of naphthalene molecules coincide so that two- and three-line spectra can be obtained but most crystal orientations give all four lines.

Part a of Fig. 7.6-8 indicates the presence of hyperfine structure on the lines for H_0 parallel to the x axis and part c shows this structure in detail as observed for two crystal temperatures, 77 and 1.65°K. The hfs appears only for this orientation. Since the x axis for the two types of naphthalene molecules are nearly 90° apart, the five-line hf structure from one molecule will be accompanied by a single line from the other. This hyperfine structure results from the electron interacting equally with the four α-protons on the molecule (intensity ratios, 1:4:6:4:1). Further splitting due to the β protons has not been observed although some additional structure is present in the 1.65°K curve. Such hyperfine structure provides unambiguous proof that naphthalene and not durene is being detected. The linewidths between maximum and minimum slopes are 3.6, 3.8, 3.8, 3.8, and 3.5 G while the spacing between points of crossover was 7.7, 7.5, 7.5, and 7.7 G for light naphthalene in light durene (H-21).

(b) Naphthalene, $\Delta M_s = 2$ Transitions. The discovery by van der Waals and De Groot (V-1) of the "forbidden transition" technique for detecting triplet-state electrons in glassy matrices provided an important step in expanding EPR techniques to many molecules for which single-crystal hosts were not readily available. In addition to simplifying the preparation of samples, this technique removes some of the tediousness in determining D values by the single-crystal technique; however, the E value cannot be determined and exact values of D have been derived only for molecules of adequate symmetry (D-3,V-1). Figure 7.6-9 (V-1) shows several half-field ($\Delta M_s = 2$) spectra for naphthalene. Spectrum a is for a single crystal of about 0.02% naphthalene in durene oriented so that H_0 and H_1 are almost parallel to the y axis of both orientations of naphthalene molecules. Theory predicts that the $\Delta M_s = 2$ transitions will appear at a magnetic field slightly less than half the strength required for the $\Delta M_s = 1$ transition (V-1).*

Spectrum b is obtained when the crystal is orientated with H_1 and H_0

---

* Here the axis of the molecules are labeled the same as in Ref. H-21 which has x and y interchanged from Refs. V-1 and D-3. When due allowance is made for the spectrometer frequencies, this absorption at 1564 G (frequency, 9425 Mc/sec) agrees closely with the predicted value:

$$(g\beta H)^2 = (h\nu/2)^2 - \tfrac{1}{4}(y - z)^2$$

where the matrix elements yz produce a small correction. The linewidth between points of maximum slope is about 10 G.

parallel to the x axis of one-half of the naphthalene molecules (the other one-half of the molecules will have magnetic fields parallel to the z axis). Although experimental conditions do not permit an accurate comparison of intensities between the spectra, the intensity of b is less than that of a, the linewidth is increased to about 20 G, and the absorption occurs at a somewhat higher field strength. Compared with the $\Delta M_s = 1$ transitions, the calculated intensity of the $\Delta M_s = 2$ transitions ranges from 25%, when $(H \parallel y)$ to 2% for $(H \parallel z)$ (V-1). The 2% value was undetectable.

The glassy sample technique succeeds because the anisotropy for the forbidden transitions is much less than that for allowed transitions; therefore, the line broadening is reduced enough to permit observations of absorption lines in a nonoriented sample. For example, in naphthalene the anisotropy for $\Delta M_s = 2$ is only about $\frac{1}{20}$ of that for $\Delta M_s = 1$. Figure 7.6-9c shows a spectrum for a glassy sample of naphthalene (0.012 mole %) in glycerol. Furthermore, for an assembly of randomly oriented molecules in a glass, the transition moment is no longer purely polarized parallel to H_0 but will have a nonvanishing component perpendicular to H_0. Therefore, the $\Delta M_s = 2$ transition can be observed in a conventional cavity. Figure 7.6-10 compares the half-field spectra for naphthalene and several other aromatic molecules with both field orientations, $H_1 \parallel H_0$ and $H_1 \perp H_0$, (G-15). For the three molecules with a threefold (or higher) symmetry axis, the $H_1 \parallel H_0$ curves have a roughly symmetrical resonance doublet while the curves for $H_1 \perp H_0$ exhibit a single asymmetrical line. De Groot and van der Waals have developed a mathematical model for glassy samples in these field orientations and find line shapes that agree well with the doublets and singlets observed experimentally (D-3). Lower-symmetry molecules like naphthalene are more difficult to handle theoretically because the parameter E is no longer zero; however, the single-line spectra for either field orientation agrees with theory (D-3).

(c) **Naphthalene Energy Level Diagram.** Figure 7.6-11 shows the energy level diagrams derived from Refs. V-1 and H-11 for triplet naphthalene in two field orientations, as indicated by the weight of the lines and the sketches of the molecules. Transitions A and A' are for H_0 along the z axis and correspond to the maximum splitting observed in Fig. 7.6-7b while B and B' are for H_0 parallel to the y axis. This diagram illustrates how the high-field portion of the energy diagram can be obtained from resonance measurements at two spectrometer frequencies or from the high and half-field transitions. The $\Delta M_s = 2$ transitions at 1602 and 1707 G fall near the half-field values for the $\Delta M_s = 1$ transitions, 1685 and 1711 G respectively. When H_0 goes to zero, both diagrams converge to the zero field splittings given by $D + E$, $D - E$, and $2E$ indicated on the left.

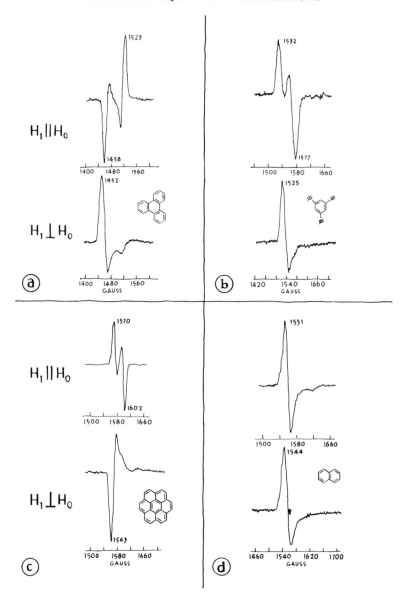

Fig. 7.6-10. Half-field spectra of phosphorescent polyaromatic hydrocarbons in a rigid glass of Alphanol 79 at 77°K. Concentrations are (a) triphenylene 0.0043 mole/kg; (b) 1,3,5-triphenylbenzene, 0.0018 mole/kg; (c) coronene, 0.0008 mole/kg; (d) naphthalene, 0.0159 mole/kg. Derivative spectra are given for two magnetic field orientations, i.e., $H_1 \| H_0$ and $H_1 \perp H_0$. Spectrometer frequency 9.422 ($H_1 \| H$) and 9.387 ($H_1 \perp H$) kMc. (Courtesy D-3.)

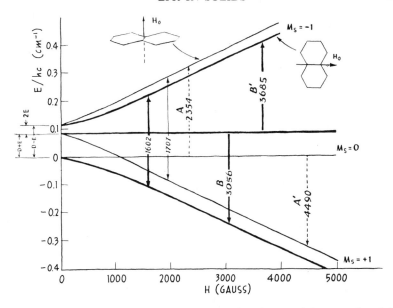

Fig. 7.6-11. Energy levels for the components of the lowest triplet state of naphtha-lene as a function of the magnetic field strength showing both $\Delta M_s = 1$ and $\Delta M_s = 2$ transitions. Observed by Hutchison and Mangum (H-21) and van der Waals and de Groot (V-1), respectively. Note that the x and y axis are interchanged in Refs. H-21 and V-1. To avoid partiality we are not including the axis.

(d) Other Photoexcited Triplets. When we look at examples other than naphthalene, the results are mostly for $\Delta M_s = 2$ transitions. Some examples were given in Fig. 7.6-10 and additional spectra are included in Fig. 7.6-12 for some of the more difficult materials (D-2). In Fig. 7.6-12 the low tem-perature not only improves the signal-to-noise ratio but in the lower two spectra the shape also changes substantially. Some typical linewidths given in Table 7.6-3 cover a range from about 7 to 20 G. As previously mentioned, some reduction in the linewidth is obtainable by deuterating the molecules. Three methods have been used to determine the zero field parameters for various materials:

1. Direct measurement with a zero field spectrometer.

2. Calculation from $\Delta M_s = 1$ transitions as given in Refs. H-21 and H-15.

3. Calculation from $\Delta M_s = 2$ transitions as given in Ref. D-3.

Some values of D and E are listed in Table 7.6-3 with the method of determination and the host material. In a few cases, naphthalene, phenan-threne, and fluorene, the values show a variation due to either the host, the field strength, or the method of measurement; however, these variations

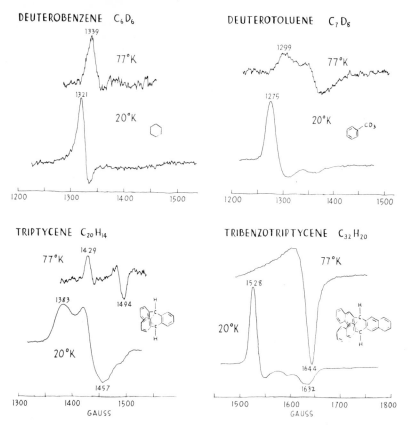

Fig. 7.6-12. Low field spectra with $H_1 \| H_0$: Spectrometer, RH1-X; frequency = 9.279 kMc; cavity, cylindrical TE_{011} (Fig. 7.6-7b); rf power level, below rf saturation level; modulation, 100 kc/sec. Samples: frozen in a rigid glass; one part by volume Spectro grade cylohexane and three parts very pure decalin; deuterobenzene, 0.0517 mole/kg; deuterotoluene, 0.0528 mole/kg; triptycene 0.0082, mole/kg; tribenzo-triptycene, 0.0026 mole/kg. (Courtesy D-2.)

are quite small. The maximum variation in D for the materials listed is only about a factor of 2.

(e) Spectroscopic Splitting Factor. Values of g have been measured for both ordinary naphthalene (H) and completely deuterated naphthalene (D) at about 22.7×10^9 cps with the following results:

	g_{xx}	g_{yy}	g_{zz}
H	2.0030 ± 0.0004	2.0030 ± 0.0012	2.0029 ± 0.0004
D	2.0030 ± 0.0004	2.0031 ± 0.0003	2.0023 ± 0.0006

Table 7.6-3

Zero-Field Parameters

Material	$D/hc,$ cm^{-1}	$E/hc,$ cm^{-1}	Linewidth $\Delta H/(Oe)$	Method	Spectrometer frequency, kMc	Ref.
Naphthalene in durene	0.1003	0.0137		2	22.7	H-19
Naphthalene in durene	0.10118	0.01408		2	9.7	H-19
Naphthalene in biphenyl	0.0994	0.0154		2	22.7	H-19
Naphthalene in biphenyl	0.09920	0.0154		2	9.7	H-19
Naphthalene	0.1049		11.2	3		S-15
Triphenylene	0.134			3		D-3
Triphenylene	0.1353		7.9	3		S-15
1,3,5-Triphenyl-benzene	0.111			3		D-3
Coronene	0.096			3		D-3
Coronene	0.0971		7.0	3		S-15
Benzene	0.1593[a]		18.1	3		S-15
Anthracene	0.0770[a]		11.9	3		S-15
Diphenyl	0.1130[a]		12.6	3		S-15
Terphenyl	0.0961[a]		9.1	3		S-15
Phenanthrene in biphenyl	0.1008	−0.0467		2	22.7	H-19
Phenanthrene in fluorene	+0.1005	−0.0445		2	22.7	H-19
Phenanthrene in fluorene	0.1335[a]		12.2	3		S-15
Fluorene in fluorene	+0.0972	−0.0134		2	22.7	H-19
Fluorene in fluorene	0.1096[a]		13.7	3		S-15
Chrysene	0.1052[a]		10.1	3		S-15
Pyrene	0.0929[a]		11.5	3		S-15
3,4-Benzpyrene	0.0758[a]		10.2	3		S-15
Benzoic acid	0.1385[a]		15.8	3		S-15
Diphenylamine	0.0994[a]		21.8	3		S-15
Indole	0.1277[a]		16.5	3		S-15
Quinoline	0.1068[a]		14.9	3		S-15
Carbaxole	0.1044[a]		11.1	3		S-15

[a] These are D_1 values, where $D_1 = [D^2 + 3E^2]^{\frac{1}{2}}$.

In all but one case g is close but slightly larger than the free electron value of 2.0023.

(f) Ion Radical Salts and Ground State Triplet Molecules. Thus far we have concentrated on triplet states produced by photoexcitation partially out of deference to history and partially to recognize the substantial effort

Table 7.6-4

Low-Field Splittings for Some Triplet States of Ion Radical Salts

Example	D/hc, cm^{-1}	E/hc, cm^{-1}	D/hc, phosphorescent state	Ref.
1. dipotassium triphenylbenzene	0.042		0.111	J-5
2. disodium decacyclene	0.021		0.05	J-5
3. diphenyldiazomethane	0.4050	0.0186		B-28
4. $(\varphi_3 PCH_3) + (TCNQ)_2{}^{-}$ [a]	0.0062	0.00098		C-8
5. $(\varphi_3 AsCH_3) + (TCNQ)_2{}^{-}$ [a]	0.0062	0.00098		C-8

[a] TCNQ = polycyanocarbon tetracyanoguinodimethane.

on such systems. However, triplet states can have other origins, e.g., chemical or thermal, as illustrated in the following discussion. Experimentally the optical problems are eliminated and the spectrometer cavity can be simplified because the triplet states are long lived. They can be prepared outside the cavity and inserted as with conventional samples. Table 7.6-4 lists some of the materials studied in this category along with their zero-field splitting parameters. Four of the five examples exhibit substantially smaller splittings than the photoexcited triplets of Table 7.6-3. With a small splitting it is necessary to establish the identity of the doublet, i.e., differentiate between the fine structure from a triplet state and

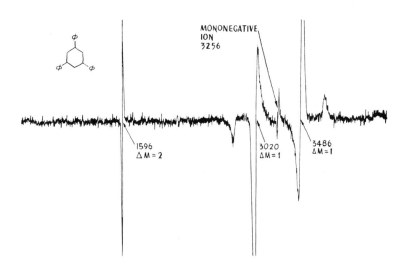

Fig. 7.6-13. Derivative EPR spectrum of a rigid solution of dipotassium triphenylbenzene in methyltetrahydrofuran: spectrometer type, RH1-X; temperature, 77°K; modulation, 100 kc, 0.1 G; sample, dinegative ion. (Courtesy J-5.)

the hyperfine structure from interactions with a nucleus. A good test for the triplet state which eliminates spurious impurity lines and hyperfine structure is the measurement of both the allowed $\Delta M_s = \pm 2$ and the $\Delta M_s = \pm 1$ transitions. Figure 7.6-13 shows such a spectra for the dinegative ion of triphenylene with both transitions indicated.

Returning to Table 7.6-4 the third example has a splitting larger than for

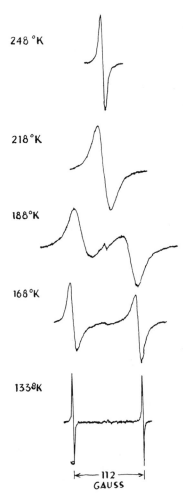

Fig. 7.6-14. Temperature dependence of the EPR absorption of a crystal of the $(\phi_3PCH_3)^+(TCNQ)_2^-$ or $(\phi_3AsCH_3)^+(TCNQ)_2^-$ salts for an arbitrary orientation. Different spectrometer gain settings were employed at the different temperatures. Spectrometer type, RH1-X; cavity, probably TE_{102} rectangular; temperature controlled with Varian gas flow system; modulation 400 cps and 100 kc. (Courtesy C-8.)

any of the photoexcited triplet states. The diphenylmethylene molecule suggested as the responsible species presumably has the two triplet electrons situated mainly on the same carbon atom so that the dipolar interaction is substantial (B-28). Example 4 in Table 7.6-4 has been examined with a thoroughness comparable to naphthalene (C-7,C-8,J-8). These thermally excited triplet states exhibit an interesting temperature-dependent EPR absorption because of temperature-dependent exchange effects. Figure 7.6-14 shows a series of spectra for the $\Delta M_s = 1$ transition at temperatures ranging from 133 to 248°K (C-8). At the lowest temperature the doublet consists of well-resolved Lorentzian shaped lines about 1–2 G in width. An increase in the temperature broadens the lines by exchange broadening until only a single line exists at 218°K. At 248°K exchange narrowing has sharpened the remaining single line. Obviously observations of the triplet state by the $\Delta M_s = 1$ transition requires low temperatures. These exchange effects also cause the $\Delta M_s = \pm 2$ transitions to disappear at the higher temperatures.

Initially the single crystals for Examples 4 and 5 of Table 7.6-4 were attached to a rotatable Teflon holder but in subsequent experiments they were cemented to a quartz rod with Duco or Epoxy cement.

7.7 BIOLOGICAL MATERIALS

The EPR spectroscopy of biological materials is a specialized extension of the observation of free radicals (see Section 7.5). Most of the observed species are radicals either natural or induced, and some biologically important examples have already been encountered in preceding sections; however, the functional biochemical and biological systems ensure a degree of complexity requiring new precautions and techniques. This complexity delayed the arrival of EPR in biology until about 1954 when Commoner et al. (C-18) reported the first evidence of EPR signals in frozen, dried tissues and suggested that free radicals were associated with metabolic activity. Despite this tardy beginning EPR has gained acceptance in many biological areas, and its use is expanding rapidly. Such features as inherent sensitivity and the nondestructive nature of the measurement make EPR an ideal tool for examining biological materials. Furthermore, a number of current theories which embrace free radicals as reactive intermediates in the chemistry of living substances need direct experimental examination. Commoner lists four such cases (C-17):

1. The Michaelis hypothesis: In biological electron transport systems of two-electron oxidation–reduction processes with a one-electron redox reaction, the reaction proceeds by two successive one-electron steps involving free radical intermediates.

2. The Szent-Györgyi suggestion: Electron transport in biological solid state systems occurs in a manner analogous to semiconductors involving physically isolated electron donors and acceptors.

3. Free radical mechanisms are involved in the biological effects of UV light, ionizing radiation, and in carcinogenesis.

4. Hinshelwood's conclusion that living cells are or contain micromolecular polyfunctional free radical systems.

Since all of these examples involve unpaired electrons, they are logical targets for EPR investigations. Despite this logic a few words of admonition from several practitioners experienced in the EPR of biological materials may help to convey the patience and determination required to cope with these systems. Gordy and Shields, who first reported EPR patterns in irradiated proteins, remark that (G-13)

"Investigators who seek to obtain specific information about molecules as complicated as those of the proteins must not be discouraged easily. After many years over a slowly unwinding course, the biochemists are just reaching the ends of some of the shorter protein chains. The x-ray analysts took 20 to 30 years to understand some of the simpler protein diffraction patterns. Encouraged by their eventual success and spurred by a little beginner's luck, we have for some years been trying to obtain information about the proteins from microwave EPR."

In commenting on the interpretation of EPR spectra Whiffen counsels, "The general procedure is by trial and error and it is very difficult to proceed with exact logic from the observations to the coupling coefficients" (W-18). Against this somber note we press on, realizing that beginner's luck plus considerable skill and persistence has resulted in substantial progress during the past 10 years.

7.7.1 Samples, Properties, and Preparation

In discussing techniques for applying EPR to biological systems Ingram (L-12) divides the materials into two main groups appropriate to the four areas of interest mentioned above:

1. Materials containing free radicals produced in: (*a*) enzyme systems; (*b*) photosynthesis, (*c*) irradiation damage, and (*d*) metabolic processes.

2. Materials containing transition metal ions.

Such diverse materials have a wide range of properties but the main problems for EPR arise from the combination of water and low radical concentration frequently encountered in functional systems, i.e., the high dielectric loss of water lowers the cavity Q and thus the spectrometer sensitivity while at the same time the low radical concentration has to be accepted as nature sees fit to provide, particularly in studies of metabolic processes and enzyme reactions. Furthermore, these materials provide an ideal situation for ambiguous results arising from paramagnetic impurities. Many biological samples are not available in a highly purified state; therefore, the experimental procedure should be designed to ferret out such impurity resonances, e.g., by controlled reactions involving the radicals or through tracer techniques.

7.7.2 EPR Considerations

Many of the complications encountered with EPR in biology arise because of the water problem. Several features of this problem have been discussed in preceding sections, e.g., in Section 3.5 water is the classical material in the "loss proportional to E^2" category and Table 4-14 gives an indication of the magnitude of this loss compared with quartz, which is one of the best high-frequency dielectrics. At X-band frequencies, water is 5000 times as lossy as quartz. We will shortly be concerned with the frequency dependence of this loss; therefore, it is well to note that the lowest value in Table 4-14 is at about 10^8 cps where water is about 700 times as lossy as quartz. Experimentally this means that a drop or two of misplaced water, i.e., in a region of modest electrical field, can ruin the Q of a cavity and make resonance measurements impossible. Turning again to Section 3.5 for guidance in dealing with the water problem we can summarize the experimental parameters available for adjustment and trade in the search for adequate sensitivity as follows:

1. In the ideal situation of no rf saturation $S \propto \eta$, Q, and $f^{3/2}$.

2. With partial saturations $S \propto \eta$, $Q^{1/2}$, and $f^{3/2}$.

3. With complete rf saturation $S \propto \eta$ and $f^{3/2}$.

With biological materials it is frequently necessary to operate with partial rf saturation and the samples definitely have a frequency-dependent loss; therefore, the filling factor emerges as the dominant parameter in controlling sensitivity. Another criterion for maximizing the signal is to load the cavity until the Q drops to two-thirds of the empty value for no rf saturation or to nearly one-half for partial saturation (F-3). Within this framework three general procedures have been followed in dealing with water:

1. Reduce the dielectric loss by freezing the H_2O.

2. Minimize the sample extension into the electric field.

3. Select the resonance frequency where the tan δ for water is a minimum.

Freezing the water avoids the problem for those materials that can tolerate the low temperatures, but for many functional biological systems this is no solution and it will not be considered further here. Most aqueous samples have been measured in systems which minimize the interaction with the electric field; therefore, more than a modicum of attention has been concerned with cavity geometry and the optimum sample thickness. For example, Stoodley (S-23) calculated values of Q as a function of sample size for both rectangular TE_{102} and cylindrical TE_{101} cavities and concluded that the rectangular cavity was more efficient by a factor of about 1.5. Figures 7.7-1 and 7.7-2 illustrate his results with plots of $Q\eta$ versus the sample thickness.* The three curves correspond to the following calculational models.

"Lossless Sample" Method. The electric and magnetic field distributions in the cavity are adjusted to allow for the perturbation by the sample assuming a refractive index of 8, but no allowance is made for field distortion due to sample losses. Such assumptions lead to the standing wave distributions shown in Fig. 7.7-3 where the magnetic field is pulled in and intensified by the sample but the effect on the electrical field is negligible.

"Empty Cavity" Solution. This model ignores the dielectric properties of the sample and uses the field distribution for the empty cavity similar to

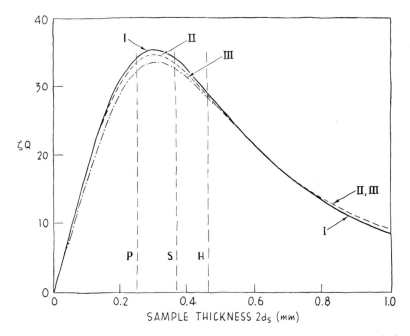

Fig. 7.7-1. Relation between ζQ and sample thickness for aqueous sample in a TE_{102} rectangular cavity, wavelength = 3.2 cm: I = curve for the "lossless sample" method; II = curve for the "empty cavity" solution; III = curve for the "empty cavity solution including the effect of the sample container. (Courtesy S-23.)

* In Refs. S-22 and S-23 ζ is used to designate the filling factor; therefore, the product ζQ in Figs. 7.7-2, 7.7-3, and 7.7-4 is equivalent to $Q\eta$ throughout the text.

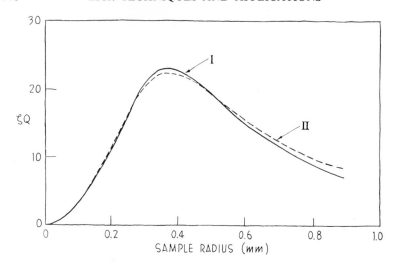

Fig. 7.7-2. Relation between ζQ and sample radius for capillary tube sample in TE_{011} cylindrical cavity, wavelength 3.2 cm: I = curve for the "lossless sample" method; II = curve for the "empty cavity" appoximation. (Courtesy S-23.)

the calculation of Fehr (F-3). This procedure leads to the "Q loaded/Q unloaded equals two-thirds" criterion for loading cavities.

"*Sample Container*" *Solution.* This is an extension of the empty cavity solution to allow for a sample in a quartz tube with 1 mm walls.

All three solutions lead to an optimum thickness of ~ 0.3 mm; however, the peak is rather broad and the $Q\eta$ factor remains nearly constant for thicknesses between 0.25 and 0.35 mm. Sample thicknesses selected by three investigators, indicated by P, S, and H in Fig. 7.7-1, ranged from 0.25 to 0.45 mm.

In Fig. 7.7-2 the lossless sample and empty cavity solutions for a cylindrical TE_{101} cavity both lead to an optimum sample diameter of 0.38 mm with a peak $Q\eta$ of 23 compared with 35 for the rectangular cavity.

Turning to Fig. 7.7-3 it is apparent that the electric field intensity is essentially proportional to the distance from the cavity center over the range of dimensions appropriate for aqueous samples, i.e., the maximum field encountered is proportional to the sample thickness. If a sample of thickness $2d$ in the TE_{102} cavity is split and mounted with a thickness $d_s/2$ at each end and d_s in the middle the losses will be cut by a factor of 4, and if the sample can be sliced in eighths and mounted on the four cavity walls, as in Fig. 4-12, the losses would be cut by a factor of approximately 16. These more involved distributions are frequently inconvenient to achieve;

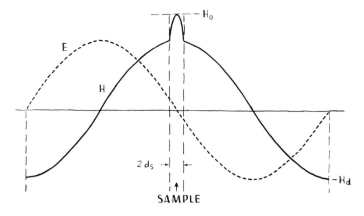

Fig. 7.7-3. Standing waves of E and H in a TE_{102} rectangular cavity. (Courtesy S-23.)

therefore, such modest signal improvements are generally of more bother than value. However, consideration for the electric field distribution suggests provisions for adjusting the cell position to center on the $E = 0$ antinode and such provisions are incorporated in some of the commercial cell holders.

In situations where thin samples are impossible or too inconvenient, prevailing practice has diverged in at least three directions:

1. Long rectangular cavities, e.g., $TE_{1,0,10}$–$TE_{1,0,12}$.
2. Low-frequency spectrometers, e.g., 100 Mc.
3. Coil elements instead of cavities.

The literature contains a few spirited remarks supporting favored approaches but a good yardstick for comparing the relative sensitivities is not available. Homemade units of all three types have been successfully used on aqueous samples and commercial models of all three arrangements are available. Following common practice, sensitivities are generally quoted in terms of detectable quantities of DPPH crystals—a yardstick that is not readily translated to aqueous samples. Under the circumstances we can only weigh the advantages and disadvantages of the several systems while deferring a judgment of relative sensitivity until comparative data appear.

In designing a long cavity a sample cell of convenient size is selected; then the cavity is lengthened until the loaded cavity Q is adequate for resonance measurements. For example, Cook and Mallard (C-20), using a quartz cell with 1 mm walls and a 1 mm thick sample space, found a $TE_{1,0,10}$ cavity to be a suitable length (see Fig. 4-30). In essence, the filling factor is being traded for Q. Unfortunately this trade is not a simple exchange, and the convenience of a large sample is purchased at a slight penalty because when the cavity is lengthened and the increased power loss to the walls is considered, the filling factor decreases faster than the Q increases (S-22). This decrease in the sensitivity factor $Q\eta$ is indicated in Fig. 7.7-4 for an X-band cavity with an optimum sample thickness as defined by curves such as Fig. 7.7-1 for each cavity length. Another convenience of the long cavity is that the sample location is not as critical as in the thin-sample short-cavity case so that elaborate adjustors or locators are not necessary.

The advocates of low-frequency spectrometers barter the Boltzmann factor of Eq. 2-1 for an inherently large sample and a minimum loss factor, tan δ. On a simple frequency basis a sample 3 mm thick at 300 Mc/sec has the same electrical length as a 0.1 mm sample at X-band frequencies. With frequencies in this megacycle range cavities are often replaced with coils which can accommodate samples of convenient size, e.g., 7 mm diam by 10 mm long.

This concept of a coil sensing element has also been extended to X-band

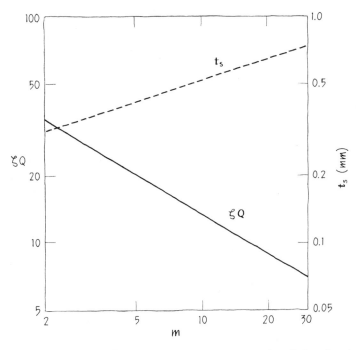

Fig. 7.7-4. Variation of the filling factor times loaded Q product (ζQ) and optimum sample thickness t_s with cavity length for TE_{1on} cavity at 9.375 kMc. (Courtesy S-22.)

frequencies, e.g., the slow "wave element" can be operated immersed in water (43). The structure can accommodate samples up to 2 cm o.d. and 4 cm long. Reported sensitivities are comparable to conventional X-band cavities. Recommendations as to the best approach to the water problem within the uncertainties of relative sensitivities must vary depending on the situation, particularly on the importance of convenience compared with sensitivity. When the spectrometer is used frequently on nonaqueous samples, the sensitivity advantages of the X band makes this frequency preferable to the low-frequency system and aqueous samples can be handled in thin sections distributed on the walls, in a slow wave structure, or in a long cavity. When aqueous samples predominate by a large margin and some control over spin concentration is available as in radiation experiments, the low-frequency spectrometer permits the largest samples coupled with advantages of magnet simplicity and initial economy. When the main problem is sensitivity and the spin concentration cannot be increased, as in the case of enzyme systems or metabolic processes, the slow wave X-band structure appears to be superior, although the relatively little comparative information makes this judgment weak.

As always, the selection of the spectrometer type involves a blending of sensitivity and convenience. The study of radicals in biological materials is virtually monopolized by X-band homodyne spectrometers with high-frequency modulation, usually 100 kc. Among biologists the passion for home-built spectrometers is well controlled and most of the investigators use commercial instruments. Such spectrometers have been quite adequate for most specimens, particularly when the spin concentration can be at least partially controlled, as for radicals generated by radiolysis or photolysis. In most functional biological materials the normally low radical concentration, the propensity for rf saturation, and the limited filling factor imposed by the water frequently strain the spectrometer sensitivity to the limit. When rf saturation limits the power to well below a milliwatt, a superheterodyne system can usually improve the signal-to-noise ratio at the expense of some added complexity. Observation with the spectrometer tuned to the dispersion phase should also avoid rf saturation, thereby enhancing the signal; however, these last two approaches are not common in the biological literature. In fact, we have encountered no dispersion measurements in this field.

Measurements of g, line shape, linewidth and hfs follow the pattern already discussed for radicals in general; however, yield or G-value determinations deserve an extra word of caution because of the complications introduced in aqueous samples. Ehrenberg (E-3) has discussed the importance of distinguishing between two effects resulting from the samples dielectric properties: (I) the field intensity inside the cavity and the cavity Q

are reduced due to losses in the sample and (2) the microwave field is distorted due to the samples high dielectric constant, as indicated in Fig. 7.7-3. Such measuring rituals as Q spoiling, dual cavities, and unobstructive yardsticks are not bothered by the change in Q when the field distortions are negligible because the Q is either reduced to a common value (Q spoiling) or the sample to yardstick signal ratio remains constant throughout the variation in Q. Unfortunately the field distortion effect can alter the sample-to-yardstick ratio in an unknown manner unless extreme care is observed in calibrating the cavity and yardsticks with standards common both in geometry and dielectric constant to the unknown samples. Furthermore, both precise sample size and location are important. Köhnlein and Müller (K-13) describe a method of calibrating a dual cavity with DPPH immersed in water. To avoid reactions with the water the DPPH was imbedded in Ceresin wax and the water was confined in thin nylon tubes. In this instance, the water reduced the DPPH resonance signal and the signal from the yardstick by the same ratio.

7.7.3 Sample Preparation and Results

(a) **Radicals by Ionizing Radiations.** Most of the radicals in this category were formed in dry biological materials where the irradiation and EPR techniques already described in Section 7.5 are applicable. Proteins and their constituent amino acids account for the lion's share of the studies. Such native fibrous proteins as silk, feathers, hair, and bone have sufficient rigidity to trap radicals at room temperature so the simple irradiation arrangements of Fig. 7.3-4 are adequate. Frequently the specimens are sealed in vials to provide a controlled atmosphere, e.g., vacuum, dry He, N_2, O_2, or water vapor, depending on the degree of isolation of reaction desired. Also, transfer techniques are convenient for many of these materials, i.e., transferring the vial from the radiation source to the cavity and sliding the sample to the nonirradiated end of the vial for EPR observations. Irradiation sources, rates, and total doses are similar to those listed for organic compounds. X-ray generators and ^{60}Co sources predominate and total doses commonly range from 10^6 to 10^8 rads. Table 7.7-1 lists the exposure conditions for typical examples.

As with other organic radicals, the splitting factors are near but always slightly greater than the free electron value, i.e., between 2.0023 and 2.01. Hyperfine structure is usually present and the resolution in native materials corresponds to that generally observed in glassy or multicrystalline materials. Despite the extreme complexity of biological materials the main features of the hfs frequently are limited to a few patterns. For example, Gordy and Shields (G-13) found that two kinds of hf patterns are very common for irradiated proteins. One is the doublet presumably resulting

Table 7.7-1

Typical Irradiation Conditions for Biological Materials

Material	Radiation	Rate	Total dose	Temp	Atmosphere	Ref.
Seeds						
Agrostis stolonifere (barley)	x-rays		0.8–3×10^5 rads	$-193°K$	Air	E-4
Dry *Agrostis stolonifere*, 4.5% H_2O	185 KV x-rays	800 R/min	1.5×10^5 rads	$293°K$	N_2	S-19
Proteins and nucleic acids						
Gelatine	100–150 KV x-rays	1000–20,000 R/min	10^6–10^7 rads	77–$300°K$	Vacuum	M-16
Human serum albumin	100–150 KV x-rays	1000–20,000 R/min	10^6–10^7 rads	77–$300°K$	Vacuum	M-16
Pepsin	100–150 KV x-rays	1000–20,000 R/min	10^6–10^7 rads	77–$300°K$	Vacuum	M-16
Casein	100–150 KV x-rays	1000–20,000 R/min	10^6–10^7 rads	77–$300°K$	Vacuum	M-16
Thiogel	100–150 KV x-rays	1000–20,000 R/min	10^6–10^7 rads	77–$300°K$	Vacuum	M-16
Hemoglobin	100–150 KV x-rays	1000–20,000 R/min	10^6–10^7 rads	77–$300°K$	Vacuum	M-16
Deoxyribonucleic acid (DNA)	100–150 KV x-rays	1000–20,000 R/min	10^6–10^7 rads	77–$300°K$	Vacuum	M-16
	^{60}Co	7×10^5 rads/hr	10^7 rads	$77°K$	Vacuum	A-4
Ribonucleic acid	100–150 KV x-rays	1000–20,000 R/min	10^6–10^7 rads	77–$300°K$	Vacuum	M-16
DNA from salmon sperm	^{60}Co	7×10^5 rads/hr	10^7 rads	$77°K$	Vacuum	O-4
	^{60}Co	6×10^6 rads/hr	to 5×10^7 rads	$77°K$	Vacuum	
DNA from herring sperm	^{60}Co	2.7×10^4 R/hr 5.6×10^5 R/hr	0.8–6×10^7 R	Room	Various atmospheres	D-10
Silk, chicken feather quill	^{60}Co		$\sim 5 \times 10^6$ R	$77°K$		P-5
Rat-tail tendon, fish fin bone						G-13
Bird leg bone, porcupine quill etc.						G-14

from electron interactions with the hydrogen at a CH bond and characteristic of glycylglycine or polyglycine. The other is characteristic of irradiated cystine (sometimes called the "sulfur pattern" because the unpaired electron is interacting with a sulfur atom). Figure 7.7-5 shows these two spectra along with spectra from native materials exhibiting similar hfs. Protein spectra are not always as clear and simple as these examples because both spectra may be superimposed, other species may exist at low temperatures, or impurity atoms either native to the sample or the environment may broaden existing or generate new lines.

When the doublet and "sulfur" patterns are superimposed, several

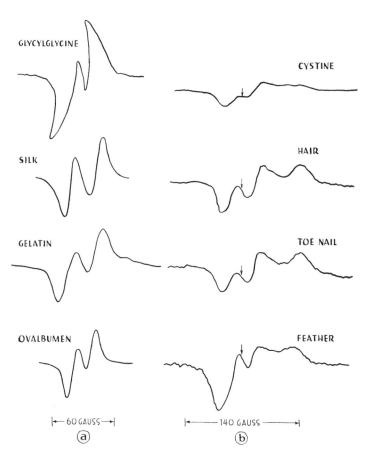

Fig. 7.7-5. Two types of hfs commonly observed in irradiated protein materials: (a) the glycylglycine pattern and (b) the sulfur pattern. [(a) After G-13, M-16, H-10; (b) Courtesy G-12.]

experimental techniques can be of assistance in unfolding the spectrum, e.g., field orientation, selective modulation amplitude, mechanical mixtures of constituent amino acids, and thermal annealing. Interestingly, the doublet in some of the fibrous proteins exhibits a field orientation dependence in the hf splitting similar to that observed in well-ordered crystals. Table 7.7-2 shows examples of this dependence ranging from a factor of 2 in well-ordered silk to nearly isotropic splitting in bone with an average ΔH of about 18 G (G-11). While the "sulfur" spectrum exhibits a larger anisotropic g factor, it is not particularly orientation dependent; therefore, sample orientation may assist in determining which lines belong to the doublet. Frequently the "sulfur" spectrum is considerably broader than the doublet pattern and the magnetic field modulation amplitude can be selected to favor either the narrow or broad lines. Under certain conditions, particularly low-temperature experiments, the protein spectrum can be duplicated with a fair degree of fit by irradiating mechanical mixtures of the constituent amino acids. If the synthesis is satisfactory, the irradiated acids can be measured to determine their contribution. At room temperature and above substantial evidence exists for the migration of radiation damage in various proteins (H-9,P-5), e.g., the hfs changes during warming or during prolonged storage at constant temperature. Figure 7.7-6 illustrates this change in both the doublet and "sulfur" spectra for samples warmed from 77°K to room temperature. Apparently this change in hfs involves the migration of unpaired spins to new sites because the total spin concentration changes only slightly. In mechanical mixtures such conversions are not observed. Figure 7.7-7 shows a similar change as it occurs slowly at constant temperature, i.e., over an 8 day period. Presumably the conversion rates depend both on the material and the temperature, e.g.,

Table 7.7-2

Dependence of the Doublet HF Splitting in Some Irradiated Native Proteins on Their Orientation in the Magnetic Field (G-13)

Specimen	Observed doublet splitting, G	
	Specimen axis $\parallel H$	Specimen axis $\perp H$
Silk	26	13
Chicken feather quill	20	16.5
Rat tail tendon	18.2	16.2
Fish fin bone	18	15.8
Bird leg bone	17.8	15.6

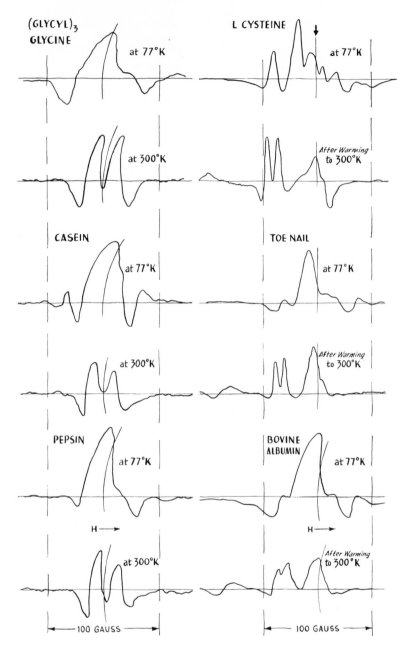

Fig. 7.7-6. Electron spin resonance patterns (second-derivative curves) of γ-irradiated natural proteins at two temperatures exhibiting the glycylglycine and sulfur patterns. The top curves represent observations of the unwarmed sample immediately after irradiation at 77°K. The bottom curves were recorded about an hour after the samples had been warmed at 300°K. The vertical lines mark the position for $g = 2.0036$ (the g factor of the DPPH reference signal). (Courtesy P-5.)

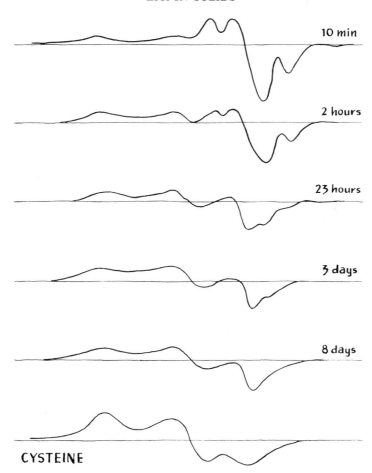

10 min

2 hours

23 hours

3 days

8 days

CYSTEINE

Fig. 7.7-7. The change with time in the qualitative EPR spectrum of reduced glutathione. The polycrystalline compound was irradiated and kept in vacuum at room temperature. First derivative spectrum; dose = 4.2×10^5 R; a comparison spectrum of cysteine is included. (Courtesy H-9.)

a 10 min heat at 100°C produced about the same results as the 8 days at room temperature (H-9).

Considerable interest and effort has been devoted to quantitative measurements of the radical yield. The interchange of standards (Table 5-5) originated in and has been carried out primarily in laboratories concerned with materials of biological interest. All studies of radiation protection systems require such quantitative data. Absolute yield measurements are difficult to make and considerable variation appears in the results reported from different laboratories. Müller (M-16) observed that irradiated dry amino acids, proteins, and nucleic acids had G values of an equal order of magnitude and excluding molecules containing aromatic rings, approximately one radical is produced per 100 eV of absorbed energy, i.e., $G = 1$. Both temperature and atmosphere influence the yield as discussed in Section 7.5; therefore, the highest yields are obtained when the material has sufficient rigidity to trap radicals, but enough flexibility to permit one molecular fragment to escape, thus avoiding recombination. Table 7.7-3 lists G values for a number of biological materials with some of the yardsticks and temperatures involved. No attempt has been made to compare all the measurements reported for a given substance, and indeed, a larger spread of values can be found, a point that is not surprising in view of the uncertainties in quantitative measurements. Furthermore, it must always be remembered that the observed G values always represent a lower limit because they correspond to the number of radicals stabilized long enough for the observation, not necessarily the number produced. Considering these circumstances and the yardstick problem, the agreement in Table 7.7-3 seems quite good.

(b) Radicals Trapped by Sudden Freezing. The radicals involved in this method are usually intermediate species in a chemical reaction that has been interrupted by sudden freezing. Generally the ritual involves (*1*) thoroughly mixing the reacting solutions, (*2*) continuing the reaction for a predetermined time, and (*3*) terminating the reaction by squirting the solution into a freezing bath. A series of samples prepared with different reaction times thus indicates the role of the radicals at various stages of the reaction. To obtain meaningful results, both the mixing and freezing times must be short compared with the reaction under study. For example, Bray (B-29) used a freezing time one-tenth the half-time of the reaction for a dilute aqueous solution. A jet diameter of 0.2 mm was calculated for a freezing time of 10 msec, assuming 20°C water squirted into −80°C hexane under conditions where the water retained a cylindrical geometry and turbulance maintained the water surface at nearly −80°C throughout the freezing process. Several factors are important in selecting the freezing bath. First, the bath should be immiscible with respect to the sample. Second, the temperature should be maintained as low as possible without causing undue viscosity. Third, the boiling point should be higher than the sample temperature to avoid the reduction in heat transfer that occurs when there is local vaporization at the sample bath interface. Liquid nitrogen has been used but not too successfully because of gassification at the point of contact with the sample (Y-1). Hexane (mp, −100°C; bp, +70°C) cooled in solid CO_2 to about −60°C and isopentane (mp, −160°C; bp, +30°C) cooled with liquid nitrogen to about −140°C have been

Table 7.7-3. Examples of *G* Values in Biological Materials

Material	Atmospheric pressure, mm Hg	Irradiation dose, R	eV/rad	G value	Temp, °K	Yardstick	Method[a]	Ref.
Bovine serum albumin	10^{-4} to 10^{-5}	3.6×10^5		4.0	295	Coal[b]	1	H-18
	10^{-4} to 10^{-5}	3.6×10^5		3.5	77	Coal	1	H-18
	10^{-4} to 10^{-5}		100	1.0			1	M-16
Human serum albumin	10^{-4} to 10^{-5}		70				3	M-16
Gelatin	10^{-4} to 10^{-5}		17	5.9	300		3	M-16
	10^{-4} to 10^{-5}		~50	~2	77		3	M-16
Ribonuclease	10^{-4} to 10^{-5}	3.6×10^5		6.7	295	Coal	1	H-10
	10^{-4} to 10^{-5}	3.6×10^5		4.5	295	Coal	1	H-10
					77			
Casein	10^{-4} to 10^{-5}		160	0.6			3	M-16
Pepsin	10^{-4} to 10^{-5}		40	2.5			3	M-16
Sperm heads			250	0.4			3	M-16
ADN (sperm of herring)	10^{-3}	2×10^7		0.067	300	Carbon		D-10
Insulin	10^{-4} to 10^{-5}	3.6×10^5		4.1	295	Coal	1	H-10
Zein	10^{-4} to 10^{-5}	3.6×10^5		5.0	295	Coal	1	H-10
	10^{-4} to 10^{-5}	3.6×10^5		2.3	77	Coal	1	H-10
Ovalbumin	10^{-4} to 10^{-5}	3.6×10^5		2.3	295	Coal	1	H-10
Papain	10^{-4} to 10^{-5}	3.6×10^5		4.1	295	Coal	1	H-10
Aldolase	10^{-4} to 10^{-5}	3.6×10^5		4.5	295	Coal	1	H-10
Thiogel			14	7.1	295	Coal	3	M-16
Hemoglobin			140	0.7			3	M-16
Deoxyribonucleic acid			170	0.6			3	M-16
Libonucleic acid			110	0.9			3	M-16

[a] (1) Graphical integrations; (2) weighing; (3) Momentum balance.   [b] Anthracite powdered carbon calibrated against DPPH.

satisfactory for aqueous solutions having a half-life of about 110 msec (B-29). Figure 7.7-8 shows the apparatus used by Bray (B-29) to measure, mix, and freeze aqueous samples. A hydrolic ram (A) forces metered amounts of the reacting constituents from the syringe (B) through the mixing chamber (C) and the reaction tube (D), out the jet (E), and into the bath (F) in sample collection times on the order of 1 sec. In working with concentrated protein solutions it was necessary to avoid all-glass syringes because denaturation on the ground glass surfaces caused the syringes to jam. Syringes with Perspex barrels and Teflon plungers were satisfactory. All polythene tubes were connected to Perspex blocks with stainless steel couplings arranged so there was no contact between liquid and metal as indicated in insert a. The polythene tubes were heated slightly over a radiant electric heater to permit forming the flanges and drawing out the jet tip as shown in insert b.

Samples were prepared according to the following procedure: (1) Fill the syringes carefully to avoid bubbles and connect them to the mixing chamber.

(2) Adjust the drive screws (H) to make contact with the Teflon plungers and move the ram slowly to fill the system to the inlet of the mixing chamber.

(3) Withdraw the ram a little way so that it will reach maximum velocity before striking the plungers, attach a suitable reaction tube-jet assembly and set the ram stop (G) for desired quantity of sample.

(4) Close the solenoid valve and apply about 4 atm pressure to the pressure chamber, i.e., the same pressure for all samples in a series.

(5) Remove the container of cooling liquid from its bath, hold it with the surface of the liquid 1–2 cm below the jet, and open the solenoid valve.

(6) After the sample has been delivered, return the container to the cooling bath and pack the frozen sample into the bottom of the silica tube with the Teflon packer shown in insert c.

(7) Transfer the tube to a liquid nitrogen bath to reduce the reaction rate to a negligible value.

The ram velocity is controlled by the needle valve and the air pressure while the reaction time is controlled both by the ram velocity and the length of the reaction tube. The delivery time was measured by electrical contacts operated by the ram. Reaction times ranging from 10 to 10^3 msec were satisfactorily covered with this apparatus. Volumes of the reaction tubes and the jet tubes were determined by weighing each tube empty then full of H_2O.

(c) **Flow Techniques.** The various flow techniques offer another approach to the detection of short-lived paramagnetic species. No attempt is made to

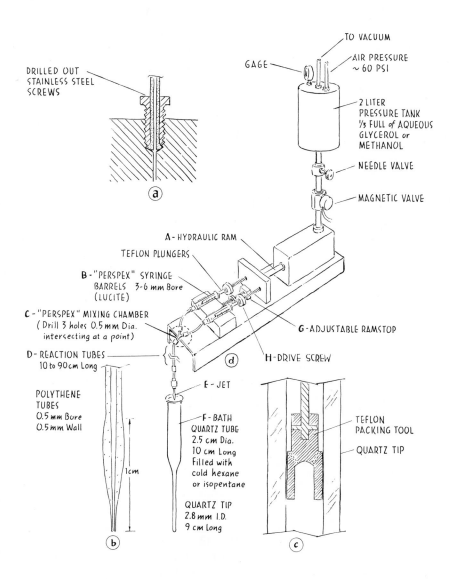

Fig. 7.7-8. Apparatus for sudden freezing of aqueous solutions: (a) connection between polythene tubes and "Perspex" block; (b) jet tip made from drawing section of polythene tube; (c) Teflon packer for compacting sample into bottom of sample tube; (d) assembled hydraulic ram. (After B-29 and B-30.)

stabilize the radicals, but on the contrary, reactions are encouraged and the radicals are observed at various stages in the course of the reaction as they flow through the EPR cavity. Herein lies one advantage of the method: since the reaction is not interrupted, there is no opportunity for the stabilizing process to alter or effect the radicals observed. Another advantage stems from the fact that flow techniques require liquids; therefore, good resolution of the hfs is possible. Of course, there are problems, particularly with biological materials. For example, most of the appropriate solutions are aqueous, necessitating the precautions of Section 7.7.2; many reactions are rapid, thereby requiring high flow rates; and particularly in the case of enzyme reactions, the sample is frequently limited both in available quantity and the concentration of unpaired electrons.

The two main variations in the flow technique are *continuous flow* and *stopped flow*. In both cases the reacting constituents are metered and mixed in a system similar to that of Fig. 7.7-8 then the solution flows into a reaction cell located in the cavity. As the names imply, the solution may be allowed to flow continuously so that the spectrometer observes radicals at a selected time after mixing or the flow may be stopped so the spectrometer follows the change in a selected group of radicals as a function of time. In the continuous flow technique the time between the start of the reaction (mixing) and the point of observation can be controlled either by varying the position of the cavity along the reaction tube, by varying the flow rate, or by a combination of position and flow rate. With aqueous solutions and thin rectangular reaction cells it is slightly more convenient to vary the flow rate than to change positions. Also the variable rate can be less extravagant in the comsumption of sample, particularly at longer times. If the signal-to-noise level permits, all the EPR characteristics can be determined, particularly the hfs and the spin concentration. Besides offering the usual opportunities for identification, the hfs indicates whether a single radical step is involved or several species are participating in the reaction. The spin concentration measurements are particularly useful because they determine the reaction rate; however, once the positions of the absorption lines are known, it is more convenient to use the stopped flow system to measure radical formation and decay rates, particularly in fast reactions. In the stopped flow technique the spectrometer is adjusted to sit on one of the absorption peaks, the flow is started and the radical formation rate is measured, then the flow is stopped while the spectrometer records the rate of radical decay. Flow control can be achieved with three microsolenoid valves, one located at each entrance to the mixing chamber and one at the exit of the reaction cell. Two advantages of stopped flow control are economic use of the sample and direct determination of decay rates.

A general requirement for all flow techniques is speed because all manipulations such as mixing and flow rate must be fast compared with the reaction rate and in stopped flow experiments the detection system must be able to faithfully follow the decay rate. A few reactions are very slow, with radical lifetimes extending up to an hour or more, in which case the speed requirement is so relaxed that samples can be mixed and sampled in conventional cells. Most reactions require the speed of flow systems which have a minimum time from mixing to measurement of about 5–10 msec (Y-1), e.g., mixing times are about 1 msec and several milliseconds are required to fill the reaction cell.

Several results obtained with continuous flow and stopped flow systems are shown in Figs. 7.7-9 and 7.7-10, respectively. When the radical formation rate is fast compared with the flow rate, the signal jumps immediately

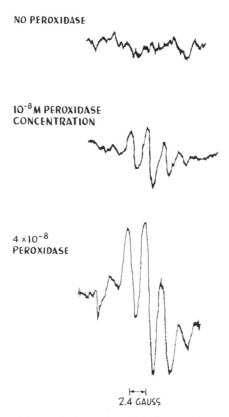

NO PEROXIDASE

10^{-8} M PEROXIDASE
CONCENTRATION

4×10^{-8}
PEROXIDASE

|←——→|
2.4 GAUSS

Fig. 7.7-9. Spectra of the semiquinone formed in the steady state during continuous flow at a flow rate of 8 ml/sec: $10^{-2}M$ hydroquinone; $10^{-2}M$ H_2O_2; pH = 4.8; and the concentrations of peroxidase are indicated. (Courtesy Y-1.)

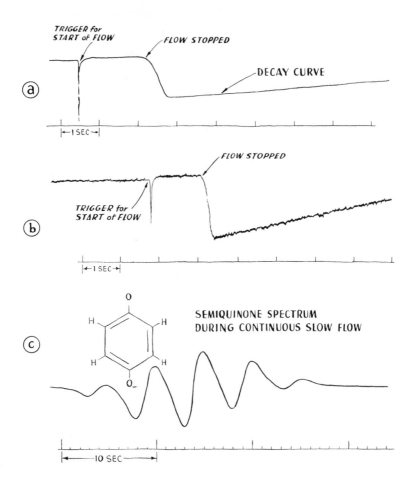

Fig. 7.7-10 Parts (a), (b), and (c) illustrate the application of stopped flow systems to studying the rate of formation of the semiquinone of hydroquinone. In (a), $10^{-3}M$ hydroquinone in alcohol and an alkaline alcohol solution with a limited concentration of O_2 were fed into the mixing chamber and then passed into the sample cell in the cavity at a flow rate of 6 cm³/sec. The trace was obtained by adjusting the magnetic field so that the signal would be at its maximum. The left-hand marker on (a) indicates where the flow was started, zero concentration of free radicals being observed in the cavity. The second marker indicates where the flow was stopped and the formation of the semiquinone begins. Subsequently the entire formation curve was traced out. The half-life for this reaction is 0.5 sec. Part (b) illustrates how the formation rate is increased when the solutions are saturated with O_2 (half-life, 0.15 sec). Part (c) shows the complete spectrum of the intermediate species obtained during continuous flow. (Courtesy V-5.)

to the steady-state level and only the decay rate is measurable. However, faster relative flow rates may permit resolution of both the formation and decay curves as shown in Fig. 7.7-10. Because of the general utility of flow systems they are available from several commercial suppliers, as indicated in the Appendix.

(d) Photosynthesis. As in other reactions EPR has been especially valuable in detecting intermediate products during photosynthesis. In reviewing the subject Calvin and Androes (C-1) point out that while the ultimate products have been known for a long time, e.g., carbohydrates, oxygen, and other plant substances, earlier steps remain to be established. The currently postulated intermediates contain unpaired electrons and are therefore ideal subjects for EPR. While optical spectroscopy gave general support to such models, EPR provided the first direct evidence that free radicals participate in the metabolic activity of living cells (C-17). Experimentally the EPR equipment and procedures parallel closely those already described under photolysis. However, the usual complexities involving H_2O in the biological samples prevail and presumably the situation is substantially different on a microscopic level. The photosynthesis organism apparently absorbs a photon and efficiently carries out an orderly chemical transformation without damage to itself while in the photolysis of Section 7.5.5 the situation is somewhat simpler in that the absorbing molecules are sacrificed directly in the reaction.

Initially, EPR measurements were made on lyophilized spinach leaves which exhibited a photosensitive resonance in addition to an overlapping spectrum with five hyperfine peaks that persisted in unilluminated material. Unfortunately such preparation techniques leave a small cloud of uncertainty surrounding the interpretation of these first results because living cells might not behave in the same manner as these leaves. Accordingly, subsequent studies have also incorporated samples of living algae and bacteria. Table 7.7-4 lists some typical examples, references, and experimental conditions.

The EPR parameters receiving the most attention are:

1. Hyperfine structure: In view of the specimens complicated structure and the rather minimal resolution of the hf lines, the radicals are not readily identified; however, it has been possible to determine the number of species present and their relative photosensitivity.

2. Spin concentration: Quantum efficiency is an important factor in photosynthesis; therefore, there is a strong interest in quantitative measurements.

3. Time response of EPR signal to the exciting light: In the absence of sufficient evidence to identify the paramagnetic species, such kinetic

Table 7.7-4

Examples of Photosensitive Materials Studied by EPR Techniques

Material	Optical absorption peak, Å	Temp, °K	Light wave-length, Å	Ref.
Chloroplasts				
Spinach leaves	6700	120 and 298	7250[a]	S-18
				C-1
Tobacco leaves			Tungsten filament lamp	S-18
Whole algae				
Chlorella			White[b]	C-17
Scenedesmus			White	S-18
Romaria			White	S-18
Nostoc			White	S-18
Anacystis			White	S-18
Photosynthetic bacteria				
Rhodospirillum rubrum	8800	120–298	5080–7200	C-1
			White	S-18
Rhodopseudomonas spheroides	4200	120–298	White	C-1
				S-18
Chromatium			White	S-18
Chromatophores from chromatium			White	S-18
Dry polycrystalline chlorophyll A	below 4000	77	Zirconium arc White	S-16
Solid β-carotene		77	White	S-16
Chlorella pyrenoidosa	6950	273	5420[c]	A-8

[a] 1.1×10^{16} quanta/sec into microwave cavity.
[b] 190–6750 Lux.
[c] 500–900 W filtered.

studies provide an additional basis for judging the feasibility of various proposed models.

The main experimental problems arise from two factors that limit the useful sample size and thus the available signal-to-noise ratio: first, the presence of water in many living samples, and second, the high optical absorption characteristics of these materials restrict the penetration of the exciting light to very thin surface layers. Other factors that influence the rate of rise or decay of the light-induced EPR signal are light intensity, temperature, pH, redox potential, the physiological state of the organisms, and the preparation and storage of the chromatophores. In comparison experiments these factors should be controlled. Some typical values listed in Ref. R-7 for *Rhodospirillum rubrum* are 10^{16} photons/cm^2-sec, $22 \pm 2°$C, 7.5 pH, $+0.30$ V, 5 days growth, and variable storage, respectively. In particular it is important to control the light and temperature so the two effects will not become confused. Tungsten filament projection lamps of 300–1000 W rating are convenient sources of visible illumination; however, they should be used in conjunction with a water filter to remove the infrared radiation and suitable optical filters to remove ineffective wavelengths. Extraneous room illumination should also be reduced to a negligible level, e.g., with simple fiber, wood, or black velvet light shields. Measurements of the sample temperature during illumination are desirable to avoid unknown temperature changes. Tungsten lamps are sufficiently stable so that no special regulation is required to avoid drifts in signal level during the measurement of a spectrum. Stability is a problem with high-pressure mercury arc lamps like the AH-6. JH1 or AN1 100 W lamps are sufficiently stable but a bit awkward and inefficient optically because of their size. The dewar, cavity, and illumination arrangements of Fig. 7.6-4 are suitable with the addition of the necessary filters and light baffles. Early kinetic studies (24) were made with tungsten filament lamps and a camera shutter to provide a light pulse. Unfortunately the signal-to-noise ratio was too small on a one-flash basis to permit reliable measurements of the EPR signal growth so that only the decay was recorded. More recent measurements have incorporated a neon lamp which emits principally between

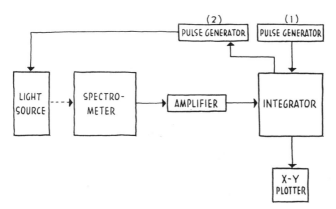

Fig. 7.7-11. Block diagram for photochemical kinetic studies. The appropriate spectrometer, i.e., either optical or EPR, was inserted as desired. (Courtesy R-7.)

5800 and 7200 Å and can be electronically modulated to provide a light pulse with a rise and decay time of about 10 μsec (R-7). When combined with a commercial multichannel analyzer so that the signal can be integrated over many pulses, the signal rise and decay rates become measurable. Figure 7.7-11 illustrates the system used in Ref. R-7. Pulse generator No. 1 determines the repetition rate and starts an event by initiating a sweep of the integrator. After a fixed time delay the integrator triggers the neon lamp and pulse generator No. 2 which controls the duration of the flash. Some typical values for *Rhodospirillum rubrum* were flash duration, 2 sec; repetition time, 16 sec; and integrator sweep times, from 1 to 16 sec, i.e., covering any fraction of the repetition time desired (R-7). Fifty to 500 events provided suitable signal-to-noise ratios.

7.7.4 Typical Results

Figure 7.7-12 shows a sampling of derivative spectra for chlorophyll-containing plant substances, whole algae, and photosynthetic bacteria. All of these materials exhibit a resonance in the dark but exposure to light increases the amplitude of the original spectrum and introduces a new component to the chloroplasts and algae spectrum. Three of the spectra

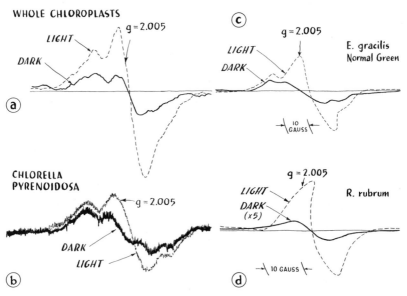

Fig. 7.7-12. EPR spectra in photosensitive plant substances, whole algae, and bacteria. (Chloroplasts, courtesy C-1; *C. pyrenoidosa*, courtesy V-5; *E. gracilis* and *R. rubrum*, curvilinear plots, courtesy C-17.)

contain a hfs of five lines separated by about 6 G in *Chlorella* while the "light" superimposed species appears to be a single line. Although all the *g* factors are close to the free electron value, their slight displacement has been useful in measuring the relative amplitudes of the "light" and "dark" components (C-1). Since only one component develops in the dark, the center of the spectrum where the derivitive crosses the base line is readily apparent and because the "light" *g* values are different, some signal (entirely due to the "light" component) will develop at this position during illumination.

The exciting light can be described by two parameters, i.e., spectral distribution and intensity, and both can influence the development and behavior of detectable spins. In addition, spin production is sensitive to the sample temperature. Figure 7.7-13 illustrates some of the observed light intensity and temperature effects with the development of spins in living algae. The spectrum can be resolved into two components. At both temperatures, component II increases rapidly with light intensity and soon saturates while component I responds to the changing light intensity only at the lower temperature where a saturation behavior is also apparent. Meaningful quantitative measurements of quantum yield must be made at the first part of the curve where the signal is almost linearly proportional to the light intensity. Here the quantum yield is described as (number of

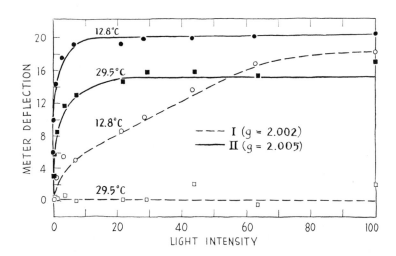

Fig. 7.7-13. EPR signals in photosensitive living algae. Spectral component I develops mostly after component II has reached its maximum value. Component II is observed in the dark, increases with light intensity and has 5 hf lines centered on *g* = 2.005. (Couresty C-17.)

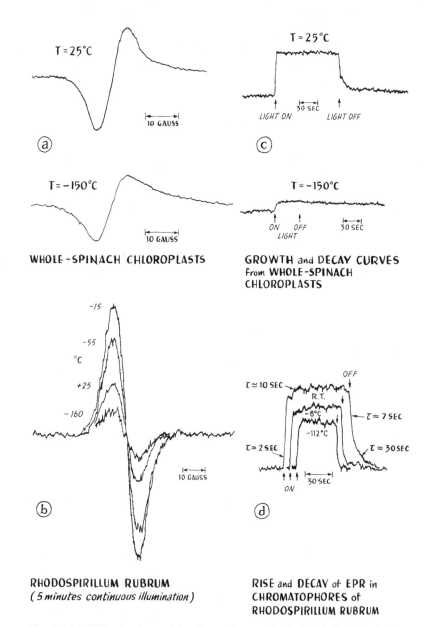

T = 25°C

10 GAUSS

(a)

T = -150°C

10 GAUSS

WHOLE-SPINACH CHLOROPLASTS

T = 25°C

30 SEC

LIGHT ON   LIGHT OFF

(c)

T = -150°C

ON   OFF   30 SEC
LIGHT

GROWTH and DECAY CURVES from WHOLE-SPINACH CHLOROPLASTS

-15
-55
°C
+25
-160

10 GAUSS

(b)

$\tau \approx 10$ SEC   OFF
R.T.
-8°C $\tau \approx 7$ SEC
-112°C
$\tau \approx 2$ SEC $\tau \approx 30$ SEC

ON   30 SEC

(d)

RHODOSPIRILLUM RUBRUM
(5 minutes continuous illumination)

RISE and DECAY of EPR in CHROMATOPHORES of RHODOSPIRILLUM RUBRUM

Fig. 7.7-14. EPR signals resulting from photosynthesis in whole-spinach chloroplasts and *Rhodospirillum rubrum*; *a* and *b* are derivative curves; *c* and *d* are rise and decay curves. (Courtesy C-1.)

unpaired spins)/(number of incident light quanta). In another example, a value of 0.03 was obtained for spinach chloroplasts exposed to about 1.1 × 10^{16} light quanta/sec in a band 400 Å wide centered at 7250 Å (S-18).

The *Chlorella* data in Fig. 7.7-13 indicate that both components are generated more efficiently at the lower temperature. A similar behavior has been observed in other materials; however, this trend does not extend indefinitely. For example, the signal in the spinach chloroplasts of Fig. 7.7-14*a* decreases somewhere between 25 and −150°C. Also the signal for *Rhodospirillum rubrum* increases as the temperatures are lowered to −15°C, then decreases at lower temperatures. Signals have been detected down to 77°K but not at 4°K. When the signal has been formed in whole-spinach chloroplasts by illumination at low temperatures, it does not decay when the light is turned off but persists until the sample is warmed. On the

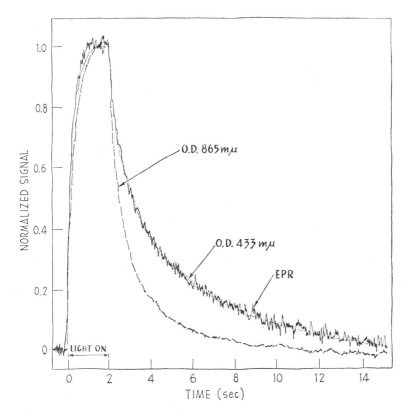

Fig. 7.7-15. Comparison of EPR and optical density signals from the same sample of *Rhodospirillum rubrum* chromatophors. (Courtesy R-7.)

contrary the signal in *R. rubrum* at low temperatures faithfully grows and decays with the light intensity, as shown in Fig. 7.7-14. At higher temperatures, particularly room temperature, the decay signal is altered by the appearance of slower components.

Because of efforts to distinguish whether the paramagnetic species are (*1*) either ordinary chemical radicals formed by the separation of atoms or diffusion of molecular particles, (*2*) unpaired electrons produced by electron transfer, or (*3*) delocalized orbitals in molecular arrays, considerable attention has been given to spin concentration growth and decay measurements as functions of temperature. Early attempts suffered from inadequate resolution at sensitivities capable of detecting the signal above the noise. This type of problem is built to order for signal-to-noise enhancement with a time-averaging computer (R-7). Figure 7.7-15 shows resolved rise and decay signals of both optical density and EPR for *R. rubrum* chromatophors at room temperature. The technique of using several wavelengths in the optical density measurements made it possible to determine which component corresponded to the EPR signal.

Appendix

This includes features and performance specifications of commercial EPR spectrometers as advertised in company literature. While the listing gives a reliable indication of the instruments available in 1967, recent arrivals or departures in the manufacturing ranks may have been overlooked because of the fairly brisk turnover.

Allgemeine Elektricitäts Gesellschaft, Frankfurt, Germany[a]

Spectrometer type (nearest)	RH1-X
Sensitivity, ΔH spins for 1 sec time constant	2×10^{11}
Resolution	~ 1 part in 10^5
Microwave features	
Resonant frequency	9.5 kMc
Klystron power output, W	0.03
Frequency control element	Locked to cavity
Bridge element	Hybrid T
Cavity	
Geometry	Rectangular
Mode	TE_{102}
Q	> 4500
Required magnet gap, in.	1.6
Modulation coils	External
Modulation frequency	125 kc
Modulation amplitude	0.01–10 Oe
Magnets	
Pole diameter, in.	4.7
Field range, Oe	5600 max.
field stability over sample vol.	> 1 part in 10^5
Sweep amplitude	
minimum, Oe	3
maximum, Oe	3000
Sweep rate	
minimum, min	1
maximum, min	100
Sweep linearity	$< 1\%$
Sample size	3.7 mm tube
Accessories	
Nuclear resonance probe	
Variable-temperature sample holder, -160 to $300°C$	

[a] Model: Z23/FMS 57 120a.

Alpha Scientific Laboratories Inc., Berkeley, Calif.[a]

Model	340[b]
Sensitivity, ΔH spins for 1 sec time constant	10^{14}
Resolution	1 part in 10^5
Microwave features	
Resonant frequency	335 Mc
Tuning range	320–350 Mc
Frequency control element	Locked to resonant structure
Frequency stability	1 part in 10^5
Cavity	
Geometry	Helix probe
Openings	Helix is exposed
required magnet gap, in.	About 1
Modulation coils	External
Modulation frequency	100 kc, 60 cps
Modulation amplitude	25G, 150G
Magnets	
Pole diameter, in.	6
Field range	0–500 G
Accessories	
X-band slow-wave structure	
X-band dielectric cavity	
Low-temperature cooling system	
Type 330 digital field control (Hall probe sensor)	
Average transient memory computer	
Digitally converted alpha numeric display, for direct computer entry	

[a] Catalog R-65.
[b] Model 341, same as Model 340 except Helmholtz coils are used for the magnet. Model 345, same as Model 340 except no magnet supplied.

Bruker-Scientific, Irvington-on-Hudson, N.Y.

Models	B-ER 418S	B-ER 414S
Sensitivity, ΔH spins for 1 sec time constant	$< 10^{11}$	$< 10^{11}$
Resolution, mG	3	3
Microwave features		
Resonant frequency, kMc	9.6 (35 available)	9.6 (35 available)
Klystron power output, W	0.25	0.04 (0.25 available)
Frequency control element	Crystal locked	
Frequency stability	$< 10^{-8}$	$< 10^{-6}$

(continued)

Bruker-Scientific, Irvington-on-Hudson, N.Y. (*continued*)

Models	B-ER 418S	B-ER 414S
Cavity		
Modulation frequency	713 cps, 100 kc	100 kc
Modulation amplitude, max G	25	25
Magnets		
Field range, max kG	15	11
(with tapered pole caps)	24	16
Field uniformity, mG	< 3	< 10
Sweep amplitude		
minimum, kG	2.8	1
maximum, kG	10	11
Accessories		
Double modulator cavities		
Cavities for irradiation		
Time-averaging computer		
Integrator		
Unit for field and frequency measurements		

Decca Radar, Wilton-on-Thames, Surrey, England[a]

Models	X-1	X-2[b]
Spectrometer type (nearest)	RH1-X	RS4-X
Sensitivity, ΔH spins for 1 sec time constant	4×10^{11}	~ 6 db better than X-1
Resolution	100 mG	100 mG
Microwave features		
Resonant frequency	9.27 kMc	9.27 kMc
Tuning range	480 Mc/sec	480 Mc/sec
Frequency control element	Crystal-controlled oscillator	Crystal-controlled oscillator
Frequency stability	Few parts in 10^7	Few parts in 10^7
Bridge element	6 db coupler	6 db coupler
Detector	Balanced mixer	Balanced mixer
Cavity		
Geometry	Rectangular	Rectangular
Mode	TE_{102}	TE_{102}
Openings	Irradiation aperture	Irradiation aperture
Q	7000	7000
Required magnet gap, in.	$2\frac{1}{4}$	$2\frac{1}{4}$
Modulation coils	External	External
Modulation frequency	100 kc	100 kc

(*continued*)

Decca Radar, Wilton-on-Thames, Surrey, England (*continued*)

Models	X-1	X-2[b]
Magnets		
Pole diameter, in.	7	11
Field range, kG	0–6	0–20
Field stability with time (30 sec)	50 mG	50 mG
Sweep amplitude		
minimum, mG	100	100
maximum, kG	6	14
Sweep rate		
minimum, mG/sec	1	1
maximum, mG/sec	50	50
Sample size	5, 8, 11 mm o.d. tubes	5, 8, 11 mm o.d. tubes
Accessories		
Aqueous sample cell		
Variable temperature insert, 85–570°K		
Liquid flow mixing cell		

[a] Nov. 26, 1965.

[b] The model X-3 is the same as the X-1 with the addition of 33 cps field modulation and detection.

Hilger and Watts Ltd., London, England[a]

Models	ESR1	ESR2	ESR3
Spectrometer type (nearest)	RH2-X	RH2-Q	RH2-X + Q
Sensitivity, ΔH spins for 1 sec time constant	2×10^{12}	2×10^{12}	2×10^{12}
Resolution	1 part in 10^5	1 part in 10^5	1 part in 10^5
Microwave features			
Resonant frequency	9.4 kMc	35 kMc	9.4 and 35 kMc
Tuning range		34.2–35.8 kMc	
Klystron power output, W	0.035	0.03	$x = 0.035$, $Q = 0.03$
Frequency control element	Reference cavity	Reference cavity	Reference cavities
Bridge element	Hybrid T	Hybrid T	Hybrid T
detector	Single crystal	Single crystal	Single crystals
Cavity			
Geometry	Rectangular	Cylindrical	
Mode	TE_{102}	TE_{012}	
Openings	Irradiation window	None	

(*continued*)

Hilger and Watts Ltd., London, England (*continued*)

Models	ESR1	ESR2
Cavity		
Q	~ 300	5000–6000
Required magnet gap, in.	1.7	0.865
Modulation coils	Internal	External
Modulation frequency	100 kc and 50 cps	100 kc and 50 cps
Modulation amplitude	1 G/Amp	0.5 G/A
Magnet gap, in.	1.77	1.38
Magnets		
Pole diameter, in.	8	8
Field range	to 9.0 kG	to 13 kG
Field stability with time ($\frac{1}{2}$ hr)	1 part in 10^5	1 part in 10^5
Sample size	6 mm o.d. tube	3 mm o.d. tube
Accessories		
W932 low-temperature cavity	Cylindrical internal modulation	
W934 aqueous solution cavity	Rectangular	
W935 liquid helium cavity	Cylindrical	
W981 single-crystal cavity		Cylindrical
W983 general purpose cavity		Cylindrical
Continuous-flow system	X band	
Double-sample cavities	X band	
Double-resonance ENDOR	X band	
Electrolysis cell	X band	

[a] Catalogs CH 424, CH 421/2.

Hitachi Ltd., Tokyo, Japan

Model	771
Sensitivity, ΔH spins for 1 sec time constant	5×10^{10}
Resolution	10^5
Microwave features	
Resonant frequency, kMc	9.2
Klystron power output, W	0.3
Frequency control element	
Frequency stability	10^{-6}

(*continued*)

Hitachi Ltd., Tokyo, Japan (*continued*)

Model	771
Cavity	
Modulation frequency, kc	100
Modulation amplitude, max G	40
Magnets	
Field range, max kG	6
Field uniformity, mG	35
Sweep amplitude	
minimum, G	0.1
maximum, kG	6
Sweep rates, min	
minimum	0.5
maximum	300
Accessories	
Variable temperature accessory	
Flow mixing equipment	
Ultraviolet source	
Integrator	
Liquid nitrogen temperature unit	

Japan Electron Optics Laboratory Co., Ltd., Tokyo, Japan[a]

Models	JES-P-10	JES-3BS-X	JES-3BS-K	JES-3BS-Q
Spectrometer type (nearest)	RH1-X	RH1-X	RH1-K	RH1-Q
Sensitivity, ΔH spins for 1 sec time constant	10^{11}	10^{11}	5×10^{10}	10^{10}
Resolution	1×10^{-5}	1×10^{-5}	1×10^{-5}	1×10^{-5}
Microwave features				
Resonant frequency, kMc	9.4	9.4	24	35
Klystron power output, W		0.3	0.03	0.02
Frequency control element	AFC locks on the sample cavity			
Frequency stability		1×10^{-6}	1×10^{-6}	1×10^{-6}
Bridge element	Hybrid T	Hybrid T	Hybrid T	Hybrid T
Detector	Single crystal	Single crystal	Single crystal	Single crystal

(*continued*)

Japan Electron Optics Laboratory Co., Ltd., Tokyo, Japan (*continued*)

Models	JES-P-10	JES-3BS-X	JES-3BS-K	JES-3BS-Q
Cavity				
Geometry	Cylindrical	Cylindrical	Cylindrical	Cylindrical
Mode	TE_{011}	TE_{011}	TE_{012}	TE_{012}
Openings	Irradiation window	Irradiation window		
Modulation coils	External	External	External	External
Modulation frequency	100 kc	100 kc and 80 cps	100 kc and 80 cps	100 kc and 80 cps
Modulation amplitude, G	0.01–20	0.01–20	0.01–10 and 0.01–20	0.01–10 and 0.01–20
Magnet gap, in.		2.36	2.36	2.36
Magnets				
Pole diameter, in.		11.8	11.8	11.8
Field range, max kG				
50 mm gap	2.8	18	18	18
60 mm gap	4.0	13	13	13
Field stability with time		1×10^{-6}	1×10^{-6}	1×10^{-6}
Field stability over sample volume		$1 \times 10^{-6}/cm^3$	$1 \times 10^{-6}/cm^3$	$1 \times 10^{-6}/cm^3$
Field setting accuracy, G		0.1	0.1	0.1
Sweep amplitude				
minimum, G	± 15	± 5	± 5	± 5
maximum, G	± 300	± 1000	± 1000	± 1000
Sweep rate, min				
minimum		7.5	7.5	7.5
maximum		120	120	120
Sweep linearity		0.5%	0.5%	0.5%
Field control		Hall plate	Hall plate	Hall plate
Sample size	5 mm o.d. tube	5 mm o.d. tube	3 mm o.d. tube	2 mm o.d. tube

Accessories

  JES-VT-2 temperature controller, $-170°C$ to $+200°C \pm 2°C$ X, K, Q band

  JES-UCT-2 variable temperature adapter X, K, Q band

  JES-UCD-2X liquid N_2 insertion type dewar, X band

  JES-UCR-2X sample angular rotation device, X band

  JES-SM-1 sample mixing kit, X band

  JES-EL-10 electrolytic cell, X band

  JES-LC-O1 aqueous solution sample cell

  JES-UV-1 ultraviolet-ray irradiator

  JES-ID-2 integrator

  JES-LHC-1X liquid helium cavity

  JES-LHD-IX liquid helium dewar

  JRA-1 spectrum accumulator

---

[a] Bulletin 642373-N8 Dd.

Magnion Inc.-Strand Laboratories, Burlington, Mass.

Models	602 B/X, 602 A/K, 602 A/Ka, 602 A/V
Spectrometer type (nearest)	RH3
Sensitivity, ΔH spins for 1 sec time constant	5×10^{10} to 10^9
Resolution	3 parts in 10^6
Microwave features	
Resonant frequency, kMc	$\sim 9.5, 25, 35, 70$
Tuning range	8.5–9.6, 23–25, 35–36
Klystron power output, W	0.5, 0.4, 0.15, 0.3
Frequency control element	Sample cavity
Bridge element	Ferrite circulator
Detector	Dual balanced mixer
Cavity	
Geometry	Cylindrical
Mode	TE_{011}
Openings	Irradiation windows in some designs
Modulation coils	External
Modulation frequency	20, 40, 80, 200, 400 cps 6, 100 kc
Magnets	
Field range, max kG	50
Field uniformity, G	10^{-5} to 10^{-6}
Accessories	
Low-temperature cavities	
Temperature control electrolytic cells	
Special purpose cavities	
Dewars	

Varian Associates, Palo Alto, Calif.

	E3	V-4502-10	V-4503-10[a]
Models			
Spectrometer type (nearest)		RH1-X RH2-X	
Sensitivity, ΔH spins for 1 sec time constant	5×10^{10}	5×10^{10}	5×10^{9}
Resolution	2 parts in 10^5	1 part in 10^6	~ 2 parts in 10^5
Microwave features			
Resonant frequency, kMc	9.5	9.5	35
Tuning range	8.8–9.6		
Klystron power output, W	0.3	0.3	0.1
Frequency control element	Sample cavity	Sample or external cavity	Sample or external cavity
Frequency stability	1 part in 10^6	1 part in 10^6	1 part in 10^6
Bridge element	Circulator	Magic T	Circulator
Detector	Single crystal	Single crystal	Single crystal
Cavity			
Geometry	Rectangular	Rectangular	Cylindrical
Mode	TE_{102}	TE_{102}	TE_{011}
Openings	Irradiation window	Irradiation window	none
Q	7000	7000	7000
Required magnet gap, in.	1.75	1.75	$1\frac{7}{8}$
Modulation coils	External	External	External
Modulation frequency	100 kc	20, 40, 80, 200, 400 cps; 100 kc	20, 40, 80, 200, 400 cps; 100 kc
Modulation amplitude max G	40	35 at 100 kc 50 at audio	35 at 100 kc 50 at audio
Magnet gap, in.		2.625	
Magnets			
Pole diameter, in.	4	6	6
Field range, max kG	6.0		
Field stability over sample volume		0.05	0.05
Field setting accuracy	0.1 G		
Sweep amplitude			
minimum, G	100	0.250	
maximum, G	5×10^3	10^4	
Sweep rate			
minimum	0.5 min	30 sec	
maximum	16 hr	1 hr 40 min	
Sweep linearity	$\pm 0.5\%$ of scan range	$\pm 0.5\%$ of scan range	$\pm 0.5\%$ of scan range
Field control	Fieldial (Hall probe)	Fieldial (Hall probe)	Fieldial (Hall probe)
Sample size	11 mm o.d. tube	11 mm o.d. tube	

(continued)

Varian Associates, Palo Alto, Calif. (*continued*)

Accessories

    V-K3525 superheterodyne, converts V-4500 homodyne bridge to super-heterodyne system

    V-4545B liquid helium dewar system, low-temperature TE_{102} rectangular cavity, X-band

    V-4546 liquid nitrogen, internal dewar insert

    V-4546-1 liquid nitrogen, internal dewar insert, offset

    V-4557 variable temperature, $-185°C$ to $+300°C \pm 3°C$

    E-4557 variable temperature, for E-3 spectrometer

    V-4548 aqueous solution sample cell, for rectangular cavity

    V-4548-1 aqueous solution sample cell, for rectangular cavity

    V-4549 liquid flow mixing chamber, for rectangular cavity

    V-4556 electrolytic cell

    Axial hole pole caps

    V-3506 flux stabilizer, concentric annular windings for poles

    V-3507 slow-sweep unit

    V-3532 field homogeneity control system to reduce spacial inhomogeneity of magnetic field

    V-4532 dual sample EPR cavity, add to V-4531

    V-4533 rotating cavity, TE_{011} cylindrical cavity

    V-4534 optical transmission cavity, add to rectangular TE_{102} cavity

    Fieldial Mark II magnetic field regulator (Hall probe sensor)

    C-1024 time-averaging computer

    V-4565 liquid helium dewar system, low-temperature TE_{011} mode cylindrical cavity, K band

    V-4535 large sample access cavity, cylindrical TE_{01n} (n may be 1, 2, 3, 4), accepts 1 in. diam sample tube

---

[a] The Varian spectrometer systems in a common series differ only in the magnet and its mount.

The V-4501-11 and V-4503-11 have a 9 in. magnet system and a fixed 45° magnet mount.

The V-4502-12 and V-4503-12 have a 9 in. magnet system and rotate about the vertical axis.

The V-4502-13 and V-4503-13 have a 9 in. magnet system, a movable base, horizontal rotation, and vertical rotation.

The V-4502-14 and V-4503-14 have a 12 in. magnet system, rotate about horizontal axis.

The V-4502-15 and V-4503-15 have a 12 in. magnet system, 45° mount, rotate about vertical axis.

The V-4502-16 and V-4503-16 have a 15 in. magnet system.

The V-4502-9 has a 6 in. magnet, and only 100 kc modulation.

Features of Various Sizes of Electromagnets

Examples of maximum fields for various air gaps

Pole diameter, in.	4	6	9	12	15	22
Air gap, in.	0.375	0.25	0.25	0.25	0.25	0.25
Maximum field, G	17,000	35,000	38,000	42,000	46,000	51,000
Air gap, in.	4.0	2.0	3.0	4.0	4.0	4.0
Maximum field, G	4000	10,000	9000	8000	15,000	20,000

Examples of field spatial uniformity

Pole face, in.	9	9	9, with tapered pole caps	9, with tapered pole caps
Field intensity, G	3550	3550	10,000	20,000
Air gap, in.	2.25	3	2.5	1
Maximum Deviation from central field value in volume, mG	100	80	50	200
Volume elements				
Diameter, in.	1	1.5	1	1
Length, in.	1.75	1.5	0.5	0.5

Pole face, in.	12	12, with tapered pole caps	12, with tapered pole caps
Field intensity, G	3500	20,000	14,000
Air gap, in.	4	1.5	2
Maximum deviation from central field value in volume, mG	50	200	100
Volume element			
Diameter, in.	2	1.5	1
Length, in.	1	0.75	0.5

References

A-1. Abkowitz, M., and A. Honig, *Rev. Sci. Instr.*, **33**, 568 (1962).

A-2. Abragam, A., and M. H. L. Pryce, *Proc. Roy. Soc. (London)*, **A205**, 135 (1951).

A-3. Adrian, F. J., E. L. Cochran, and V. A. Bowers, "ESR Spectrum and Structure of the Formyl Radical," BuWeps, NOrd 7386, Johns Hopkins Applied Physics Lab., Silver Springs, Md.

A-4. Alexander, P., J. T. Lett, and M. G. Ormerod, *Biochim. Biophys. Acta*, **51**, 207 (1961).

A-5. Alger, R. S., "Radiation Effects in Polymers," *Physics and Chemistry of the Organic Solid State*, Vol. II, D. Fox, M. N. Lebes, and A. Weissberger, Eds., Interscience, New York, 1965.

A-6. Alger, R. S., T. H. Anderson, and L. A. Webb, *J. Chem. Phys.*, **30**, 695 (1959).

A-7. Allen, L. C., H. M. Gladney, and S. H. Glarum, *J. Chem. Phys.*, **40**, 3135, (1964).

A-8. Allen, M. B., L. H. Piette, and J. C. Murchio, *Biochim. Biophys. Acta*, **60**, 539 (1962).

A-9. Al'tshuler, S. A., and B. M. Kozyrev, *Electron Paramagnetic Resonance*, Academic Press, New York, 1964.

A-10. Anderson, R. S., "Electron Spin Resonance," in *Methods of Experimental Physics*, Vol. 3, Dudley Williams, Ed., Academic Press, New York, 1962.

A-11. Andrews, E. R., *Phys. Rev.*, **91**, 425 (1953).

A-12. Arnold, E., and A. Patterson, Jr., "Calculation of Conductivity in Sodium, Liquid Ammonia Solutions," in *Metal–Ammonia Solutions*, G. Lepoutre and M. J. Sienko, Eds., Benjamin, New York, 1964.

A-13. Assenheim, H. M., *Chemical Products and Aerosol News* (July and Aug. 1962).

A-14. Atkins, P. W., N. Keen, and M. C. R. Symons, *J. Chem. Soc.*, **1963**, 250.

A-15. Ayscough, P. B., and C. Thomson, *Trans. Faraday Soc.*, **58**, 1477 (1962).

B-1. Bagguley, D. M. S., and J. H. E. Griffiths, *Nature*, **162**, 538 (1948).

B-2. Baker, J. M., and N. C. Ford, Jr., *Phys. Rev.*, **136**, A1692 (1964).

B-3. Bauer, C. L., and R. B. Gordon, *Phys. Rev.*, **126**, 73 (1962).

B-4. Baum, W. A., and L. Dunkelman, *J. Opt. Soc. Am.*, **40**, 782 (1950).

B-5. Beckman, T. A., and K. S. Pitzer, *J. Phys. Chem.*, **65**, 1527 (1961).

B-6. Bennett, J. E., D. J. E. Ingram, and J. G. Tapley, *J. Chem. Phys.*, **23**, 215 (1955).

B-7. Bennett, R. G., and A. Henglein, *J. Chem. Phys.*, **30**, 1117 (1959).

B-8. Bennett, W. R., *Electrical Noise*, McGraw-Hill, New York, 1960.

B-9. Beringer, R., and J. G. Castle, *Phys. Rev.*, **81**, 82 (1951).

B-10. Beringer, R., and J. G. Castle, *Phys. Rev.*, **78**, 581 (1950).

B-11. Beringer, R., and M. A. Heald, *Phys. Rev.*, **95**, 1474 (1954).

B-12. Beringer, R., E. B. Rawson, and A. F. Henry, *Phys. Rev.*, **94**, 343 (1954).

B-13. Berkowitz, R. S., *Modern Radar, Analysis, Evaluation, and System Design*, Interscience, New York, 1965.

B-14. Bienenstock, A., and H. Brooks, *Phys. Rev.*, **136**, A784 (1964).

B-15. Bleaney, B., *Phil. Mag.*, **42**, 441 (1951).

B-16. Bleaney, B., J. H. N. Loubser, and R. P. Penrose, *Proc. Phys. Soc. (London)*, **59**, 185 (1947).

B-17. Bleaney, B., and K. W. H. Stevens, *Reps. Progr. Phys.*, **16**, 108 (1953).

B-18. Bloembergen, N., E. M. Purcell, and R. V. Pound, *Phys. Rev.*, **73**, 679 (1948).

B-19. Bloembergen, N., and S. Wang, *Phys. Rev.*, **93**, 72 (1954).

B-20. Blois, M. S., H. W. Brown, and J. E. Maling, "Precision g-Value Measurements on Free Radicals of Biological Interest," in *Free Radicals in Biological Systems*, M. S. Blois, H. W. Brown, R. M. Lemmon, R. O. Lindblom, and M. Weissbluth, Eds., Academic Press, New York, 1961.

B-21. Blois, M. S., H. W. Brown, R. M. Lemmon, R. O. Lindblom, and M. Weissbluth, Eds., *Free Radicals in Biological Systems*, Academic Press, New York, 1961.

B-22. Blume, R. J., *Phys. Rev.*, **109**, 1867 (1958).

B-23. Boag, J. W., "Electron Spin Resonance in Biology," in *Radiation Effects in Physics, Chemistry and Biology*, M. Ebert, and A. Howard, Eds., Proc. Intern. Congr. Radiation Research, 2nd, North-Holland, Amsterdam (1963).

B-24. Bolton, J. R., and G. K. Fraenkel, *J. Chem. Phys.*, **40**, 3307 (1964).

B-25. Bowers, K. D., and W. B. Mims, *Phys. Rev.*, **115**, 285 (1959).

B-26. Bowers, K. D., and J. Owen, *Rept. Progr. Phys.*, **18**, 304 (1955).

B-27. Bradshaw, W. W., D. G. Cadena, Jr., G. W. Crawford, and H. A. W. Spetzler, *Radiation Res.*, **17**, 11 (1962).

B-28. Brandon, R. W., G. L. Closs, and C. A. Hutchison, Jr., *J. Chem. Phys.*, **37**, 1878 (1962).

B-29. Bray, R. C., *J. Biochem.*, **81**, 189 (1961).

B-30. Bray, R. C., and R. Pettersson, *J. Biochem.*, **81**, 194 (1961).

B-31. Bridge, N. K., *Nature*, **185**, 31 (1960).

B-32. Brivati, J. A., N. Keen, and M. C. R. Symons, *J. Chem. Soc.*, **1962**, 237.

B-33. Bron, W. E., *Phys. Rev.*, **125**, 509 (1962).

B-34. Burgess, V. R., *J. Sci. Instr.*, **38**, 98 (1961).

B-35. Bussey, H. E., *IRE Trans. Instr.*, **9**, No. 2, 171 (1960).

B-36. Bussey, H. E., "Table of Attenuator Settings for Measuring the Q of an Absorption Resonator," Radio Standards Laboratory, National Bureau of Standards, Boulder, Col.

C-1. Calvin, M., and G. M. Androes, *Science*, **138**, 867 (1962).

C-2. Carr, H. Y., and E. M. Purcell, *Phys. Rev.*, **94**, 630 (1954).

C-3. Castle, J. G., Jr., P. F. Chester, and P. E. Wagner, *Phys. Rev.*, **119**, 953 (1960).

C-4. Castle, J. G., Jr., D. W. Feldman, P. G. Klemens, and R. A. Weeks, *Phys. Rev.*, **130**, 577 (1963).

C-5. Castner, T. G., Jr., *Phys. Rev.*, **130**, 58 (1963).

C-6. Castner, T. G., Jr., *Phys. Rev.*, **115**, 1506 (1959).

C-7. Chesnut, D. B., and P. Arthur, Jr., *J. Chem. Phys.*, **36**, 2969 (1962).

C-8. Chesnut, D. B., and W. D. Phillips, *J. Chem. Phys.*, **35**, 1002 (1961).

C-9. Chesnut, D. B., and G. J. Sloan, *J. Chem. Phys.*, **35**, 443 (1961).

C-10. Chesnut, D. B., and G. J. Sloan, *J. Chem. Phys.*, **33**, 637 (1960).

C-11. Chester, P. F., P. E. Wagner, and J. G. Castle, Jr., *Phys. Rev.*, **110**, 281 (1958).

C-12. Chester, P. F., P. E. Wagner, J. G. Castle, Jr., and G. Conn, *Rev. Sci. Instr.*, **30**, 1127 (1959).

C-13. Chu, T. L., G. E. Pake, J. Townsend, and S. I. Weissman, *J. Phys. Chem.*, **57**, 504 (1953).

C-14. Cochran, E. L., F. J. Adrian, and V. A. Bowers, "ESR Detection of the Cyanogen and Methylene Imino Free Radical," Applied Physics Laboratory, Johns Hopkins University, Silver Spring, Md.

C-15. Cochran, E. L., F. J. Adrian, and V. A. Bowers, "Anisotopic hf Interaction in the ESR Spectra of Alkyl Radicals," Applied Physics Laboratory of Johns Hopkins University, Silver Spring, Md.

C-16. Collins, R. L., M. D. Bell, and G. Kraus, *J. Appl. Phys.*, **30**, 56 (1959).

C-17. Commoner, B., "ESR Studies of Biochemical and Biological Systems, Application à la Biochemie et à la Chimie Structurale de la Spectroscopie des Radiofréquences," Compte Rend. Colloq., Brussels, April 6 and 7 (1961).

C-18. Commoner, B., J. Townsend, and G. E. Pake, *Nature*, **174**, 689 (1954).

C-19. Cook, A. R., L. M. Matarrese, and J. S. Wells, *Rev. Sci Instr.*, **35**, 114 (1964).

C-20. Cook, P., and J. R. Mallard, *Nature*, **198**, 145 (1963).

C-21. Cook, R. P., and L. G. Stoodley, "An ESR Spectrometer for Use While Irradiating Wet Biological Systems," Royal Military College of Science, Shrivenham, Swindon, Wiltshire.

C-22. Corbett, J. W., and G. D. Watkins, *Phys. Rev.*, **138**, A555 (1965).

D-1. de Boer, J. H., *Rec. Trav. Chim.*, **56**, 301 (1937).

D-2. de Groot, M. S., and J. H. van der Waals, *Mol. Phys.*, **6**, 545 (1963).

D-3. de Groot, M. S., and J. H. van der Waals, *Mol. Phys.*, **3**, 190 (1960).

D-4. Dehmelt, H. G., *Phys. Rev.*, **99**, 527 (1955).

D-5. Delbecq, C. J., B. Smaller, and P. H. Yuster, *Phys. Rev.*, **104**, 599 (1956).

D-6. Diebel, R. N., and D. R. Kalkwarf, "Kinetic Studies of Organic Radicals formed in Irradiated Aqueous Solutions," HW-SA-3066, Radiological Chemistry Operation, Chemical Research, Hanford Laboratories Operation, Richland, Washington (June 1963).

D-7. Douthit, R. C., and J. L. Dye, *J. Am. Chem. Soc.*, **82**, 4472 (1960).

D-8. Doyle, W. T., *Phys. Rev.*, **126**, 1421 (1962).

D-9. Dresselhaus, G., A. F. Kip, and C. Kittel, *Phys. Rev.*, **98**, 368 (1955).

D-10. Duchesne, J., "Résonance de Spin Électronique et Radicaux Libres induits Par Irradiation Gamma Dans L'Acide Désoxyribonucléique,"

Biological Effect of Ionizing Radiation at the Molecular Level, International Atomic Energy Agency, Vienna (1962).

D-11. Duchesne, J., J. Depireux, and J. M. van der Kaa, *Geochim. Cosmochim. Acta*, **23**, 209 (1961).

D-12. Dyson, F. J., *Phys. Rev.*, **98**, 349 (1958).

E-1. Eastman, R. S., and R. A. Miller, Jr., in Final Report on the Relay I Program, NASA SP-76, prepared by Goddard Space Flight Center, Scientific and Technical Information Division, Greenbelt, Md. (1965).

E-2. Edelstein, N., A. Kwok, and A. H. Maki, *J. Chem. Phys.*, **41**, 3473 (1964).

E-3. Ehrenberg, A., "Research on Free Radicals in Enzyme Chemistry and in Radiation Biology," in *Free Radicals in Biological Systems*, M. S. Blois, H. W. Brown, R. M. Lemmon, R. O. Lindblom, and M. Weissbluth Eds., Academic Press, New York, 1961.

E-4. Ehrenberg, A., L. Ehrenberg, and G. Lofroth, *Abhandl. Deut. Akad. Wiss. Berlin, Kl. Med.*, No. 1, 229 (1962).

E-5. Ehrenberg, A., L. Ehrenberg, and G. Lofroth, "Chemical Changes Produced by Ionizing Radiations in Solid Carbohydrates," RISO Rept. No. 16, Nobel Medical Institute, Biochemical Dept., Stockholm, and Institute of Organic Chemistry and Biochemistry, University of Stockholm (1960).

E-6. Eisinger, J., and G. Feher, *Phys. Rev.*, **109**, 1172 (1958).

E-7. Elion, H. A., and L. Shapiro, "Application of ESR Spectroscopy" in *Analytical Chemistry*, Series IX, Vol. II, C. E. Crouthamel, Ed., Pergamon Press, New York, 1961.

E-8. Elliott, R. J., *Phys. Rev.*, **96**, 266 (1955).

E-9. Estle, T. L., and G. K. Walters, *Rev. Sci. Instr.*, **32**, 1058 (1961).

F-1. Feher, G., "Review of Electron Spin Resonance Experiments in Semiconductors," in *Paramagnetic Resonance*, Vol. II, W. Low, Ed., Academic Press, New York, 1963.

F-2. Feher, G., *Phys. Rev.*, **114**, 1219 (1959).

F-3. Feher, G., *Bell System Tech. J.*, **36**, 449 (1957).

F-4. Feher, G., R. C. Fletcher, and E. A. Gere, *Phys. Rev.*, **100**, 1784 (1955).

F-5. Feher, G., and E. A. Gere, *Phys. Rev.*, **114**, 1245 (1959).

F-6. Feher, G., J. C. Hensel, and E. A. Gere, *Phys. Rev. Letters*, **5**, 309 (1960).

F-7. Feher, G., and A. F. Kip, *Phys. Rev.*, **98**, 337 (1955).

F-8. Feher, G., D. K. Wilson, and E. A. Gere, *Phys. Rev. Letters*, **3**, 25 (1959).

F-9. Feldman, D. W., R. W. Warren, and J. G. Castle, Jr., *Phys. Rev.*, **135**, A470 (1964).

F-10. Fessenden, R. W., and R. H. Schuler, RRL 112, Radiation Research Laboratories, Mellon Institute, Pittsburgh, Pa. (1963); *J. Chem. Phys.*, **39**, 2147 (1963).

F-11. Firth, I. M., *J. Sci. Instr.*, **39**, 131 (1962).

F-12. Fletcher, R. C., W. A. Yager, G. L. Pearson, A. N. Holden, W. T. Read, and F. R. Merritt, *Phys. Rev.*, **94**, 1392 (1954).

F-13. Fletcher, R. C., W. A. Yager, G. L. Pearson, and F. R. Merritt, *Phys. Rev.*, **95**, 844 (1954).

F-14. Foner, S. N., E. L. Cochran, V. A. Bowers, and C. K. Jen, *J. Chem. Phys.*, **32**, 963 (1960).

F-15. Fujimoto, M., and D. J. E. Ingram, *Trans. Faraday Soc.*, **54**, 1304 (1958).

G-1. Galt, J. K., W. A. Yager, F. R. Merritt, B. B. Cetlin, and H. W. Dail, Jr., *Phys. Rev.*, **100**, 748 (1955).

G-2. Garstens, M. A., and A. H. Ryan, *Phys. Rev.*, **81**, 888 (1951).

G-3. Geske, D. H., and A. H. Maki, *J. Am. Chem. Soc.*, **82**, 2671 (1960).

G-4. Gibson, J. F., D. J. E. Ingram, M. C. R. Symons, and M. G. Townsend, *Trans. Faraday Soc.*, **53**, 914 (1957).

G-5. Gillam, A. E., and E. S. Stern, *An Introduction to Electronic Absorption Spectroscopy in Organic Chemistry*, Edward Arnold Ltd., London, 1954.

G-6. Ginzton, E. L., *Microwave Measurements*, McGraw-Hill, New York, 1957.

G-7. Giordmaine, J. A., L. E. Alsop, F. R. Nash, and C. H. Townes, *Phys. Rev.*, **109**, 302 (1958).

G-8. Gold, M., and W. L. Jolly, *Inorganic Chemistry*, **1**, 818 (1962).

G-9. Goldsborough, J. P., and M. Mandel, *Rev. Sci Instr.*, **31**, 1044 (1960).

G-10. Gordon, J. P., *Rev. Sci. Intr.*, **32**, 658 (1961).

G-11. Gordy, W., "Radiation Chemistry in the Solid State as Studied with Electron Paramagnetic Resonance," in *Radiation Research*, Proc. Intern. Conf., F. R. Fisher, Ed., U.S. Army Natick Labs., Natick, Mass. (Jan. 1963).

G-12. Gordy, W., W. B. Ard, and H. Shields, *Proc. Natl. Acad. Sci. U.S.*, **41**, 983 (1955).

G-13. Gordy, W., and H. Shields, "ESR Investigations of the Proteins, Application à la Biochimie et à la Chimie Structurale de la Spectroscopie des Radiofréquences," Compte Rend. Colloq., Brussels, April 6 and 7 (1961).

G-14. Gordy, W., and H. Shields, *Proc. Natl. Acad. Sci.*, **46**, 1124 (1960).

G-15. Gordy, W., W. V. Smith, and R. F. Trambarulo, *Microwave Spectroscopy*, Wiley, New York, 1953.

G-16. Gorter, C. J., "Exposé Introductif Applications of Electron Spin Resonance," in Application à la Biochimie et à la Chimie Structurale de la Spectroscopie des Radiofréquences, Compt. Rend. Colloq., Brussels, April 6 and 7 (1961).

G-17. Graves, C. T., and M. G. Ormerod, *Polymer,* **4**, 81 (1963).

G-18. Gray, J. E., and H. E. Bussey, "Table of Attenuator Settings for Measuring the Q of an Absorption Reasonator," Radio Standards Laboratory, National Bureau of Standards, Boulder, Col.

G-19. Grimes, C. C., and A. F. Kip, *Phys. Rev.*, **132**, 1991 (1963).

H-1. Hahn, E. L., *Phys. Rev.*, **80**, 580 (1950).

H-2. Harrah, L. A., R. E. Rondeau, S. Zakanycz, D. Hale, and D. Dunbar, ASD-TDR 63-785 ESR Study of γ-Irradiated Solid Acetonitrile, AF Materials Laboratory, Research and Technology Division, Air Force Systems Command, Wright-Patterson Air Force Base, Ohio, (1963).

H-3. Hausser, K. H., "High Resolution ESR," Proc. Colloq. Spectroscopicum Internationale, 10th, College Park Md. (1962).

H-4. Hausser, K. H., *Radiation Research Supplement*, **2**, 480 (1960).

H-5. Heller, C., and H. M. McConnell, *J. Chem. Phys.*, **32**, 1535 (1960).

H-6. Henning, J. C. M., *Rev. Sci. Instr.*, **32**, 35 (1961).

H-7. Henning, J. C. M., "On the Nitrogen-14 Hyperfine Structure in the Electron Spin Resonance Spectra of Heterocyclic Anions," Zeeman Laboratorium, Universiteit Van Amsterdam, Amsterdam, the Netherlands (1964); also *J. Chem. Phys.*, **44**, 2139 (1966).

H-8. Henriksen, T., "ESR Studies on the Formation and Properties of Free Radicals in Irradiated Sulfur-Containing Substances," Norsk Hydro's Institute for Cancer Research, Oslo, Norway (1963).

H-9. Henriksen, T., and A. Pihl, *Intern. J. of Radiation Biol.*, **3**, 351 (1961).

H-10. Henriksen, T., T. Sanner, and A. Pihl, *Radiation Res.*, **18**, 147 (1963).

H-11. Hershenson, H. M., *Nuclear Magnetic Resonance and Electron Spin Resonance Spectra*, 1958–1963 Index, Academic Press, New York, 1965.

H-12. Herve, J., "Measurement of Electronic Spin–Lattice Relaxation Times by Rapid Modulation of the Saturation Factor," in *Paramagnetic Resonance*, W. Low., Ed., Vol. II, Academic Press, New York, 1963.

H-13. Hollocher, T. C., W. H. From, and N. S. Bromberg, *Phys. Med. Biol.*, **9**, 65 (1964).

H-14. Holton, W. C., and H. Blum, *Phys. Rev.*, **125**, 89 (1962).

H-15. Hornig, A. W., and J. S. Hyde, *Mol. Phys.*, **6**, 33 (1963).

H-16. Horsfield, A., J. R. Morton, and D. G. Moss, *J. Sci. Instr.*, **38**, 322 (1961).

H-17. Hoskins, R. H., and R. C. Pastor, *J. Appl. Phys.*, **31**, 1506 (1960).

H-18. Hughes, F., and J. G. Allard, *Phys. Rev.*, **125**, 173 (1962).

H-19. Hutchison, C. A., Jr., *J. Phys. Soc. Japan*, **17**, 458 (1962).

H-20. Hutchison, C. A., Jr., *J. Phys. Chem.*, **57**, 546 (1953).

H-21. Hutchison, C. A., Jr., and B. W. Mangum, *J. Chem. Phys.*, **34**, 908 (1961).

H-22. Hutchison, C. A., Jr., and B. W. Mangum, *J. Chem. Phys.*, **32**, 1261 (1960).

H-23. Hutchison, C. A., Jr., and B. W. Mangum, *J. Chem. Phys.*, **29**, 952 (1958).

H-24. Hutchison, C. A., Jr., and D. E. O'Reilly, *J. Chem. Phys.*, **34**, 1279 (1961).

H-25. Hutchison, C. A., Jr., and R. C. Pastor, *J. Chem. Phys.*, **21**, 1959 (1953).

H-26. Hutchison, C. A., Jr., and R. C. Pastor, *Phys. Rev.*, **81**, 282 (1951).

H-27. Hyde, J. S., "Evaluation of an EPR Superheterodyene Spectrometer," 6th Annual NMR-EPR Workshop, Nov. 5–9, Varian Associates Instrument Division, Palo Alto, Calif. (1962).

H-28. Hyde, J. S., "Experimental Techniques in EPR," 6th Annual NMR-EPR Workshop, Nov. 5–9, Varian Associates Instrument Division, Palo Alto, Calif. (1962).

H-29. Hyde, J. S., "Principles of EPR Instrumentation," 5th Annual NMR-EPR Varian Workshop, Oct., Varian Associates Instrument Division, Palo Alto, Calif. (1961).

H-30. Hyde, J. S., *Phys. Rev.*, **119**, 1483 (1960).

I-1. Ingram, D. J. E., *Lab. Pract.*, **12**, 518 (June 1963).

I-2. Ingram, D. J. E., *Free Radicals as Studied by Electron Spin Resonance*, Butterworths, London, 1958.

I-3. Ingram, D. J. E., *Spectroscopy at Radio and Microwave Frequencies*, 2nd ed., Butterworths, London, 1955.

I-4. Ingram, D. J. E., and J. E. Bennett, *Phil. Mag.*, **45**, 545 (1954).

I-5. Ingram, D. J. E., W. G. Hodgson, C. A. Parker, and W. T. Rees, *Nature*, **176**, 1227 (1955).

I-6. Ingram, D. J. E., J. G. Tapley, R. Jackson, R. L. Bond, and A. R. Murnaghan, *Nature*, **174**, 797 (1954).

J-1. Jarrett, H. S., "ESR Spectroscopy in Moleculic Solids," in *Solid State Physics*, Vol. 14, F. Seitz and D. Turnbull, Eds., Academic Press, New York, 1963, p. 215.

J-2. Jen, C. K., S. N. Foner, E. L. Cochran, and V. A. Bowers, *Phys. Rev.*, **112**, 1169 (1958).

J-3. Jen, C. K., and N. W. Lord, *Phys. Rev.*, **96**, 1150 (1954).

J-4. Jérome, D., and J. M. Winter, *Phys. Rev.*, **134**, A1001 (1964).

J-5. Jesse, R. E., P. Biloen, R. Prins, J. D. W. van Voorst, and G. J. Hoijtink, *Mol. Phys.*, **6**, 633 (1963).

J-6. Johnson, W. C., and A. W. Meyer, *Chem. Rev.*, **8**, 273 (1931).

J-7. Jolly, W. L., "Metal-Ammonia Solutions," in *Progress in Inorganic Chemistry*, Vol. I, F. Cotton, Ed., Interscience, New York, 1959, p. 235.

J-8. Jones, M. T., and D. B. Chesnut, *J. Chem. Phys.*, **38**, 1311 (1963).

J-9. Jung, W., and G. S. Newell, *Phys. Rev.*, **132**, 648 (1963).

K-1. Känzig, W., *J. Phys. Chem. Solids*, **17**, 88 (1960).

K-2. Känzig, W., *J. Phys. Chem. Solids*, **17**, 80 (1960).

K-3. Kaplan, D. E., M. E. Browne, and J. A. Cowen, *Rev. Sci. Instr.*, **32**, 1182 (1961).

K-4. Kaplan, J., and C. Kittel, *J. Chem. Phys.*, **21**, 1429 (1953).

K-5. Kasai, P. H., *J. Phys. Chem.*, **66**, 674 (1962).

K-6. Kelly, E. J., H. V. Secor, C. W. Keenan, and J. F. Eastham, *J. Am. Chem. Soc.*, **84**, 3611 (1962).

K-7. King, G. J., B. S. Miller, F. F. Carlson, and R. C. McMillan, *J. Chem. Phys.*, **32**, 940 (1960).

K-8. Kinzer, J. P., and I. G. Wilson, *Bell System Tech. J.*, **26**, 31 (1947).

K-9. Kip, A. F., C. Kittel, R. A. Levy, and A. M. Portis, *Phys. Rev.*, **91**, 1066 (1953).

K-10. Kip, A. F., D. N. Langenberg, and T. W. Moore, *Phys. Rev.*, **124**, 359 (1961).

K-11. Kneubühl, F. K., *J. Chem. Phys.*, **33**, 1074 (1960).

K-12. Koch, J. F., R. A. Stradling, and A. F. Kip, *Phys. Rev.*, **133**, A240 (1964).

K-13. Köhnlein, W., and A. Müller, *Phys. Med. Biol.*, **6**, 599 (1962).

K-14. Köhnlein, W., and A. Müller, "A Double Cavity for Precision Measurements of Radical Concentrations," in *Free Radicals in Biological Systems*, M. S. Blois, Jr., H. W. Brown, R. M. Lemmon, R. O. Lindblom, and M. Weissbluth, Eds., Academic Press, New York, 1961.

K-15. Kravitz, L. C., "ESR and Optical Experiments on Deep-Lying Impurities in Germanium and Silicon," Tech. Rept. HP-9, Gordon McKay Laboratory, Division of Engineering and Applied Physics, Harvard University, Cambridge, Mass. (1963).

K-16. Kroh, J., and J. W. T. Spinks, *J. Chem. Phys.*, **35**, 760 (1961).
K-17. Krongelb, S., and M. W. P. Strandberg, *J. Chem. Phys.*, **31**, 1196 (1959).

L-1. Larson, G. H., and C. D. Jeffries, *Phys. Rev.*, **141**, 461 (1966).
L-2. Lebedev, Y. S., D. M. Chernikova, N. N. Tikhomirova, and V. V. Voevodskii, *Atlas of Electron Spin Resonance Spectra*, Consultants Bureau, New York, 1963.
L-3. Lebedev, Y. S., V. V. Voevodskii, and N. N. Tikhomirova, *Atlas of Electron Spin Resonance Spectra*, Vol. 2, Consultants Bureau, New York, 1963.
L-4. Levinthal, E. C., E. H. Rogers, and R. A. Ogg, Jr., *Phys. Rev.*, **83**, 182 (1951).
L-5. Levy, R. A., *Phys. Rev.*, **102**, 31 (1956).
L-6. Lewis, G. N., and M. Calvin, *J. Am. Chem. Soc.*, **67**, 1232 (1945).
L-7. Lewis, G. N., and M. Kasha, *J. Am. Chem. Soc.*, **66**, 2100 (1944).
L-8. Lewis, G. N., and D. Lipkin, *J. Am. Chem. Soc.*, **64**, 2801 (1942).
L-9. Lewis, W. B., and F. E. Pretzel, *J. Phys. Chem. Solids*, **19**, 139 (1961).
L-10. Livingston, R., H. Zeldes, and E. H. Taylor, *Discussions Faraday Soc.*, **19**, 166 (1955).
L-11. Lord, N. W., *Phys. Rev.*, **105**, 756 (1957).
L-12. Low, W., *Paramagnetic Resonance*, Vol. II, Academic Press, New York, 1963.
L-13. Low, W., "Paramagnetic Resonance in Solids," in *Solid State Physics*, Suppl. 2, F. Seitz and D. Turnbull, Eds., Academic Press, New York, 1960.
L-14. Ludwig, G. W., *Phys. Rev.*, **137**, A1520 (1965).
L-15. Ludwig, G. W., and H. H. Woodbury, "E.S.R. in Semiconductors," in *Solid State Physics*, Vol. 13, F. Seitz and D. Turnbull, Eds., Academic Press, New York, 1962, p. 223.
L-16. Ludwig, G. W., and H. H. Woodbury, *Phys. Rev.*, **113**, 1014 (1959).

M-1. Mangiaracina, R., and S. Mrozowski, "Trapped Radicals in Organic Deposits," *Proc. Carbon Conf., 5th*, **2** (1963).
M-2. Mariner, P. F., *Introduction to Microwave Practice*, Academic Press, New York, 1961.
M-3. McAndrews, J. I., T. H. Anderson, and S. B. Martin, "Radical Yields in Irradiated Aromatics," USNRDL-TR-718, U.S. Naval Radiological Defense Laboratory, San Francisco, Calif. (1964).
M-4. McAvoy, B. R., *Rev. Sci. Instr.*, **32**, 745 (1961).
M-5. McConnell, H. M., and D. B. Chesnut, *J. Chem. Phys.*, **28**, 107 (1958)
M-6. McDonald, C. C., *J. Chem. Phys.*, **39**, 2587 (1963).
M-7. McMillan, R. C., *J. Phys. Chem. Solids*, **25**, 773 (1964).
M-8. Mikkelson, R. C., and H. J. Stapleton, *Phys. Rev.*, **140**, A1968 (1965).
M-9. Minkoff, G. J., *Frozen Free Radicals*, Interscience, New York, 1960.
M-10. M.I.T. Radar School Staff, *Principles of Radar*, McGraw-Hill, New York, 1946.
M-11. Molin, Y. N., A. T. Koritskii, A. G. Semenov, N. Y. Buben, and V. N. Shamshev, *Pribory i Tekhn. Eksperim.*, **6**, 73 (1960).
M-12. Montgomery, C. G., Ed., *Technique of Microwave Measurements* (Vol. 11, Radiation Lab. Series), McGraw-Hill, New York, 1947.

M-13. Moos, H. W., and R. H. Sands, *Phys. Rev.*, **135**, A591 (1964).

M-14. Moran, P. R., S. H. Christensen, and R. H. Silsbee, *Phys. Rev.*, **124**, 442 (1961).

M-15. Morton, J. R., *Chem. Rev.*, **64**, 453 (1964).

M-16. Müller, A., "Efficiency of Radical Production by X-rays in Substances of Biological Importance," in *Biological Effects of Ionizing Radiation at the Molecular Level*, International Atomic Energy Agency, Vienna, 1962.

N-1. Nisenoff, M., and H. Y. Fan, *Phys. Rev.*, **128**, 1605 (1962).

N-2. Noble, G. A., "Paramagnetic Resonance in Additively Colored Alkali Halides," Ph.D. Thesis No. 2682, Univ. Chicago, 1955.

N-3. Norman, I., and G. Porter, *Proc. Roy. Soc. (London)*, **A230**, 399 (1955).

O-1. Ohlsen, W. D., *Rev. Sci. Instr.*, **33**, 492 (1962).

O-2. Ohlsen, W. D., and D. F. Holcomb, *Phys. Rev.*, **126**, 1953 (1962).

O-3. O'Reilly, D. E., and J. H. Anderson, "Magnetic Properties," in *Physics and Chemistry of the Organic Solid State*, Vol. II, D. Fox, M. M. Labes, and A. Weissberger, Eds., Interscience, New York, 1965.

O-4. Ormerod, M. G., and P. Alexander, *Radiation Res.*, **18**, 495 (1963).

O-5. Orton, J. W., *Rept. Progr. Phys.*, **22**, 204 (1959).

O-6. Ovenall, D. W., and D. H. Whiffen, *Mol. Phys.*, **4**, 135 (1961).

P-1. Pake, G. E., *Paramagnetic Resonance*, Benjamin, New York, 1962.

P-2. Pake, G. E., *Am. J. Phys.*, **18**, 438 (1950).

P-3. Pake, G. E., S. I. Weissmann, and J. Townsend, *Discussions Faraday Soc.*, **19**, 147 (1955).

P-4. Pastor, R. C., and R. H. Hoskins, *J. Chem. Phys.*, **32**, 264 (1960).

P-5. Patten, F., and W. Gordy, *Proc. Natl. Acad. Sci., U.S.*, **46**, 1137 (1960).

P-6. Paul, D. E., D. Larkin, and S. I. Weissmann, *J. Am. Chem. Soc.*, **78**, 116 (1956).

P-7. Penrose, R. P., and K. W. H. Stevens, *Proc. Phys. Soc. (London)*, **63A**, 29 (1950).

P-8. Piette, L. H., "Chemical Applications of EPR," in *NMR and EPR Spectroscopy*, NMR-EPR Staff of Varian Associates, Eds., Pergamon Press, New York, 1960.

P-9. Piette, L. H., F. A. Johnson, K. A. Booman, and C. B. Colburn, *J. Chem. Phys.*, **35**, 1481 (1961).

P-10. Pimentel, G. C., "Radical Formation and Trapping in the Solid Phase," in *Formation and Trapping of Free Radicals*, A. M. Bass and H. P. Broida, Eds., Academic Press, New York, 1960.

P-11. Pippard, A. B., "Metallic Conduction at High Frequencies and Low Temperatures," *Advan. Electron. Electron Phys.*, **6**, 11 (1954).

P-12. Poole, C. P., *Electron Spin Resonance, A Comprehensive Treatise on Experimental Techniques*, Interscience, New York, 1967.

P-13. Poole, C. P., and D. E. O'Reilly, *Rev. Sci. Instr.*, **32**, 460 (1961).

P-14. Portis, A. M., *Phys. Rev.*, **91**, 1071 (1953).

P-15. Portis, A. M., A. F. Kip, and C. Kittel, *Phys. Rev.*, **90**, 988 (1953).

P-16. Pound, R. V., *Rev. Sci. Instr.*, **17**, 490 (1946).

P-17. Pressley, R. J., and H. L. Berk, *Bull. Am. Phys. Soc.*, **8**, 345 (1963).

R-1. Radford, H. E., *Phys. Rev.*, **122**, 114 (1961).

R-2. Randolph, M. L., *Rev. Sci. Instr.*, **31**, 949 (1960).

R-3. Rexroad, H. N., and W. Gordy, *Phys. Rev.*, **125**, 242 (1962).

R-4. Roberts, A., Y. Beers, and A. Hill, *Phys. Rev.*, **70, 112** (1946).

R-5. Rotblat, J., and J. A. Simmons, *Phys. Med. Biol.*, **7**, 489 (1963).

R-6. Rowan, L. G., E. L. Hahn, and W. B. Mims, *Phys. Rev.*, **137**, A61 (1965).

R-7. Ruby, R. H., I. D. Kuntz, Jr., and M. Calvin, *Proc. Natl. Acad. Sci. US*, **51**, 515 (1964).

R-8. Rupp, L. W., Jr., and P. H. Schmidt, "High Q Cavities For Microwave Spectroscopy," MM 62-1115-24, Technical Memorandum, Bell Telephone Laboratories (1962).

S-1. Saraceno, A. J., D. T. Fanale, and N. D. Coggeshall, *Anal. Chem.*, **33**, 500 (1961).

S-2. Schneider, E. E., *Discussions Faraday Soc.*, **19**, 158 (1955).

S-3. Schneider, E. E., *Phys. Rev.*, **93**, 919 (1954).

S-4. Schwartz, M., *Information, Transmission, Modulation, and Noise*, McGraw-Hill, New York, 1959.

S-5. Scott, P. L., and C. D. Jeffries, *Phys. Rev.*, **127**, 32 (1962).

S-6. Segal, B. G., M. Kaplan, and G. K. Fraenkel, *J. Chem. Phys.*, **43**, 4191 (1965).

S-7. Seitz, F., *The Modern Theory of Solids*, McGraw-Hill, New York, 1940.

S-8. Sibley, W. A., *Phys. Rev.*, **133**, A1176 (1963).

S-9. Siegman, A. E., "Traveling-Wave Techniques for Microwave Resonance Measurements," Tech. Rept. No. 155-3, Signal Corps Contract DA 36(039) SC-73178, Electron Devices Laboratory, Stanford Electronics Laboratories, Stanford University, Stanford, Calif. (Oct. 12, 1959).

S-10. Singer, L. S., *J. Appl. Phys.*, **30**, 1463 (1959).

S-11. Singer, L. S., W. A. Smith, and G. Wagoner, *Rev. Sci. Instr.*, **32**, 213 (1962).

S-12. Slater, J. C., *Quantum Theory of Matter*, McGraw-Hill, New York, 1951.

S-13. Smakula, A., *Z. Physik.*, **59**, 603 (1930).

S-14. Smaller, B., "Electron and Nuclear Magnetic Interaction in Triplet States of Various Organic Phosphors," Argonne National Laboratory, Argonne, Ill.

S-15. Smaller, B., "Recent Advances in EPR Spectroscopy," Argonne National Laboratory, Argonne, Ill.

S-16. Smaller, B., "Photo-Induced Free Spin Species in Plant Pigments," in *Free Radicals in Biological Systems*, M. S. Blois, Jr., H. W. Brown, R. M. Lemmon, R. O. Lindblom, and M. Weissbluth, Eds., Academic Press, New York, 1961.

S-17. Smith, W. V., P. P. Sorokin, I. L. Gelles, and G. J. Lasher, *Phys. Rev.*, **115**, 1546 (1959).

S-18. Sogo, P. B., L. A. Carter, and M. Calvin, "Electron Spin Resonance Studies on Photosynthetic Materials," in *Free Radicals in Biological Systems*, M. S. Blois, Jr., H. W. Brown, R. M. Lemmon, R. O. Lindblom, and M. Weissbluth, Eds., Academic Press, New York, 1961.

S-19. Sparrman, B., L. Ehrenberg, and A. Ehrenberg, *Acta Chem. Scand.*, **13**, 199 (1959).

S-20. Spong, F. W., and A. F. Kip, *Phys. Rev.*, **137**, A431 (1965).

S-21. Squires, T. L., *Introduction to Microwave Spectroscopy*, George Newnes Limited, London, 1963.

S-22. Stoodley, L. G., *Nature*, **198**, 1077 (1963).

S-23. Stoodley, L. G., *J. Electron. Control*, **14**, 531 (1963).

S-24. Strand Laboratories, Inc., "Microwave Cavities for Electron Magnetic Resonance Applications," Burlington, Mass.

T-1. Thompson, M. C., Jr., F. E. Freethey, and D. M. Waters, "Effects of End-Plate Modification on Q of X-Band Cylindrical TE_{011} Resonant Cavities," NBS Rept. 5049, Boulder Laboratories; IRE Trans. Microwave Theory Tech. MTT-7 No. 3, July 1959.

T-2. Thompson, M. C., Jr., F. E. Freethey, and D. M. Waters, "Fabrication Techniques for X-Band Cavity Resonators," NBS Report 5514, Boulder Laboratories.

T-3. Tinkham, M., and A. F. Kip, *Phys. Rev.*, **83**, 657 (1951).

T-4. Tinkham, M., and M. W. P. Strandberg, *Phys. Rev.*, **97**, 951 (1955).

T-5. Townes, C. H., and A. L. Schawlow, *Microwave Spectroscopy*, McGraw-Hill, New York, 1955.

T-6. Townsend, J., "Magnetic Resonance," in *Methods of Experimental Physics*, Vol. 2, E. Bleuler and R. O. Haxby, Eds., Academic Press, New York, 1964.

T-7. Turkevich, J., and Y. Fujita, *Phys. Today*, **18**, 26 (1965).

U-1. Uebersfeld, J., A. Étienne, and J. Combrisson, *Nature*, **174**, 614 (1954).

U-2. Ultee, C. J., *J. Phys. Chem.*, **64**, 1873 (1960).

V-1. van der Waals, J. H., and M. S. de Groot, *Mol. Phys.*, **2**, 333 (1959).

V-2. Van Gerven, L., A. Van Itterbeek, and L. de Laet, "Low Field EPR Measurements in DPPH at Low Temperatures," in *Paramagnetic Resonance*, Vol. II, W. Low, Ed., Academic Press, New York, 1963.

V-3. Van Gerven, L., A. Van Itterbeek, and E. De Wolf, *J. Phys. Radium*, **17**, 140 (1956).

V-4. van Wieringen, J. S., and J. G. Rensen, "Paramagnetic Resonance at High Temperatures," Proc. Colloq. Ampère Electron. Magnetic Resonance Solid Dielectrics, 12th, Bordeaux (1963).

V-5. Varian EPR At Work Ser., No. 18, Varian Associates, Palo Alto, Calif.

V-6. Varian EPR At Work Ser., No. 26, Varian Associates, Palo Alto, Calif.

V-7. Varian EPR At Work Ser., No. 28, Varian Associates, Palo Alto, Calif.

V-8. Varian C-1024 Time Averaging Computer Specifications INS 1534, Varian Associates, Palo Alto, Calif.

V-9. Vescial, F., N. S. VanderVen, and R. T. Schumacher, *Phys. Rev.*, **134**, A1286 (1964).

V-10. Voevodskii, V. V., and Y. N. Molin, *Radiation Res.*, **17**, 366 (1962).

V-11. Von Baeyer, H. C., *Microwave J.*, **3**, 47 (1960).

W-1. Walker, S., and H. Straw, *Spectroscopy*, Vol. II, Macmillan, New York, 1962.

W-2. Wall, L. A., D. W. Brown, and R. E. Florin, *J. Phys. Chem.*, **63**, 1762 (1959).

W-3. Warshawsky, I., *J. Inorg. Nucl. Chem.*, **25**, 601 (1963).

W-4. Watkins, G. D., and J. W. Corbett, *Phys. Rev.*, **138**, A543 (1965).

W-5. Watkins, G. D., and J. W. Corbett, *Phys. Rev.*, **134**, A1359 (1964).

W-6. Watkins, G. D., and J. W. Corbett, *Discussions Faraday Soc.*, **31**, 86 (1961).

W-7. Watkins, G. D., and J. W. Corbett, *Phys. Rev.*, **121**, 1001 (1961).

W-8. Webb, R. H., *Rev. Sci. Instr.*, **33**, 732 (1962).

W-9. Weeks, R. A., and E. Sonder, "The Relation between the Magnetic Susceptibility, Electron Spin Resonance, and the Optical absorption of the E_1' Center in Fused Silica," in *Paramagnetic Resonance*, Vol. II, W. Low, Ed., Academic Press, New York, 1963.

W-10. Weger, M., *Bell System Tech. J.*, **39**, 1013 (1960).

W-11. Wertz, J. E., *Chem. Rev.*, **55**, 829 (1955).

W-12. Wertz, J. E., P. Auzins, R. A. Weeks, and R. H. Silsbee, *Phys. Rev.*, **107**, 1535 (1957).

W-13. Wertz, J. E., J. W. Orton, and P. Auzins, "ESR Studies of Radiation Effects in Inorganic Solids," AFOSR-194, University of Minnesota.

W-14. West, W., *Fluorescence and Phosphorescence in Chemical Applications of Spectroscopy*, Interscience, New York, 1956.

W-15. Westenberg, A. A., and N. de Haas, *J. Chem. Phys.*, **40**, 3087 (1964).

W-16. Westenberg, A. A., and R. M. Fristrom, "H and O Atom Profiles Measured by ESR in C_2 Hydrocarbon-O_2 Flames," Johns Hopkins University, Applied Physics Lab., Silver Spring, Md.

W-17. Weyl, W., *Ann. Physik*, **121**, 601 (1864).

W-18. Whiffin, D. H., "ESR of Oriented Organic Radicals," in *Free Radicals in Biological Systems*, M. S. Blois, Jr., H. W. Brown, R. M. Lemmon, R. O. Lindblom, and M. Weissbluth, Eds., Academic Press, New York, 1961.

W-19. Willenbrock, F. K., and N. Bloembergen, *Phys. Rev.*, **91**, 1281 (1953).

W-20. Williams, W. L., *Phys. Rev.*, **125**, 82 (1962).

W-21. Wilmshurst, T. H., W. A. Gambling, and D. J. E. Ingram, *J. Electron. Control.*, **13**, 339 (1962).

W-22. Wilson, D. K., and G. Feher, *Phys. Rev.*, **124**, 1068 (1961).

W-23. Wilson, I. G., C. W. Schramm, and J. P. Kinzer, *Bell System Tech. J.* **25**, 408 (1946).

W-24. Wind, M., and H. Rapaport, Eds., *Handbook of Microwave Measurements*, Vol. I, Polytechnic Press of the Polytechnic Institute of Brooklyn, distributed by Interscience, New York, 1958.

W-25. Wood, R. F., and H. W. Joy, *Phys. Rev.*, **136**, 451A (1946).

W-26. Woodbury, H. H., and G. W. Ludwig, *Phys. Rev.*, **126**, 466 (1962).

W-27. Woodbury, H. H., and G. W. Ludwig, *Phys. Rev.*, **124**, 1083 (1961).

W-28. Woodbury, H. H., and G. W. Ludwig, *Phys. Rev.*, **117**, 102 (1960).

W-29. Wyard, S. J., *J. Sci. Instr.*, **42**, 769 (1965).

Y-1. Yamazaki, I., H. S. Mason, and L. Piette, *J. Biol. Chem.*, **235**, 2444 (1960).

Y-2. Yariv, A., and J. P. Gordon, *Rev. Sci. Instr.*, **32**, 462 (1961).

Z-1. Zeldes, H., and R. Livingston, *J. Chem. Phys.*, **30**, 40 (1959).

Z-2. Zimmer, K. G., *Radiation Res. Suppl.*, **1**, 519 (1959).

Laboratory References*

1. Air Force Materials Laboratory, RTD, Wright Patterson Air Force Base, Ohio, Dr. L. A. Harrah.
2. Radiation Research Laboratory, Mellon Institute, Pittsburgh, Pa., Dr. R. W. Fessenden.
3. Harvard University, Cambridge, Mass., Prof. N. Bloembergen.
4. Massachusetts Institute of Technology, Cambridge, Mass., Prof. M. W. P. Strandberg.
5. Brandeis University, Waltham, Mass., Prof. T. C. Hollocher.
6. Massachusetts Institute of Technology, Magnet Laboratory, Cambridge, Mass., Prof. W. Low.
7. Bell Telephone Laboratories, Murray Hill, New Jersey, Dr. R. C. Fletcher.
8. Central Research Department, Experimental Station, E. I. Du Pont de Nemours and Company, Wilmington, Delaware, Dr. D. B. Chesnut.
9. Hilger and Watts Ltd., London, Mr. P. J. Clowes.
10. Basic Physics Division, National Physics Laboratory, Teddington, Great Britain, Dr. D. H. Whiffen.
11. Decca Radar, Hersham, Great Britain, Mr. P. M. Butcher.
12. Royal Military College of Science, Shrivenham, Great Britain, Prof. A. Charlesby and Dr. M. G. Ormerod.
13. The University of Leicester, Leicester, Great Britain, Prof. M. C. R. Symons.
14. Chester Beaty Research Institute, Royal Cancer Hospital, London, Great Britain, Dr. R. C. Bray.
15. Physics Department, the Medical College of St. Bartholomew's Hospital, London, Great Britain, Dr. J. A. Simmons.
16. University of Nottingham, Nottingham, Great Britain, Prof. K. J. Standley.
17. University of Keele, Keele, Great Britain, Prof. D. J. E. Ingram.
18. University of Leeds, Leeds, Great Britain, Dr. P. B. Ayscough.
19. Clarendon Laboratory, Oxford University, Oxford, Great Britain, Dr. J. H. E. Griffiths, Department of Physical Chemistry, Dr. B. Coles.
20. University of Bristol, Bristol, Great Britain, Dr. J. C. Gill.
21. Norsk Hydro's Institute for Cancer Research, The Norwegian Radium Hospital, Oslo, Norway, Dr. T. Henriksen.
22. University of Uppsala, Uppsala, Sweden, Prof. T. Vänngärd.

---

* Only the principal contacts are listed; however, techniques and information also were received from many other members of these laboratories.

23. Biochemical Department, Nobel Medical Institute, Stockholm, Sweden, Dr. A. Ehrenberg.
24. Aarhus University, Aarhus, Denmark, Prof. L. T. Muus.
25. Zeeman Laboratory, University of Amsterdam, Amsterdam, the Netherlands, Dr. J. C. M. Henning; Laboratory for Physical Chemistry, Prof. G. J. Hoijtink.
26. Koninklijkel/Shell-Laboratorium, Amseterdam, Netherlands, Dr. J. H. van der Waals.
27. Kamerlingh Onnes Laboratory, Leiden, Netherlands, Dr. G. W. J. Drewes.
28. Institute of Low Temperature and Technical Physics, University of Leuven, Leuven, Belgium, Prof. A. Van Itterbeck and Dr. L. Van Gerven.
29. Belgem Institut D'Astrophysique, University of Liege, Cointe-Sclessin, Belgium, Prof. J. Duchesne.
30. Max Planck-Institut Für Biophysik, Frankfurt, Germany, Drs. A. Redhart and H. Reitböck.
31. Max Planck-Institut, Heidelberg, Germany, Dr. P. Fisher.
32. Institut für Strehlenbiology Kernforschongezentrum, Karlsruhe, Germany, Dr. A. Müller.
33. Trüb Tauber and Co., Zurich, Switzerland, Dr. F. E. Furrer.
34. Department of Chemistry, University of California, Berkeley, Calif., Prof. W. L. Jolly; Department of Physics, Prof. A. F. Kip.
35. National Bureau of Standards, Boulder, Colorado, Dr. L. M. Matarrese.
36. University of Minnesota, Minneapolis, Minn., Prof. J. E. Wertz.
37. Duke University, Durham, N. C., Prof. W. Gordy.
38. The Johns Hopkins University, Applied Physics Laboratory, Silver Spring, Md., Dr. E. L. Cochran.
39. University of Michigan, Ann Arbor, Mich., Prof. R. H. Sands.
40. Argonne National Laboratory, Lemont, Ill., Dr. B. Smaller.
41. Enrico Fermi Institute of Nuclear Studies, University of Chicago, Chicago, Ill., Prof. C. A. Hutchison, Jr.
42. Washington University, St. Louis, Mo., Dr. J. Townsend.
43. Alpha Scientific Co., Berkeley, California.
44. Stanford University, Palo Alto, California.
45. Varian Associates, Palo Alto, California, Dr. J. S. Hyde.

Author Index

Numbers in parentheses are reference numbers and show that an author's work is referred to although his name is not mentioned in the text. Numbers in *italics* indicate the pages on which the full references appear.

A

Abkowitz, M., 168(A-1), *543*

Abragam, A., 17, 20, 296(A-2), *543*

Adrian, F. J., 43(A-3,C-14,C-15), 432 (C-14), 464(A-3), *543, 545*

Alexander, P., 511(A-4,O-4), *543, 551*

Alger, R. S., 434(A-5), 457(A-6), 458 (A-6), *543*

Allard, J. G., 371(H-18), 384(H-18), 517(H-18), *548*

Allen, L. C., 92(A-7), 93(A-7), 95 (A-7), 97(A-7), *543*

Allen, M. B., 524(A-8), *543*

Alsop, L. E., 11(G-7), 12(G-7), *547*

Al'tshuler, S. A., 2(A-9), 3(A-9), 18 (A-9), 33(A-9), 107(A-9), 244 (A-9), 256(A-9), 257(A-9), 370 (A-9), 387(A-9), 404(A-9), 412 (A-9), 414(A-9), *543*

Anderson, J. H., 2(O-3), 42(O-3), *551*

Anderson, R. S., 16(A-10), 18(A-10), 19(A-10), 40(A-10), 42(A-10), 45 (A-10), 46(A-10), *543*

Anderson, T. H., 411(M-3), 443(M-3), 446(M-3), 457(A-6), 458(A-6), *543, 550*

Andrews, E. R., 217, *543*

Androes, G. M., 523, 524(C-1), 526–528(C-1), *544*

Ard, W. B., 464(G-12), 512(G-12), *547*

Arnold, E., *543*

Arthur, P., Jr., 502(C-7), *545*

Assenheim, H. M., 100(A-13), *543*

Atkins, P. W., 371(A-14), 456(A-14), *543*

Auzins, P., 395(W-12), 396(W-13), 397(W-12), *554*

B

Ayscough, P. B., 457(A-15), 459 (A-15), *543*

Bagguley, D. M. S., 207(B-1), *543*

Baker, J. M., 224(B-2), 226, *543*

Bauer, C. L., 374(B-3), *543*

Baum, W. A., 477(B-4), *543*

Beckman, T. A., 290(B-5), 297(B-5), *543*

Beers, Y., 244(R-4), 257(R-4), *552*

Bell, M. D., 416(C-16), 419(C-16), 421(C-16), 422(C-16), *545*

Bennett, J. E., 416(I-4), 417(B-6), *543, 549*

Bennett, R. G., 412(B-7), 413(B-7), *544*

Bennett, W. R., 74(B-8), 76(B-8), 77 (B-8), 87(B-8), *544*

Beringer, R., 244, 246(B-9), 247 (B-9), 252(B-11), 254(B-9), 256 (B-9), 257(B-12), *544*

Berk, H. L., 315, 320(P-17), 321(P-17), 468(P-17), *551*

Berkowitz, R. S., 74(B-13), *544*

Bielski, J. H. B., 91

Bienenstock, A., 225(B-14), *544*

Biloen, P., 500(J-5), *549*

Bleaney, B., 3(B-17), 16(B-17), 29, 32(B-17), 35(B-17), 71(B-17), 404 (B-17), 408, *544*

Bloch, F., 22

Bloembergen, N., 42(B-18), 46, 48 (B-18), 49(B-18), 54(B-18), 55 (B-18), 71(B-18), 322(W-19), 326, 327, 331(W-19), 415, *544, 554*

Blois, M. S., 74(B-21), 278(B-21), 409, 458(B-21), *544*

557

Subject Index